Accident and Emergency
Diagnosis and Management

Fourth edition

ANTHONY F.T. BROWN
MBChB (Bristol), FRCP, FRCS(Ed), FACEM, FFAEM
*Senior Staff Specialist, Department of Emergency Medicine,
Royal Brisbane Hospital
Clinical Associate Professor, Department of Anaesthesiology and
Critical Care, School of Medicine, University of Queensland,
Brisbane, Australia*

A member of the Hodder Headline Group
LONDON   NEW YORK   NEW DELHI

First published in Great Britain in 2002 by
Arnold, a member of the Hodder Headline Group,
338 Euston Road, London NW1 3BH

http://www.hoddereducation.com

Distributed in the United States of America by
Oxford University Press, Inc.,
198 Madison Avenue, New York, NY10016
Oxford is a registered trademark of Oxford University Press

British Library Cataloguing in Publication Data
A catalogue record for this book is available from the British Library

Library of Congress Cataloging-in-Publication Data
A catalogue record for this book is available from the Library of Congress

ISBN-10: 0 340 80720 2
ISBN-13: 978 0 340 80720 0

3 4 5 6 7 8 9 10

1 U MAY 2006

Commissioning Editor: Nick Dunton
Production Editor: Anke Ueberberg
Production Controller: Bryan Eccleshall
Cover Design: Terry Griffiths

Typeset in 10 on 11 pt Sabon by Charon Tec Pvt. Ltd, Chennai, India
Printed and bound by Replika Press Pvt. Ltd, India

Dedication

To Chris, who showed such dignity and spirit in his long fight with illness, but died suddenly leaving his beloved wife and children Alison, Clare and Peter with a lifetime of memories.

Contents

Preface

This new edition is again written primarily for senior house officers in the A&E department. It provides didactic, practical advice in an easily read format on the important points in the history, examination, investigation and immediate management of every patient, however unusual, complex or unexpected the presentation.

The book will also benefit general practitioners, accident and emergency and critical care area nurses, paramedics and senior medical students, helping develop teamwork based on shared knowledge as a foundation for quality emergency care.

The entire text has been extensively revised and updated to include the latest European Resuscitation Council guidelines for adult and paediatric advanced life support, tetanus prophylaxis guidelines, an entirely new section on environmental emergencies, and many new topics, such as acute coronary syndromes, hyponatraemia, hypercalcaemia, dengue, purpura, triage and inter-hospital transfers, to name but a few. In addition, risk management and incident reporting are featured to impress upon all of us that the need to remain in the forefront of developments in acute care is tempered by the propriety of practising good medicine at every opportunity.

Accident and emergency medicine is now a major specialty at the leading edge of acute care delivery, setting the highest standards for its practitioners to follow. A practical, up-to-date core handbook is essential. It is with this in mind that I offer this new edition to my colleagues.

Anthony F.T. Brown
October 2001

Acknowledgements

I am again indebted to my emergency medicine colleagues for making many helpful comments and astute suggestions for this new edition: Dr Mike Beckett and Mr John Heyworth in the UK; Dr Ian Rogers and Dr Geoff Hughes in Australia/New Zealand; and the peripatetic Dr Chris McLauchlan, who made an enormous contribution in his own inimitable style. Thank you all for sharing your knowledge and expertise so readily to enrich this book.

Thanks also to Dr Geoff Smaldon of Butterworth-Heinemann in Oxford for his vision, enthusiasm and encouragement, and Nick Dunton of Arnold for continuing this support and commitment.

Finally, my greatest debt is to Monique Cichocki, who typed all the drafts with outstanding accuracy and reliability, meeting every deadline calmly and successfully. Thank you.

Anthony F.T. Brown
October 2001

MEDICAL EMERGENCIES

CARDIOPULMONARY RESUSCITATION

DIAGNOSIS

Cardiopulmonary resuscitation (CPR) is required if a collapsed person is unconscious, not breathing and has no pulse in a large artery such as the carotid or femoral, although the following may also be present:
  (1) a brief tonic grand mal fit
  (2) gasping breathing
  (3) pallor or cyanosis
  (4) dilated pupils.

MANAGEMENT

  (1) This is based on the European Resuscitation Council guidelines 2000.[1]
    (i)   The first person on the scene stays with the patient and commences resuscitation, making a note of the time.
    (ii) The second person summons help and organises the arrival of equipment, then assists with the resuscitation.
  (2) *Immediate actions*. The aim is to maintain oxygenation of the brain and heart until a stable cardiac output is achieved.
    (i)   Lay the patient flat on a hard surface such as a trolley. If the patient is on the floor and enough people are available, lift the patient onto a trolley to facilitate the resuscitation procedure.
    (ii) Give a single thump to the precordium in witnessed or monitored arrests, where the rhythm is ventricular fibrillation or pulseless ventricular tachycardia.
    (iii) Open the airway by tilting the head and lifting the chin to prevent the tongue from occluding the larynx.
    (iv) Remove any obvious obstruction including loose dentures from the mouth, but leave well-fitting dentures in place.

(v)   Commence assisted ventilation.

(vi)   Commence external cardiac massage.

(3) *Assisted ventilation*

(i)   Start mouth-to-mouth/nose or mouth-to-mask respiration using a Laerdal Pocket Mask without delay.

(ii)   An Ambu or Laerdal bag with oxygen reservoir attached and face mask may be used by a trained person after first inserting an oropharyngeal (Guedel) airway.

(iii) If the chest fails to inflate, check for leaks around the mask or airway then consider obstruction of the upper airway (see p. 33).

Note: adequate oxygenation is achieved by the above measures. Attempts at endotracheal intubation should only be made by doctors experienced in the technique.

(4) *External cardiac massage*

(i)   Place the heel of the hand over the lower half of the sternum. Place the other hand on top, keeping the arms straight and applying a vertical compression force.

(ii)   Depress the sternum 4–5 cm at a rate of about 100 compressions per minute.

(iii) It is unnecessary to synchronise massage with ventilation if there are two operators. If still alone, perform 15 compressions to every two ventilations. This should create a palpable femoral pulse.

(iv) In small children, only one hand should be used, at a rate of 100 compressions per minute. In infants, use the tips of two fingers at a rate of 100 compressions per minute.

Note: avoid using excessive force causing rib fractures, flail chest, liver lacerations, etc.

(5) *Definitive treatment*

(i)   After confirming the diagnosis of cardiac arrest, give the patient an immediate 200-J shock.

(ii)   *Defibrillation*

      (a) This is an emergency situation. Do not await electrocardiogram (ECG) confirmation at this crucial stage in re-establishing the circulation.

      (b) Place one paddle on the right parasternal area over the second intercostal space, and the other on the mid-anterior axillary line over the fifth left intercostal space.

      (c) Avoid positioning paddles over ECG electrodes, medication patches or implanted devices, e.g. pacemaker.

      (d) Charge the paddles once on the patient's chest.

      (e) Ensure good contact is made using electrode jelly (never KY jelly) or gel pads and firm pressure.

      (f) Make sure that no one is touching the patient or bed. Give a 'stand clear' warning when the shock is about to be delivered.

(6) Connect the ECG monitor and observe one of four possible traces:

    (i)   ventricular fibrillation (see p. 5);

    (ii)   ventricular tachycardia (see p. 5);

    (iii)   asystole (see p. 7);

    (iv)   electromechanical dissociation (see p. 7).

(7) Establish an initial intravenous line in the antecubital fossa, and commence a normal saline infusion giving at least 20 ml to flush any drugs administered towards the heart.

(8) Unless the cardiac resuscitation is rapidly successful, establish a second intravenous line.

    (i)   Ideally, the line should be inserted into a central vein, either the external or internal jugular or the subclavian.

    (ii)   This central line should be inserted only by a skilled doctor, as inadvertent arterial puncture, haemothorax or pneumothorax may invalidate further resuscitation attempts.

    (iii)   Also, the central venous route poses additional serious hazards should thrombolytic therapy be indicated.

    (iv)   All drugs are then given via this central line.

(9) *Endotracheal intubation.* A skilled doctor with airway training should now insert a cuffed endotracheal tube. This improves oxygenation and prevents inhalation of vomit or blood from the mouth or stomach.

    (i) Use an 8.5–9.5-mm diameter endotracheal tube in adult males and a 7.5–8.5-mm diameter tube in adult females.

    (ii) Pass the tube between the vocal cords under direct vision, using a curved-blade laryngoscope.

    (iii) Inflate the cuff, connect the oxygen supply, and check the correct position of the tube by auscultation or end tidal carbon dioxide measurement. Tie the tube in place.

    (iv) Never delay CPR for more than 20 s to secure the airway.

(10) Subsequent management depends on the cardiac rhythm and the patient's condition. Keep the ECG monitor attached to the patient at all times.

(11) *Ventricular fibrillation (VF)/pulseless ventricular tachycardia (VT).* See Table 1 for a rapid overview of treatment.

    (i) VF is asynchronous, chaotic ventricular activity producing no cardiac output.

    (ii) Pulseless VT is a wide-complex, regular tachycardia associated with no clinically detectable cardiac output.

    (iii) Treat with immediate DC shocks:

        (a) start at 200 J (2 J/kg in small children);

        (b) if unsuccessful, repeat 200 J;

        (c) if unsuccessful, give further DC shock at 360 J;

        (d) do not remove paddles from the chest wall between shocks.

    (iv) If VF/VT recur, perform CPR for 1 min and correct reversible causes (see p. 8):

        (a) give 10 ml of 1:10 000 adrenaline (1 mg);

        (b) give further 1:10 000 adrenaline 10 ml (1 mg) every 3 min until return of spontaneous circulation (ROSC).

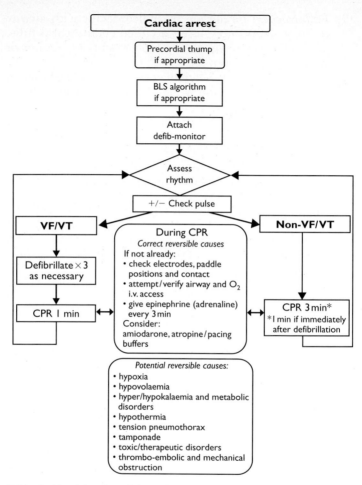

Table 1. Algorithm for adult cardiorespiratory arrest (reproduced by kind permission of *Resuscitation*[1])

(12) Re-assess ECG rhythm and presence of a pulse.
   (i)   If VF or pulseless VT are still present, repeat a set
         of three DC shocks at 360 J.
      (a)   Do not remove paddles from chest wall
            between shocks.

          (b)   Do not perform CPR between shocks provided defibrillator recharges in under 20 s.

     (ii)   Follow set of shocks with 1 min of CPR before repeating above cycle.

(13) During this period of CPR:
     (i)   If not already done:
          (a)   check paddle position and contact;
          (b)   attempt/verify endotracheal tube position, and successful intravenous access.
     (ii)   Consider the following antiarrhythmics:
          (a)   *Lignocaine*. Give initial bolus of 1 mg/kg i.v., followed by 0.5 mg/kg if necessary.
          (b)   *Amiodarone*. Give initial bolus of 300 mg, which may be repeated at a dose of 150 mg.
          (c)   *Magnesium*. Give 8 mmol or 4 ml of 49.3% magnesium sulphate i.v., particularly in torsades de pointes and suspected hypomagnesaemia.
    (iii)   Consider buffering agent:
          (a)   *8.4% sodium bicarbonate*. Give 50 mmol (50 ml) i.v., then as guided by arterial blood gases (ABG).
          (b)   Particular indications are for hyperkalaemia, tricyclic antidepressant overdose (see p. 77), protracted arrest greater than 15 min and documented metabolic acidosis.

(14) *Non-VF/VT, i.e. asystole or electromechanical dissociation*
     (i)   Asystole is absence of any cardiac electrical activity.
          (a)   Make sure the ECG leads are not disconnected or broken by observing compression artefact on the ECG screen during CPR.
          (b)   Check appropriate ECG lead selection and sensitivity.
          (c)   If there is any difficulty in diagnosis, always treat as for VF/VT.
     (ii)   Electromechanical dissociation (EMD) or pulseless electrical activity (PEA). This is the presence of a coordinated electrical rhythm without detectable cardiac output.

    (iii)   Asystole and EMD have a poor prognosis as defibrillation is of no use. See Table 1 for a rapid overview of treatment.

        (a)   Perform CPR for up to 3 min correcting reversible causes (see point 15 below), and give 1:10 000 adrenaline 10 ml (1 mg) every 3 min until ROSC.

        (b)   Give atropine 3 mg once.

Note: if venous access is impossible, give atropine, adrenaline and lignocaine via the endotracheal tube at twice the intravenous dosage, diluted with normal saline or water to a total volume of 10 ml.

(15)   Always look out for the following conditions, which may precipitate cardiorespiratory arrest or decrease the chances of successful resuscitation ('4 Hs and 4 Ts').

    (i)   *Hypoxaemia*

        (a)   Make sure maximal oxygen is being delivered at 15 l/min.

        (b)   Confirm ventilation at 400–600 ml tidal volume is creating a visible rise and fall of the chest.

    (ii)   *Hypovolaemia*

        (a)   Severe blood loss following trauma, gastrointestinal haemorrhage, ruptured aortic aneurysm or ruptured ectopic pregnancy may cause cardiovascular collapse and cardiac arrest.

        (b)   This must always be considered in cases of unexplained cardiovascular collapse.

        (c)   Get senior accident and emergency (A&E) department help, and search for the source of bleeding.

        (d)   Give judicious fluid replacement and call the surgical/vascular/obstetrics and gynaecology (O&G) team.

    (iii)   *Hypothermia*

        (a)   Check the core temperature with a low-reading thermometer.

        (b)   Moderate (32–29°C) or severe (under 29°C) hypothermia will require heroic measures such as active core rewarming with warmed pleural, peritoneal or gastric lavage, or even extracorporeal rewarming (see p. 125).

(c) Get senior A&E help, and do not cease CPR until the temperature is at least 33°C or the team leader determines futility.

(iv) *Hyper/hypokalaemia and metabolic disorders*

(a) Rapidly check the potassium and calcium initially.

(b) Give a bolus of 5 mmol potassium i.v. for hypokalaemia.

(c) Give 5–10 ml of 10% calcium chloride for hyperkalaemia, hypocalcaemia or calcium-channel blocking drug overdose.

(v) *Tamponade*

(a) Cardiac tamponade may follow trauma, myocardial infarction, dissecting aneurysm or pericarditis.

(b) There is hypotension, tachycardia, pulsus paradoxus and engorged neck veins that rise on inspiration (Kussmaul's sign). The heart sounds are quiet, the apex beat is impalpable, and EMD may ensue.

(c) If the patient is in extremis, perform pericardiocentesis. Insert a cardiac needle between the angle of the xiphisternum and the left costal margin at 45 degrees to the horizontal, aiming for the left shoulder (see Fig. 1). Sometimes aspirating as little as 50 ml restores the cardiac output, although immediate thoracotomy is usually indicated in cases resulting from trauma (see p. 155).

(vi) *Tension pneumothorax*

(a) Tension usually follows a traumatic rather than a spontaneous pneumothorax, particularly if positive pressure ventilation is used. It results in extreme respiratory distress and circulatory collapse.

(b) The patient becomes increasingly breathless and cyanosed, and develops a tachycardia

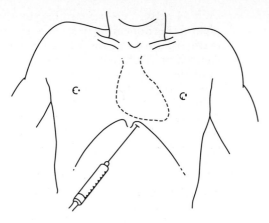

Fig. 1. Pericardial aspiration.

with hypotension. There is decreased chest expansion on the affected side, a hyper-resonant percussion note, and absent or diminished breath sounds. The trachea is displaced towards the other side, and the neck veins usually distended.

(c) This is a life-threatening situation requiring immediate relief, without waiting for a chest X-ray (CXR).

(d) Insert a wide-bore needle or cannula through the second intercostal space in the midclavicular line. This will be followed by a whistle of air outwards.

(e) Insert an intercostal drain (see p. 26).

(vii) *Toxins/poisons/drugs*

(a) Many conditions cause cardiorespiratory arrest, such as tricyclic antidepressant (see p. 77), calcium-channel blocking drug (see p. 82) or beta-blocker (see p. 82) poisoning, and hydrofluoric acid burns (see p. 186).

(b) All must be recognised early and treated specifically.

(viii) *Thromboembolism/mechanical obstruction*
   (a) Perform external cardiac massage, which may break up a massive pulmonary embolism (PE), and give a fluid load of 20 ml/kg.
   (b) If clinical suspicion is high and there are no absolute contraindications, give thrombolysis such as alteplase (rt-PA) 100 mg i.v.

(16) If still in asystole, the prognosis is usually hopeless. However, if P waves or any other electrical activity, such as severe bradycardia, are present with poor perfusion, consider pacing:
   (i) Use an external (transcutaneous) pacemaker to maintain the cardiac output until a transvenous wire is inserted.
   (ii) A temporary transvenous pacemaker wire may then be inserted blind via a central vein, but ideally should be passed under X-ray guidance.

(17) *Subsequent action.* It is important to continue effective external cardiac massage until the heartbeat is strong enough to produce a peripheral pulse.
   (i) If there is persistent hypotension, and treatable causes such as hypoxia, hypovolaemia, tension pneumothorax, etc. have been excluded, give 1:10 000 adrenaline 1 ml (100 µg) i.v. repeated to maintain a blood pressure (BP) equal to the patient's usual BP, or at least a systolic BP greater than 100 mm Hg. As soon as possible, the adrenaline and other vasoactive drugs should be given via a dedicated central venous line.
   (ii) If ventricular fibrillation has been reverted successfully, continue the same drug as an infusion, or if no drug was used commence lignocaine to prevent recurrent VF. Usual infusion rates are lignocaine 2–4 mg/min or amiodarone 1 mg/min for 6 h, then 0.5 mg/min to a maximum of 2 g over 24 h.
   (iii) Transfer the patient to the intensive care unit or coronary care unit. The following investigations will be required, but should not delay transfer:
      (a) CXR to look for pneumothorax, pulmonary oedema and pulmonary collapse; confirm

correct positioning of the endotracheal tube and central line;
- (b) blood gases;
- (c) serum sodium, potassium and glucose;
- (d) 12-lead ECG.

(iv) The patient must be transferred with a trained nurse and doctor in attendance. A portable cardiac monitor, defibrillator, oxygen and suction should be available on the trolley.

(18) *When to stop.* The decision to cease further attempts at resuscitation is difficult and should be made only by the senior A&E doctor. Survival from cardiac arrest is greatest when:
- (i) the event is witnessed;
- (ii) a bystander starts resuscitation;
- (iii) the heart arrests in VF or VT.
- (iv) defibrillation is carried out at an early stage, with successful cardioversion achieved in 2–3 min, and not more than 8 min.

Note: special consideration is given to near-drowning, hypothermia and acute poisoning (especially with tricyclic antidepressants). Full recovery has followed in apparently hopeless cases (fixed dilated pupils, non-VF/VT) with resuscitation prolonged for several hours.

CHEST PAIN

DIFFERENTIAL DIAGNOSIS

Consider the life-threatening diagnoses first:
- (i) acute coronary syndromes, such as myocardial infarction or unstable angina
- (ii) pulmonary embolus
- (iii) aortic dissection.

These may present with a normal CXR and ECG, and may therefore need to be referred on clinical suspicion alone. Always establish venous access, give 35% oxygen, and attach a cardiac monitor and pulse oximeter to the patient.

Other causes to consider include:
(iv) pericarditis
(v)   pleurisy
(vi) pneumonia
(vii) pneumothorax
(viii) abdominal – oesophagitis, oesophageal rupture, gall-
       bladder disease, etc.
(ix) musculoskeletal and chest wall pain.

ACUTE CORONARY SYNDROME

The term acute coronary syndrome (ACS) encompasses the
spectrum of patients presenting with chest pain or other
symptoms due to myocardial ischaemia, ranging from unstable
angina, non-Q-wave myocardial infarction (MI) to transmural
Q-wave MI.

DIAGNOSIS

(1) Predisposing factors include cigarette smoking, hyper-
    tension, diabetes, hypercholesterolaemia and a positive
    family history.
(2) There may be a prior history of angina, myocardial
    infarction or heart failure.
(3) Typical pain is central, heavy, burning, crushing or tight
    retrosternal, usually lasting for several minutes or
    longer, unrelieved by sublingual nitrates and associated
    with anxiety, dyspnoea, nausea and vomiting.
(4) The pain radiates to the neck, jaw, one or both arms, the
    back and occasionally the epigastrium, or may present
    at these sites alone.
(5) The patient may be clammy, sweaty, breathless and
    pale.
(6) The spectrum of possible underlying diagnoses includes:
    (i)   Unstable angina with ischaemic pain that is severe
          and of recent onset, or has become abruptly worse,
          occurs at rest or follows a recent MI.
    (ii) Non-Q-wave MI is a retrospective diagnosis based
          on raised cardiac enzymes in the absence of classic
          ST elevation on the ECG. Other ECG changes of

ST depression and T-wave inversion may be seen in either unstable angina or non-Q-wave MI.

(iii)   Q-wave MI usually causes persistent ST elevation, raised cardiac enzymes and the development of Q waves.

(7) The patient may present atypically with the complications of heart failure, cardiac arrhythmia, hypotension, systemic embolism or collapse. Alternatively, the patient may look deceptively well.

(8) Investigations that subsequently establish the underlying diagnosis include:

(i)   *ECG.* This essential investigation must be performed immediately.

(a)   Acute changes include convex ST elevation (acute injury), T-wave inversion (ischaemia) and the formation of Q waves (infarction).

(b)   Inferior MI causes changes in leads II, III and aVF.

(c)   Anterior MI causes changes in I, aVL and V1–V3 (anteroseptal) or V4–V6 (anterolateral).

(d)   True posterior MI causes mirror-image changes of tall R waves and ST depression in leads V1–V4.

(ii)   Raised cardiac enzymes such as creatine kinase (CK), creatine kinase MB (CK-MB) and cardiac troponin I or T (cTnI, cTnT).

(iii)   CXR to look for pulmonary oedema, cardiomegaly and atelectasis. Request a portable X-ray in the A&E department, providing this does not delay admission to the ward.

MANAGEMENT

(1) Establish venous access with an intravenous cannula and attach a cardiac monitor and pulse oximeter to the patient.

(2) Give high-dose 40–60% oxygen unless there is a prior history of obstructive airways disease, in which case give 28% oxygen. Aim for an oxygen saturation over 94%.

(3) Give aspirin 150–300 mg orally unless contraindicated by known hypersensitivity.

(4) Maximise pain relief:

   (i) Give glyceryl trinitrate (GTN) 150–300 µg sublingually, avoiding excessive hypotension (see point 5(ii)).

   (ii) Add morphine 2.5–5 mg i.v. with an antiemetic, e.g. metoclopramide 10 mg i.v. if pain persists.

(5) Treat left heart failure (see p. 32):

   (i) Sit the patient upright and give a diuretic such as frusemide 40 mg i.v. or twice their usual oral daily dose intravenously if already on frusemide.

   (ii) If not improving, give glyceryl trinitrate 300 µg sublingually. Remove the tablet if excessive hypotension (systolic BP less than 100 mm Hg) occurs.

   (iii) In refractory cases, repeat the frusemide and commence a GTN infusion.

      (a) Add GTN 200 mg to 500 ml of 5% dextrose, i.e. 400 µg/ml, using a glass bottle and low-absorption polyethylene infusion set.

      (b) Infuse initially at 1 ml/h, maintaining systolic BP above 100 mm Hg. Gradually increase to over 20 ml/h, avoiding hypotension.

   (iv) Commence mask continuous positive airways pressure (CPAP) respiratory support.

      (a) Use a dedicated high-flow fresh gas circuit with variable resistor valve.

      (b) A trained nurse must remain in attendance at all times.

(6) *Thrombolysis*. Consider thrombolytic therapy in consultation with the senior A&E doctor. Aim to commence thrombolysis within a maximum of 30 min of the patient's arrival in hospital. Do not cause delay by transferring to coronary care.

   (i) Thrombolysis is indicated within 12 h of the onset of myocardial ischaemic pain in patients with ECG evidence of ST elevation MI (ST elevation of at least 1 mm in two contiguous limb leads and 2 mm in two contiguous precordial leads) or new bundle branch block, particularly left bundle branch block (LBBB).

(ii)   Absolute contraindications to thrombolysis include:

    (a)   active gastrointestinal bleeding, major surgery or trauma, including prolonged CPR in previous 2 weeks;

    (b)   intracerebral or subarachnoid haemorrhage ever;

    (c)   thrombotic stroke in previous 6 months;

    (d)   pregnancy, proliferative diabetic retinopathy, known bleeding diathesis, or uncontrolled hypertension (systolic BP over 200 mm Hg, diastolic BP over 110 mm Hg);

    (e)   aortic dissection (see p. 21).

(iii)   Relative contraindications (thrombolysis may still be considered in those at highest risk of death, or with greatest net clinical benefit, e.g. large anterior infarction presenting early) include:

    (a)   arterial puncture or central line;

    (b)   past history of gastrointestinal bleeding;

    (c)   current use of warfarin;

    (d)   menstruation;

    (e)   severe hepatic or renal disease.

(iv)   Give streptokinase 1.5 million units over 45–60 min in 100 ml normal saline.

    (a)   Continue ECG monitoring throughout for reperfusion arrhythmias.

    (b)   Slow or stop the infusion if hypotension or rash occur. Restart the infusion as soon as they have resolved.

    (c)   Occasionally, severe hypotension and anaphylaxis may occur, requiring colloids, adrenaline, etc. (see p. 102).

(v)   Use alteplase (rt-PA), reteplase (r-PA) or tenecteplase (TNKase) if the patient has ever had streptokinase before (except within the previous 5 days), if the patient is allergic, or preferably in patients under 75 years presenting early with anterior MI:

    (a)   Give a bolus of alteplase 15 mg (15 ml), followed by an infusion of 0.75 mg/kg over 30 min (not to exceed 50 mg), then 0.5 mg/kg over 60 min (not to exceed 35 mg).

(b) Or give reteplase 10 u as a bolus over no more than 2 min, followed after 30 min by a further 10-u bolus.

(c) Or give tenecteplase 30 mg (for patients less than 60 kg) up to 50 mg (for patients 90 kg or over) as a single bolus over 10 s.

(d) Commence unfractionated heparin 5000 u i.v. as a bolus, followed by an infusion at 1000 u/h for patients over 80 kg, or 800 u/h for patients less than 80 kg.

(7) In the absence of ST elevation on ECG, patients with suspected unstable angina and non-Q-wave MI should receive heparin.

(i) Give unfractionated heparin 5000 u i.v. as a bolus, followed by an infusion at 1000 u/h for patients over 80 kg, or 800 u/h for patients less than 80 kg, titrated to an activated partial thromboplastin time (APTT) of 50–75 s by 6-h post-infusion start.

(ii) Alternatively, use low-molecular-weight heparin (LMWH) such as enoxaparin 1 mg/kg s.c. or dalteparin 120 IU s.c. 12-hourly if this is preferred hospital policy.

(8) Treat cardiac arrhythmias. Similar treatment principles apply in non-ACS situations.

(i) *Bradycardia*. This may be sinus, junctional (nodal) or due to atrioventricular block:

(a) Give a bolus of atropine 0.5–0.6 mg i.v.

(b) If it persists, repeat the atropine for sinus or junctional bradycardia.

(c) If it persists with atrioventricular block, consider inserting a temporary transvenous pacemaker wire. An external (transcutaneous) pacemaker may be used until X-ray guidance is available.

(d) Avoid using an isoprenaline infusion immediately following acute MI, as this may provoke ventricular fibrillation.

(ii) *Ventricular tachycardia (VT)*

(a) If the patient is hypotensive or collapsed, give a 100-J synchronised DC shock, ideally after a senior doctor with airway experience has given a short-acting general anaesthetic or intravenous midazolam in the conscious patient.

(b) If the patient is not hypotensive, give lignocaine up to 100 mg i.v. as a bolus and then start an infusion of lignocaine at 2–4 mg/min.

(c) If the lignocaine fails, or as the alternative, give amiodarone 150 mg i.v. over 5–10 min up to twice, then 300 mg over 1 h as required, and repeat a synchronised DC shock.

Note: frequent ventricular ectopics do not require treatment, unless they are multifocal or arrive on the T wave of the preceding complex.

(iii) *Supraventricular tachycardia*

(a) If the patient is shocked or hypotensive, proceed directly to synchronised DC cardioversion starting at 100 J after a senior doctor with airway experience has given a short-acting anaesthetic.

(b) In the absence of shock, continue oxygen, and check that pain, anxiety or heart failure have been treated.

(c) Then use a vagal stimulus such as carotid sinus massage: press firmly at the upper border of the thyroid cartilage against the vertebral process with a circular motion, or get the patient to perform a Valsalva manoeuvre.

(d) If this fails, give adenosine 6 mg rapidly over 2–5 s i.v., followed by 12 mg rapidly after 1–2 min, then a further 12 mg rapidly twice more if still no response. Warn the patient to expect transient facial flushing, dyspnoea, chest pressure and nausea. Give a reduced initial dose if the patient is on dipyridamole.

(e) An alternative is verapamil 5–10 mg i.v. as a bolus over 30 s to 2 min. Verapamil may cause hypotension and bradycardia, particularly in elderly patients, who should be pretreated with calcium gluconate 10 ml given slowly i.v.

- (f) Never use verapamil after a beta blocker, or if digitalis toxicity is suspected, or the patient has a wide complex tachycardia.
- (g) Adenosine may be used in wide complex tachycardia, due to either supraventricular tachycardia with aberrant conduction or ventricular tachycardia. Persistence of the arrhythmia suggests VT, therefore treat as in point 8 (ii).

- (iv) *Atrial flutter and fibrillation*
  - (a) If the patient is shocked or hypotensive, proceed directly to synchronised DC cardioversion starting at 50 J. In patients on digoxin therapy, a temporary transvenous pacemaker may be required as asystole may follow DC shock.
  - (b) Otherwise, give verapamil 5–10 mg i.v. to slow the ventricular rate providing the QRS complexes are not widened. Follow this by digitalising the patient with digoxin 500 μg orally or slowly i.v.
  - (c) Alternatively, give amiodarone 300 mg i.v. over 1 h, then 900 mg in next 23 h to achieve sinus rhythm. Beware precipitating bradycardia in patients already on beta blockers, calcium antagonists or digoxin.

(9) Discuss every patient with suspected ACS with the senior A&E doctor.
  - (i) Admit immediately to coronary care all patients with ECG changes, heart failure, hypotension, arrhythmias, persistent pain, raised cardiac enzymes or unstable angina.
  - (ii) Refer for coronary care high-risk patients with known ischaemic heart disease, two or more cardiac risk factors, aged over 65 years or typical cardiac pain.
  - (iii) All remaining patients with possible cardiac pain, or atypical pain without a definite alternate diagnosis must be admitted for observation for at least 6–9 h.

Note: never send home any patient after a single cardiac enzymes result, as you are committed to repeating them at least once, or more usually at 3 h, 6 h and 9 h post-arrival.

PULMONARY EMBOLUS

DIAGNOSIS

(1) Predisposing factors include pre-existing cardiovascular or respiratory disease, malignancy, deep vein thrombosis (DVT) or previous thromboembolism, immobilisation, trauma or recent surgery, pregnancy, the oral contraceptive pill, obesity and long-distance travel.

(2) A small pulmonary embolism (PE) causes sudden dyspnoea, pleuritic pain and possibly haemoptysis, with few physical signs; but look for a low-grade pyrexia (37.5°C), tachypnoea over 20/min, tachycardia and a pleural rub.

(3) A major PE causes dyspnoea, chest pain and collapse, associated with cyanosis, tachycardia, hypotension, a parasternal heave, raised jugular venous pressure (JVP), and a loud delayed pulmonary second sound.

(4) The CXR may be normal or may show a blunted costophrenic angle, raised hemidiaphragm, an area of infarction or linear atelectasis, or an area of oligaemia.

(5) The ECG may show a tachycardia alone or possibly right axis deviation, right heart strain, right bundle branch block (RBBB) and atrial fibrillation.

(6) Blood gases will reflect hypoxia and hypocapnia from hyperventilation, but may be normal.

MANAGEMENT

(1) Give high-dose oxygen through a face mask. Aim for an oxygen saturation above 94%.

(2) Establish venous access with an intravenous cannula, send blood for full blood count (FBC), coagulation profile, urea and electrolytes (U&E), and liver function tests (LFTs), and attach a cardiac monitor and pulse oximeter to the patient.

(3) Relieve pain if it is severe with morphine 5 mg i.v., and give an antiemetic such as metoclopramide 10 mg i.v.

(4) Commence unfractionated heparin 5000 u i.v. as a bolus, followed by 1000 u/h in the high- or intermediate-probability patient without contraindications unless diagnostic tests are imminently available. Alternatively, give LMWH such as enoxaparin 1 mg/kg s.c. or dalteparin 100 IU/kg s.c. 12-hourly if this is preferred hospital policy for a suspected small PE.

(5) Discuss investigation options with the senior A&E doctor:

  (i) A ventilation perfusion (V/Q) lung scan, lower limb ultrasound (to look for an embolic source), computerised tomography pulmonary angiogram (CTPA) or pulmonary angiography may be used to make the diagnosis.

  (ii) The validity of any of the above tests is dependent on the pretest probability determined by the risk factor profile, clinical features and initial investigations.[2]

(6) Admit all patients with a positive diagnosis or indeterminate tests for continued heparin i.v., followed by warfarin orally, or alternative management if the diagnosis is finally excluded.

AORTIC DISSECTION

DIAGNOSIS

(1) Predisposed to by hypertension, Marfan's syndrome or trauma.

(2) The pain is sudden, sharp or tearing, retrosternal or in the back, migratory, and may be severe and resistant to opiates.

(3) Look for absent pulses, a difference of blood pressure in the arms, or the complications of the dissection:

  (i) myocardial ischaemia, aortic incompetence and haemopericardium with pericardial rub or cardiac tamponade (see p. 9);

  (ii) pleural rub or effusion;

  (iii) altered consciousness, syncope, hemiplegia or
         paraplegia;
  (iv)   oliguria and haematuria;
  (v)   intestinal ischaemia or bowel infarction.
(4) The CXR may show a widened mediastinum, blurred
    aortic knob and a left pleural effusion.
(5) The ECG remains remarkably normal despite the
    severity of the pain, but often shows left ventricular
    hypertrophy.

MANAGEMENT

(1) Give high-dose oxygen via a face mask. Aim for an
    oxygen saturation above 94%.
(2) Establish venous access with a large-bore (14 or 16
    gauge) intravenous cannula, send blood for group and
    cross-match, and attach a cardiac monitor and pulse
    oximeter to the patient.
(3) Relieve the pain with morphine 5 mg i.v. and give an
    antiemetic.
(4) Reduce the systolic BP to below 110 mm Hg using a
    labetalol infusion or sodium nitroprusside plus propra-
    nolol in consultation with the senior A&E doctor.
(5) Organise an urgent transoesophageal echocardiogram,
    helical CT scan or aortogram to confirm the diagnosis.
    Contact the cardiothoracic surgeons.

PERICARDITIS

DIAGNOSIS

(1) This may be post-viral or follow a myocardial infarc-
    tion, pericardiotomy, connective tissue disorder,
    uraemia, trauma, tuberculosis or a neoplasm.
(2) The pain is sharp, pleuritic, retrosternal and relieved by
    sitting forward.
(3) A pericardial friction rub is best heard along the left ster-
    nal edge with the patient sitting forward, and is usually
    present at some stage.

(4) An ECG may show tachycardia alone, widespread con-
    cave ST elevation or atrial fibrillation.
(5) The CXR is usually normal, even if a pericardial effu-
    sion is present.

MANAGEMENT

(1) Give the patient a nonsteroidal anti-inflammatory agent
    such as diclofenac (Voltarol) 50 mg orally t.d.s. or
    ibuprofen 400 mg orally t.d.s.
(2) Send blood for FBC, U&E, cardiac enzymes and viral
    serology.
(3) Refer the patient to the medical team for bed rest and
    cardiac monitoring if there are widespread ECG changes
    or raised cardiac enzymes. Echocardiography and peri-
    cardiocentesis are indicated for signs of cardiac tampon-
    ade, such as tachycardia, hypotension, pulsus paradoxus
    and a raised JVP that rises on inspiration, known as
    Kussmaul's sign (see p. 9).

PLEURISY

DIAGNOSIS

(1) Pleurisy or pleuritic pain occurs in association with
    pneumonia, pulmonary infarction, neoplasia, TB, con-
    nective tissue disorders, uraemia or following trauma.
(2) It may also be due to viruses, especially enteroviruses,
    and may be mimicked by a pneumothorax or epidemic
    myalgia (Bornholm disease).
(3) The pain is sharp, localised and exacerbated by moving,
    coughing or breathing, which tends to be shallow.
    Radiation to the shoulder or abdomen occurs with
    diaphragmatic involvement.
(4) A pleural rub is heard, although it may be inaudible if
    pain limits deep breathing, and disappears as an effusion
    develops.
(5) The CXR may reveal the underlying cause or may be
    quite normal.

MANAGEMENT

(1) Give the patient oxygen and a nonsteroidal anti-inflammatory agent such as diclofenac (Voltarol) 50 mg orally t.d.s. or ibuprofen 400 mg orally t.d.s.

(2) Send arterial blood gases if there are significant signs of pulmonary parenchymal disease, and perform an ECG.

(3) If there are associated sudden dyspnoea, tachypnoea and risk factors for thromboembolism, exclude a pulmonary embolus, which is possible even with a normal CXR and ECG (see p. 20).

(4) Refer the patient to the medical team for treatment of the underlying cause.

COMMUNITY-ACQUIRED PNEUMONIA (CAP)

DIAGNOSIS

(1) Fever, dyspnoea, productive cough, haemoptysis and pleuritic chest pain are present.

(2) Less obvious presentations include septicaemia with shock, acute confusional state particularly in the elderly, and referred upper abdominal pain.

(3) Examination may reveal signs of lobar infection, with a dull percussion note and bronchial breathing, but usually there are only localised moist crepitations with diminished breath sounds.

(4) The CXR shows diffuse shadowing unless there is lobar consolidation.

(5) Features of severe CAP include one or more of the following:
  (i)   respiratory rate over 30/min;
  (ii) systolic BP less than 90 mm Hg;
  (iii) diastolic BP less than 60 mm Hg;
  (iv) multilobar CXR changes;
  (v)   white cell count (WCC) less than 4×10^9/l or more than 30×10^9/l;
  (vi) F_iO_2 more than 35% to maintain S_aO_2 of more than 90%.

MANAGEMENT

(1) Give the patient high-dose oxygen, unless there is a known history of obstructive airways disease (use 28%). Aim for an oxygen saturation above 94%.

(2) Take blood for blood culture, WCC, U&E, LFTs and blood sugar. Check the blood gases, particularly if the S_aO_2 is under 92% despite oxygen.

(3) Commence benzylpenicillin 1.2 g i.v. or erythromycin 500 mg orally if atypical pneumonia is suspected, and refer the patient to the medical team.

(4) Severe patients must be referred to intensive therapy unit (ITU) and started on erythromycin 500 mg i.v. and cefuroxime 750 mg.

(5) Young, fit adults with single lobe involvement may be well enough to return home on amoxycillin 500 mg orally t.d.s. or erythromycin 500 mg orally q.d.s. both for 5 days. Inform the patient's general practitioner (GP) by telephone or a letter if the patient is not admitted.

PNEUMOTHORAX

DIAGNOSIS

(1) This may occur spontaneously (especially in Marfan's syndrome, or in tall, asthenic body types), from trauma, and in association with chronic lung disease, e.g. asthma, emphysema or cystic fibrosis.

(2) It may cause only slight dyspnoea and pleuritic chest pain, even when the whole lung is collapsed. Significant dyspnoea with loss of usual exercise tolerance is common in chronic lung disease.

(3) Examination shows reduced chest expansion on the affected side, increased resonance on percussion, and diminished breath sounds.

(4) Request a CXR in all cases. Do not wait for this if there are signs of tension, but proceed immediately to insertion of a wide-bore cannula or intercostal drain (see p. 26).

MANAGEMENT

(1) Patients with a small to moderate (lung collapsed less than halfway to heart border) pneumothorax and with no significant dyspnoea and no chronic lung disease may go home. Arrange immediate follow-up with the GP and A&E review in 1 week. Advise against air travel until changes on the CXR have resolved.

(2) Simple aspiration is appropriate for patients under 50 years without chronic lung disease, with complete collapse or significant dyspnoea.[3]

    (i) Infiltrate local anaesthetic down to the pleura in the second intercostal space in the mid-clavicular line.

    (ii) Insert a 16 gauge cannula into the pleural cavity, withdraw the needle, and connect to a 50-ml syringe with three-way tap.

    (iii) Aspirate air until resistance is felt, the patient coughs excessively, or more than 2500 ml is aspirated.

    (iv) Repeat the CXR; if the lung has re-expanded, observe and repeat the CXR again after 6 h:

        (a) if the lung remains expanded, discharge and arrange follow-up with the GP as above;

        (b) if the lung has collapsed again, insert an intercostal drain.

(3) An intercostal drain is thus only indicated for:

    (i) tension pneumothorax;

    (ii) traumatic pneumothorax or haemothorax;

    (iii) a pneumothorax causing significant dyspnoea, if there is pre-existing chronic lung disease or age over 50 years;

    (iv) any pneumothorax prior to anaesthesia or positive pressure ventilation;

    (v) failed simple aspiration, e.g. more than just a small residual rim of air around the lung.

(4) *Insertion of an intercostal drain*

    (i) Insert the drain into the fifth intercostal space in the mid-axillary line after infiltration with local anaesthetic down to the pleura.

(ii) Use a scalpel blade to incise the skin and subcutaneous fat, followed by blunt dissection down to and through the parietal pleura.

(iii) Slide the drain in gently with a pair of curved artery forceps having removed the trocar.

(iv) Use a size 20–24 French gauge directed apically for a simple pneumothorax, or a larger 28–32 French gauge directed basally for a haemothorax. Connect the drain to an underwater seal.

ABDOMINAL CAUSES OF CHEST PAIN

DIAGNOSIS AND MANAGEMENT

(1) *Oesophagitis*
   (i) This is suggested by burning retrosternal or epigastric pain, worse on stooping, exacerbated by hot drinks or food, and relieved by antacids.
   (ii) It may mimic cardiac pain and be relieved by sublingual glyceryl trinitrate, so consult the senior A&E doctor if there is doubt about the diagnosis, even if the ECG is normal.
   (iii) Otherwise give an antacid and metoclopramide 5 mg orally t.d.s.

(2) *Oesophageal rupture.* See p. 153.

(3) *Acute cholecystitis, pancreatitis and peptic ulceration* can cause chest pain, but other diagnostic features should be present.

MUSCULOSKELETAL AND CHEST WALL PAIN

DIAGNOSIS AND MANAGEMENT

(1) Musculoskeletal disorders cause pain that is worse with movement and breathing. There may have been preceding strenuous exercise, a bout of coughing, or a history of minor trauma.

(2) Pain is localised on palpation and the ECG is normal. A CXR may show a fractured rib but is otherwise normal.

(3) Give the patient a nonsteroidal anti-inflammatory analgesic such as diclofenac 50 mg orally t.d.s. or ibuprofen 400 mg orally t.d.s., and refer back to the GP.

(4) Two specific causes are:

  (i)   *costochondritis (Tietze's syndrome):* causes localised pain and tenderness typically around the second costochondral junction. Prescribe diclofenac 50 mg orally t.d.s. or ibuprofen 400 mg orally t.d.s., and refer the patient back to the GP;

  (ii) *shingles:* causes pain localised to a dermatome, unaffected by breathing, associated with an area of hyperaesthesia preceding the characteristic rash.

    (a) Give the patient (usually elderly) with severe pain a narcotic analgesic and aciclovir 800 mg orally five times a day or famciclovir 250 mg orally t.d.s., if seen within 72 h of vesicle eruption.

    (b) Admit to a suitable isolation area if unable to be nursed at home.

THE BREATHLESS PATIENT

DIFFERENTIAL DIAGNOSIS

Consider the following, some of which were covered in the preceding section on chest pain:

(1) acute asthma
(2) pulmonary oedema
(3) pulmonary embolus
(4) pneumonia and exacerbation of bronchitis
(5) pneumothorax
(6) acute upper airway obstruction
(7) metabolic causes, such as acidosis in diabetic ketosis or salicylate poisoning
(8) muscular weakness from myasthenia gravis or Guillain–Barre syndrome.

ACUTE ASTHMA

DIAGNOSIS

(1) Ascertain the precipitating factors in the present attack, its duration, treatment given including steroids and theophylline derivatives, and the response to treatment.

(2) Ask about previous attacks, hospital admissions, ventilation in an intensive care unit, and the regular use of steroids.

(3) The highest risk categories for a severe attack are:
   (i) the 'morning dipper' – the patient who wakes breathless in the early morning;
   (ii) a recent acute attack within the last month, especially if the patient required steroids;
   (iii) the 'brittle' asthmatic prone to sudden catastrophic attacks;
   (iv) any prior ITU admissions.

(4) Assess the severity of the present attack by carefully examining the patient before any nebuliser therapy is given. A severe attack is indicated by any of the following:[4]
   (i) inability to complete sentences in one breath;
   (ii) respiratory rate of 25 or more breaths/min;
   (iii) tachycardia of 110 or more beats/min;
   (iv) peak expiratory flow (PEF) or forced expiratory volume (FEV_1) 50% or less of predicted or known best (see Fig. 2).

(5) A life-threatening attack is indicated by any of the following:
   (i) PEF under 33% of predicted or best;
   (ii) silent chest, cyanosis or feeble respiratory effort;
   (iii) bradycardia or hypotension;
   (iv) exhaustion, confusion or coma.

MANAGEMENT

(1) Commence high-dose oxygen via a face mask. Maintain the oxygen saturation above 94%.

(2) Give salbutamol 5 mg via an oxygen-driven nebuliser, diluted with 3 ml normal saline.

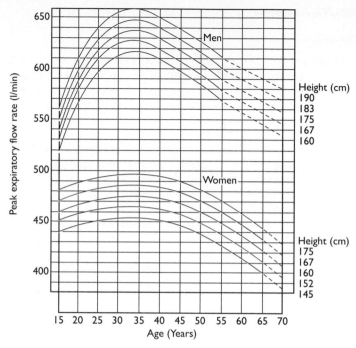

Fig. 2. Predicted normal peak expiratory flow rate in adult males and females (reproduced by kind permission of *Clement Clark International Ltd*).

(3) If there is no response or there is a severe attack, add ipratropium (Atrovent) 500 µg to a second dose of salbutamol 5 mg via the nebuliser.

(4) If the patient is still wheezy, involve the senior A&E doctor and perform the following:

    (i)   Give prednisolone 50 mg orally or hydrocortisone 200 mg i.v. if unable to swallow. Repeat the salbutamol 5 mg via the nebuliser up to every 15–30 min.

    (ii)   Send blood for WCC, U&E and blood sugar, and commence an i.v. infusion of normal saline if the patient is dehydrated.

(iii)   Perform CXR to look for a pneumothorax or an area of consolidation.

(iv)   Arterial blood gases only if the patient is not improving. Markers of a very severe, life-threatening attack are:

    (a)   normal 5–6 kPa (38–45 mm Hg) or high P_aCO_2;

    (b)   severe hypoxia with P_aO_2 under 8 kPa (60 mm Hg);

    (c)   a low pH (or high hydrogen ion concentration);

    (d)   also check K, which may be low.

(v)   Commence an i.v. bronchodilator under ECG control.

    (a)   Give salbutamol 250 μg i.v. over 10 min, followed by an infusion of 5 mg salbutamol in 500 ml of 5% dextrose, i.e. 10 μg/ml at 5 μg/min (30 ml/h or 0.5 ml/min) initially.

    (b)   Or consider a slow bolus of aminophylline 5 mg/kg over 20 min followed by an infusion of 500 mg aminophylline in 500 ml of 5% dextrose, i.e. 1 mg/ml at 0.5 mg/kg/h (35 ml/h or 0.58 ml/min for 70-kg patient).

    (c)   Omit the bolus if the patient is already taking oral theophylline, and send blood for a theophylline level.

(vi)   Admit the patient under the medical team if patient stabilises with a PEF over 50%.

(vii)   Otherwise call the anaesthetist for a deteriorating patient with hypoxia (P_aO_2 less than 8 kPa or 60 mm Hg), hypercapnia (P_aCO_2 over 6 kPa or 45 mm Hg), or any features of a life-threatening attack, and admit to the intensive care unit.

(5)   Meanwhile, in the patient with a mild attack (PEF over 75% predicted) or moderate attack (PEF 50–75% predicted) that improves with nebuliser therapy alone to a PEF over 75%:

    (i)   discharge if the GP can provide early follow-up and the patient has salbutamol and beclomethasone inhalers (and knows how to use them), and prednisolone 50 mg orally daily reduced over 7 days;

(ii)   if there is any doubt about discharging the patient, admit for overnight observation.

PULMONARY OEDEMA

DIAGNOSIS

(1) Pulmonary oedema is usually caused by left ventricular failure due to myocardial infarction, hypertension, an arrhythmia, fluid overload or valvular disease.

(2) Occasional non-cardiac causes include septicaemia, uraemia, head injury, intracranial haemorrhage, and inhalation of smoke or noxious gases.

(3) The patient is clammy, distressed and dyspnoeic, prefers to sit upright, and may have a tachycardia, basal crepitations and a triple rhythm.

(4) The CXR shows engorged upper-lobe veins, a perihilar haze, cardiomegaly, septal Kerley B lines, and small bilateral pleural effusions.

(5) The ECG may help indicate the aetiology.

MANAGEMENT

(1) Sit the patient upright and give 40–60% oxygen, unless the patient is known to have chronic bronchitis, in which case 28% oxygen should be used. Aim for an oxygen saturation above 94%.

(2) Give frusemide 40 mg i.v., or twice their usual oral daily dose i.v. if already on frusemide.

(3) Give glyceryl trinitrate (GTN) 150–300 μg sublingually, which may be repeated. Remove the tablet if excessive hypotension (systolic BP less than 100 mm Hg) occurs.

(4) In refractory cases, get senior A&E doctor help, repeat the frusemide, and commence a GTN infusion, providing the patient is not hypotensive.

(i)   Add GTN 200 mg to 500 ml of 5% dextrose, i.e. 400 μg/ml, using a glass bottle and low-absorption polyethylene infusion set.

    (ii)   Infuse initially at 1 ml/h, maintaining systolic BP above 100 mm Hg. Gradually increase to 20 ml/h or more, avoiding hypotension.

(5) Commence mask CPAP respiratory support:

    (i)   Use a dedicated, high-flow fresh gas circuit, tight-fitting mask and variable resistor valve.

    (ii)   A trained nurse must remain in attendance at all times, as some patients will not tolerate the mask.

    (iii) Never simply use wall oxygen with a black anaesthetic mask and head harness, as this may asphyxiate the patient.

(6) Morphine 1–2.5 mg i.v. with an antiemetic such as metoclopramide 10 mg i.v. is rarely helpful, as it may further obtund the patient.

(7) Admit the patient under the medical team.

PULMONARY EMBOLUS

See p. 20.

PNEUMONIA

See p. 24.

PNEUMOTHORAX

See p. 25.

ACUTE UPPER AIRWAY OBSTRUCTION

DIAGNOSIS

(1) Acute upper airway obstruction may be due to croup, epiglottitis, inhaled foreign body, smoke inhalation, angioneurotic oedema, trauma, carcinoma or retropharyngeal abscess.

(2) There is severe distress, ineffective respiratory efforts, stridor and cyanosis, followed by unconsciousness. There may also be wheeze, coughing, hoarseness or complete aphonia.

MANAGEMENT

This depends on the suspected cause.

(1) Sit the patient up and give 100% oxygen via a face mask. Attach a cardiac monitor and pulse oximeter to the patient. Aim for an oxygen saturation above 94%.

(2) *If inhalation of a foreign body is suspected:*

    (i)   Perform the Heimlich manoeuvre. Stand behind the patient, place your arms around the upper abdomen with your hands clasped in the epigastrium, and give thrusts upwards to expel the obstruction.

    (ii)   In older children and adults, perform up to five back blows and chest thrusts with the victim lying on the side if the Heimlich manoeuvre fails.

    (iii)   In an infant or small child, hold head-down and deliver up to five back blows with the heel of the free hand.

    (iv)   If this fails, perform up to five chest thrusts using the same landmark as for cardiac compression to dislodge foreign material in the airway.

    (v)   If the foreign body is still present, attempt removal under direct vision using a laryngoscope and a pair of long-handled Magill forceps.

    (vi)   If the patient is in extremis and all else has failed, proceed to cricothyrotomy (see Fig. 3).

        (a)   Extend the patient's neck and identify the cricothyroid membrane between the lower border of the thyroid cartilage and the upper border of the cricoid cartilage.

        (b)   Achieve rapid access by inserting a large-bore 14 gauge intravenous cannula through the cricothyroid membrane.

        (c)   Attach this to wall oxygen at 15 l/min using a Y-connector. Insufflate oxygen by intermittent occlusion of the open end of the Y-connector for 1 s in every 5 s.

        (d)   Alternatively, make an incision through the cricothyroid membrane with a scalpel blade, and insert a 4–6-mm ET tube (or small tracheostomy tube) and connect this to an Ambu or Laerdal bag and the oxygen supply.

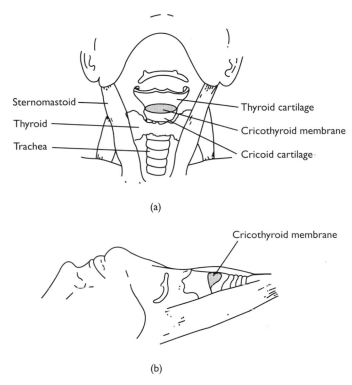

Fig. 3. Cricothyrotomy. The anatomical relationships of the cricothyroid membrane are shown. (a) Anteroposterior view; (b) oblique lateral view.

(3) *Croup.* See p. 288. A child with croup will have a barking cough, harsh stridor and hoarseness, and will be frightened and miserable but not systemically ill. Refer to the paediatric team.

(4) *Epiglottitis.* See p. 289. Inflammation of the epiglottis presents with sudden onset of difficulty in breathing, soft inspiratory stridor, dysphagia and drooling. The child looks toxic and unwell.

    (i)   Do not examine further, i.e. no rectal temperature, BP, or X-ray. Do not attempt to visualise the throat.

    (ii)   Leave the parent holding the child upright with an oxygen mask held near the child's face.

    (iii)   Call for senior emergency department (ED), paediatric, anaesthetic and ENT assistance immediately.

(5) *Smoke inhalation.* See p. 177.

    (i)   Give 100% oxygen and nebulised salbutamol, and refer to intensive care or specialist burns unit if there is an associated respiratory burn. Be prepared to intubate if gross laryngeal oedema occurs.

    (ii)   Send blood for blood gases and a carboxyhaemoglobin level.

(6) *Angioedema.* See p. 101.

    (i)   Give high-dose oxygen and 0.3–0.5 ml of 1:1000 adrenaline intramuscularly, repeated as necessary.

    (ii)   Change to 0.75–1.5 μg/kg, i.e. 50–100 μg or 0.5–1.0 ml of 1:10 000, 5–10 ml of 1:100 000 adrenaline for a 70-kg patient given slowly i.v. if circulatory collapse occurs.

    (iii)   Intubation may still be required, performed by a skilled doctor with airway training.

UPPER GASTROINTESTINAL HAEMORRHAGE

DIAGNOSIS

(1) This presents as:

    (i)   haematemesis and/or melaena

    (ii)   haematochezia – bright red rectal bleeding

    (iii)   collapse and shock

    (iv)   syncope and postural hypotension

    (v)   fatigue, dyspnoea, angina, etc.

(2) Causes include:

    (i)   peptic ulceration (over 50% of cases)

    (ii)   gastritis

        (a)   post-alcohol

      (b)   drug-induced (salicylates, nonsteroidal anti-inflammatory drugs)

(iii)   Mallory–Weiss tear – oesophageal tear following vomiting or retching

(iv)   bleeding oesophageal or gastric varices associated with portal hypertension (usually due to alcoholic cirrhosis)

(v)   reflux oesophagitis

(vi)   others, including gastric neoplasm, blood coagulation disorders, or a connective tissue disorder.

MANAGEMENT

(1) If the patient is shocked, give oxygen and attach a pulse oximeter and cardiac monitor to the patient. Establish venous access with a large-bore 14 gauge intravenous cannula.

(2) (i)   Take blood for haemoglobin (Hb), packed cell volume (PCV), U&E, blood sugar, LFTs, clotting studies including a prothrombin index (PTI) and cross-match from 2 to 4 units of blood, according to the presumed aetiology and degree of shock. As transfusion will preclude further investigation, consider taking blood for later vitamin B_{12} and folate levels.

    (ii)   If liver disease is suspected, examine for jaundice, bruising, gynaecomastia, spider naevi, palmar erythema, clubbing, hepatomegaly and encephalopathy. If portal hypertension is suspected, examine for splenomegaly and ascites.

(3) Commence a transfusion:

    (i)   Start with normal saline 1–2 l.

    (ii)   If the patient is still shocked, use polygeline (Haemaccel), or O-negative blood if the situation is desperate.

    (iii)   Give cross-matched blood when it is available.

(4) Arrange for an urgent endoscopy, particularly in patients who continue to bleed, have suspected varices or are aged over 60 years.

(i)   Endoscopy will differentiate the cause of the bleeding and allow immediate thermal or injection therapy where appropriate.

(ii)   Start octreotide 50 µg i.v bolus followed by 50 µg/h infusion if variceal bleeding is possible.

(5) Refer every case to the medical team for admission. A surgical opinion is indicated if endoscopic therapy fails or is unavailable and bleeding is continuous.

Note: inserting a central venous pressure (CVP) line in a hypotensive, shocked patient is difficult and dangerous, and is best left until initial transfusion is under way for a skilled doctor to perform.

DIABETIC COMA AND PRECOMA

Hypoglycaemia rapidly produces coma in diabetics, compared with the slower onset of altered consciousness in diabetic ketoacidosis and hyperosmolar non-ketotic coma.

DIABETIC KETOACIDOSIS

DIAGNOSIS

(1) Diabetic ketoacidosis (DKA) may occur in a known diabetic, precipitated by trauma, infection, myocardial infarction, cerebral infarction, pancreatitis or inadequate insulin therapy (e.g. insulin stopped in an unwell diabetic patient 'because he is not eating').

(2) Alternatively, it may arise de novo in an undiagnosed diabetic, heralded by polyuria, polydipsia, weight loss, abdominal pain, lethargy or coma.

(3) The predominant features arise from salt and water depletion and acidosis, hence there is dry skin, tachycardia, hypotension (especially postural) and deep sighing respirations (Kussmaul breathing). The ketones may be detected on the breath as a sickly sweet smell.

Note: every patient who presents with abdominal pain, vomiting or thirst must have urine tested for sugar and ketones.

MANAGEMENT

(1) Attach a cardiac monitor and pulse oximeter to the patient, give oxygen and aim for an oxygen saturation above 94%.

(2) Establish venous access and send blood urgently for U&E and blood sugar, blood cultures and FBC.

(3) Start an i.v. infusion and run in 500 ml–1 l normal saline, followed by a further 500 ml/h for the next 4 h if the diagnosis is confirmed.

(4) Send blood for blood gases and organise a CXR, ECG and midstream specimen of urine (MSU).

(5) If the patient is unconscious, pass a nasogastric tube and catheterise the bladder.

(6) (i) Give soluble insulin 10 units i.v. stat.

    (ii) Commence an insulin infusion: add 50 units soluble insulin to 500 ml Haemaccel, i.e. 1 u/10 ml, and run at 5 u/h or 50 ml/h.

    (iii) Continue the i.v. normal saline resuscitation until the blood sugar is 15 mmol/l or less, then change to 5% dextrose but continue the insulin infusion.

(7) Add potassium (K) to the i.v. fluid when the plasma K level is known (this should be within 30 min).

    (i) If K is less than 3.0 mmol/l, give 40 mmol potassium chloride (KCl) per hour (3 g KCl).

    (ii) If K is 3.0–4.0 mmol/l, give 26.8 mmol KCl/h (2 g KCl).

    (iii) If K is 4.0–5.0 mmol/l, give 20 mmol KCl/h (1.5 g KCl).

    (iv) If K is 5.0–6.0 mmol/l, give 13.4 mmol KCl/h (1 g KCl).

    (v) Stop the potassium if:
        (a) the patient is anuric;
        (b) the level is over 6.0 mmol/l;
        (c) the ECG shows peaked T waves or QRS complex widening.

(8) Refer the patient to the medical team or intensive care.
(9) Do not give i.v. sodium bicarbonate except on the advice of the senior A&E doctor. It may be considered if the pH remains below 7.0 with incipient circulatory failure.

HYPEROSMOLAR NON-KETOTIC COMA

DIAGNOSIS

(1) Hyperosmolar non-ketotic coma is more common in the elderly, non-insulin-dependent patient.
(2) It is precipitated by thiazide diuretic use, steroids, infection, myocardial infarction or a stroke.
(3) The patient presents with an altered level of consciousness and focal neurological signs. Mortality is 50%.
(4) Blood glucose and serum osmolarity tend to be higher than in DKA. The osmolarity usually exceeds 350 mosmol/l. It may be estimated by $2(Na + K) +$ urea + glucose (all units in mmol/l).

MANAGEMENT

(1) This is comparable to DKA (see p. 38).
(2) Give i.v. normal saline or half-normal saline if the serum sodium exceeds 150 mmol/l at a similar or slower rate to DKA.
(3) Similar insulin but lower potassium replacement rates are usually required than in DKA.
(4) Commence a prophylactic heparin infusion at 1000 units/h.

ACID–BASE AND ELECTROLYTE DISTURBANCES

Metabolic or respiratory acidosis or alkalosis, hypokalaemia or hyperkalaemia, hyponatraemia and hypercalcaemia may all present as life-threatening emergencies, sometimes with minimal preceding clinical features.

METABOLIC ACIDOSIS

DIAGNOSIS

(1) Causes may be associated with an increased anion gap over 15, calculated from $Na + K - (Cl + HCO_3)$ (all units in mmol/l). These include:
- (i) increased acid production:
  - (a) ketoacidosis, e.g. diabetic, alcoholic, starvation;
  - (b) lactic acidosis (serum lactate >2.5 mmol/l), e.g. cardiac arrest, shock, hypoxia, severe anaemia, liver failure, sepsis, pancreatitis, and drugs such as phenformin, iron and cyanide;
- (ii) exogenous acid ingestion:
  - (a) salicylate
  - (b) ethanol
  - (c) methanol
  - (d) ethylene glycol;
- (iii) decreased acid excretion, as in renal failure.

(2) Or causes may be associated with a normal anion gap under 15. The loss of bicarbonate is balanced by an increase in chloride, resulting in hyperchloraemia. These include:
- (i) loss of alkali:
  - (a) diarrhoea
  - (b) small bowel fistula
  - (c) ureterosigmoidostomy
  - (d) carbonic anhydrase inhibitors;
- (ii) decreased hydrogen ion excretion:
  - (a) hypoadrenalism
  - (b) distal renal tubular acidosis;
- (iii) administration of cationic acids:
  - (a) synthetic amino acid solutions
  - (b) ammonium chloride.

(3) There is a primary fall in plasma bicarbonate below 22 mmol/l.

Table 2. Primary acid–base disturbances with expected compensatory response

Disorder	Primary change	Compensatory response
Metabolic acidosis	↓Bicarbonate	Rapid ↓ P_aCO_2
Metabolic alkalosis	↑Bicarbonate	Variable ↑ P_aCO_2
Respiratory acidosis		
Acute	↑P_aCO_2	Immediate, small ↑ bicarbonate
Chronic	↑P_aCO_2	Slow, larger ↑ bicarbonate
Respiratory alkalosis		
Acute	↓P_aCO_2	Immediate ↓ bicarbonate
Chronic	↓P_aCO_2	Slow, larger ↓ bicarbonate

(4) There is a compensatory fall in the P_aCO_2 (see Table 2).
    (i) Predicted P_aCO_2 (mm Hg) = $1.25\,HCO_3$ (mmol/l) + 10.
    (ii) To convert predicted P_aCO_2 in mm Hg to kPa, multiply by 0.133.
(5) There are few specific clinical features in acute metabolic acidosis other than hyperventilation.

MANAGEMENT

(1) Give oxygen and commence i.v. fluid to maintain the circulation.
(2) Correct any reversible underlying disorders, such as diabetic ketoacidosis.
(3) Refer the patient to the medical team. Dialysis will be necessary for renal failure, and severe salicylate or methanol poisoning.

METABOLIC ALKALOSIS

DIAGNOSIS

(1) Causes are due to a loss of hydrogen ions or a gain of bicarbonate ions, usually in association with an extracellular fluid deficit, hyperaldosteronism or severe hypokalaemia.
    (i) Loss of hydrogen ions:
        (a) vomiting, gastric aspiration

      (b)   diuretics, steroids, carbenoxolone
      (c)   Cushings, Conn's, or Bartter's syndromes.
   (ii)   Gain of bicarbonate ions:
      (a)   excess bicarbonate, including antacids
      (b)   metabolism of lactate, citrate, acetate.

(2) There is a primary increase in plasma bicarbonate above 28 mmol/l.

(3) There is a compensatory rise in P_aCO_2 (see Table 2).
   (i)   Predicted P_aCO_2 (mm Hg) = [HCO_3 (mmol/l)/2] + 30.
   (ii)   To convert predicted P_aCO_2 in mm Hg to kPa, multiply by 0.133.

(4) There are no specific clinical features.

MANAGEMENT

(1) Correct any reversible underlying disorder.
(2) Give normal saline i.v. with potassium if low.

RESPIRATORY ACIDOSIS

DIAGNOSIS

(1) Causes are due to ventilatory failure.
   (i)   *Acute ventilatory failure*
      (a)   sedative drugs e.g. opiates, barbiturates, benzo-diazepines
      (b)   head injury, thoracic or high spinal trauma
      (c)   stroke, meningitis
      (d)   critical asthma, pneumonia
      (e)   neuromuscular disorders, e.g. Guillain–Barre, myasthenia gravis.
   (ii)   *Chronic ventilatory failure*
      (a)   exacerbation of chronic obstructive pulmonary disease (COPD), pulmonary fibrosis
      (b)   marked obesity.

(2) There is a primary increase in P_aCO_2 above 44 mm Hg.

(3) There is a compensatory rise in plasma bicarbonate (see Table 2).

(i)   To convert P_aCO_2 in kPa to mm Hg, multiply by 7.518.

(ii)   In acute respiratory acidosis, predicted HCO_3 (mmol/l) = $[P_aCO_2 \text{ (mm Hg)}/10] + 20$.

(iii) In chronic respiratory acidosis, predicted HCO_3 (mmol/l) = $[P_aCO_2 \text{ (mm Hg)}/2] + 2$.

(4) Hypercapnia leads to confusion, coma and a bounding pulse, although associated hypoxia may dominate the clinical picture.

MANAGEMENT

(1) Give oxygen and commence assisted ventilation by bag-mask ventilation or endotracheal intubation. Call for senior A&E help.

(2) Correct any reversible underlying disorder, e.g. naloxone for opiate poisoning.

(3) Remember that the pulse oximeter may record a normal oxygen saturation in a patient receiving supplemental oxygen, despite the presence of dangerous hypoventilation.

RESPIRATORY ALKALOSIS

DIAGNOSIS

(1) Causes include:

    (i)   Hypoxia:

        (a) acute, e.g. asthma, pneumonia, pulmonary oedema

        (b) chronic, e.g. pulmonary fibrosis, altitude, anaemia.

    (ii)   Respiratory centre stimulation:

        (a) fever, thyrotoxicosis

        (b) head injury, CNS disease

        (c) salicylate poisoning

        (d) pain, fear, anxiety

        (e) pregnancy

        (f) sympathomimetics.

    (iii) Excessive artificial ventilation.

(2) There is a primary decrease in P_aCO_2 below 36 mm Hg.
(3) There is a compensatory fall in plasma bicarbonate (see Table 2).
   (i)   To convert P_aCO_2 in kPa to mm Hg, multiply by 7.518.
   (ii)   In acute respiratory alkalosis, predicted HCO_3 (mmol/l) = $[P_aCO_2$ (mm Hg)/4] + 14.
   (iii) In chronic respiratory alkalosis, predicted HCO_3 (mmol/l) = $[P_aCO_2$ (mm Hg)/2] + 4.
(4) Light-headedness, paraesthaesiae, tingling and numbness with tetany occur, due to decreased ionised calcium.

MANAGEMENT

(1) Look for and correct any reversible underlying disorder.
(2) Never diagnose 'hysterical hyperventilation' until subtle presentations of pneumonia, PE, pneumothorax, fever, etc. have been excluded. Otherwise reassure the patient and ask them to re-breathe into a paper bag if hyperventilation is likely.

HYPOKALAEMIA

DIAGNOSIS

(1) Causes include:
   (i)   Inadequate intake, e.g. alcoholism, starvation.
   (ii)   Abnormal gastrointestinal (GI) losses: vomiting, diarrhoea, laxative abuse.
   (iii) Abnormal renal losses:
       (a) Cushing's, Conn's and Bartter's syndromes
       (b) ectopic adrenocorticotropic hormone (ACTH) production
       (c) drugs, e.g. diuretics, steroids, carbenoxolone
       (d) hypomagnesaemia.
   (iv)   Compartmental shift:
       (a) alkalosis
       (b) insulin
       (c) salbutamol, terbutaline, aminophylline.
(2) Weakness, lassitude, paralytic ileus and eventually thirst, polyuria and rhabdomyolysis occur.

(3) Nonspecific ECG changes include:
  (i)   flat or inverted T waves, prominent U waves;
  (ii)   prolonged PR interval;
  (iii)   ventricular arrhythmias, including torsades de
          pointes.

MANAGEMENT

(1) Attach an ECG monitor, gain i.v. access and replace
    potassium immediately in the following:
  (i)   serum potassium below 3.0 mmol/l;
  (ii)   serum potassium 3.0–3.5 mmol/l in patients with
          chronic heart failure or cardiac arrhythmias, par-
          ticularly if on digoxin or following myocardial
          infarction.
(2) Give potassium 10–20 mmol/h i.v. (never exceed
    40 mmol/h) under ECG control.
(3) Change to oral supplements or maintenance i.v. replace-
    ment when the serum potassium is above 3.5 mmol/l.
(4) Refer the patient to the medical team for treatment of
    the underlying condition.

HYPERKALAEMIA

DIAGNOSIS

(1) Causes include:
  (i)   Spurious, e.g. haemolysed specimen, thrombo-
          cytosis.
  (ii)   Excessive exogenous or endogenous intake:
          (a)   potassium supplements, blood transfusion;
          (b)   rhabdomyolysis, burns.
  (iii)   Decreased excretion:
          (a)   renal failure, Addison's disease;
          (b)   drugs, e.g. potassium-sparing diuretics,
                angiotensin-converting enzyme (ACE) inhi-
                bitors, nonsteroidal anti-inflammatory drugs
                (NSAIDs).
  (iv)   Compartmental shift:
          (a)   acidosis

     (b)   digoxin poisoning, suxamethonium.
(2) Weakness, flaccid paralysis and paraesthesia occur.
(3) ECG changes are characteristic:
    (i)   tall peaked T waves;
    (ii)   ST depression, prolonged PR interval;
    (iii)   QRS widening, absent P waves, sine wave pattern;
    (iv)   ventricular tachycardia, fibrillation or asystole.

MANAGEMENT

(1) Attach an ECG monitor to the patient, gain i.v. access and give 10% calcium chloride 5–10 ml slowly i.v. repeated until life-threatening ECG changes normalise.
(2) Lower the serum potassium rapidly with:
    (i)   50% dextrose 50 ml i.v. with 10 units of soluble insulin;
    (ii)   8.4% sodium bicarbonate 50 ml i.v. providing there is no danger of sodium overload;
    (iii)   salbutamol 10–20 mg nebulised or 5 μg/kg i.v. bolus over 5–10 min.
(3) Refer the patient to the medical team. Urgent haemodialysis or peritoneal dialysis may be necessary, particularly in known renal failure.

HYPONATRAEMIA

DIAGNOSIS

(1) Spurious hyponatraemia occurs in hyperglycaemia. Adjust serum sodium up by 1 mmol/l per 3-mmol/l increase in blood sugar.
(2) True causes are considered according to the patient's underlying volume status.
    (i)   Hypovolaemic hyponatraemia:
        (a)   renal losses – diuretics, Addison's disease, glycosuria, ketonuria;
        (b)   extrarenal losses – vomiting, diarrhoea, burns, pancreatitis.

(ii)   Normovolaemic hyponatraemia:
   (a) syndrome of inappropriate antidiuretic hormone secretion (SIADH) – head injury, meningoencephalitis, cerebrovascular accident (CVA), pneumonia, COPD, neoplasia, HIV infection;
   (b) iatrogenic – transurethral resection of the prostate (TURP) irrigation fluid, hypotonic i.v. fluids postoperative;
   (c) drugs – carbamazepine, NSAIDs, antidepressants, Ecstasy;
   (d) psychogenic polydipsia.
(iii) Hypervolaemic hyponatraemia:
   (a) congestive cardiac failure
   (b) chronic renal failure
   (c) cirrhosis with ascites
   (d) nephrotic syndrome.

(3) Clinical features progress as the serum sodium level drops:
   (i)   anorexia, nausea, vomiting, lethargy
   (ii)   weakness, cramps, headache
   (iii) confusion, seizures, coma (sodium <120 mmol/l).

MANAGEMENT

(1) Assess the underlying volume status. Look at the skin turgor, JVP, measure lying and sitting BP, listen for basal crackles.
(2) Send blood for FBC, U&E, LFTs, thyroid function and osmolarity. Send urine for sodium and osmolarity.
(3) Request a CXR and ECG, and seek senior A&E doctor help.
(4) Treatment is based on the acuity and severity of symptoms and actual sodium level:
   (i)   Commence 1 l normal saline i.v. for acute hypovolaemia.
   (ii)   Treat underlying medical conditions, e.g. antibiotics for sepsis.
   (iii) Otherwise discontinue implicated drug therapy and restrict fluid in more chronic cases.

(iv) Discuss with ITU the use of hypertonic 3% saline
      i.v. in patients with fits or coma. Excessively rapid
      serum sodium repletion and the underlying disease
      process itself are linked to the development of cen-
      tral pontine myelinolysis.

HYPERCALCAEMIA

Minor levels are frequently asymptomatic, but should still be
investigated.

DIAGNOSIS

(1) Causes include malignancy, hyperparathyroidism, drugs
    such as thiazides and vitamin D, sarcoid and TB, thyro-
    toxicosis, Addison's disease and renal failure.
(2) Anorexia, nausea, vomiting, abdominal pain and consti-
    pation occur, with lethargy, polydipsia, polyuria, weak-
    ness, psychosis, confusion and coma (serum calcium >
    3.5 mmol/l).
(3) A CXR may show an underlying cause. ECG may show
    bradycardia and a shortened QT interval.

MANAGEMENT

(1) Insert a large-bore i.v. cannula, send blood for FBC,
    U&E, LFTs, lipase and thyroid function, and commence
    rehydration with 0.9% normal saline i.v. at 500 ml/h.
(2) Give frusemide 20–40 mg i.v. once urine output is estab-
    lished to maintain a diuresis.
(3) Refer the patient to the medical team for longer-term
    therapy with steroids, biphosphonates or dialysis.

THE COLLAPSED OR UNCONSCIOUS PATIENT

The aim is to resuscitate the patient, treat urgent precipitating
conditions, and build up a picture of the situation. The definitive diagnosis may not be made in the A&E department.

MANAGEMENT

(1) (i)   If the patient is unconscious, clear the airway by tilting the head and lifting the chin and remove dentures, vomit or blood with a quick sweep round the mouth with a Yankauer sucker.

  (ii)   In trauma cases, open the airway with the jaw thrust only, avoiding movement of the neck.

  (iii)   Insert an oropharyngeal airway and give oxygen. Attach a cardiac monitor and pulse oximeter to the patient. Aim for an oxygen saturation above 94%.

  (iv)   If there is a reduced or absent gag reflex, urgently call an airway skilled doctor to insert an endotracheal tube.

(2) If no pulse is felt, commence cardiopulmonary resuscitation (see p. 2).

(3) Otherwise:

  (i)   if there is any suggestion of face, head or neck trauma, apply a semi-rigid collar before moving the patient;

  (ii)   remove all the patient's clothing.

(4) (i)   Insert an i.v. cannula and take blood for FBC, coagulation profile, blood sugar, electrolytes, LFTs, blood culture and drug screen for salicylate and paracetamol. Perform arterial blood gases (ABG).

  (ii)   Give 50 ml of 50% dextrose i.v. if the Glucostix is low. Remember that dextrose can precipitate Wernicke's encephalopathy in alcoholic or malnourished patients, who require thiamine 100 mg i.v. immediately.

(5) Record the pulse, BP, temperature (if 35°C, repeat with a low-reading thermometer to exclude hypothermia) and the pupil size and reaction.

(6) If there are pinpoint pupils with hypoventilation, give naloxone 0.4–2 mg i.v. to reverse narcotic poisoning.

(7) Consider other conditions requiring immediate action:

  (i)   *Tension pneumothorax*

(a)   This usually follows trauma, especially if positive pressure ventilation is being given.

(b)   Insert a large-bore cannula or intercostal drain without waiting for an X-ray (see p. 9).

(ii)   *Cardiac arrhythmia.* Treat as necessary after recording a formal 12-lead ECG (see p. 17).

(iii)   *Exsanguination*

(a)   Bleeding may be obvious or concealed, coming from the gastrointestinal tract, an aortic aneurysm or a ruptured ectopic pregnancy.

(b)   Cross-match blood, give i.v. fluids and refer the patient for an urgent surgical opinion.

(iv)   *Anaphylaxis*

(a)   This may follow drug therapy or food ingestion, a bee sting or i.v. contrast administration.

(b)   Give 0.3–0.5 ml of 1:1000 adrenaline intramuscularly repeated as necessary.

(c)   If there is circulatory collapse, give 1:10 000 or 1:100 000 adrenaline 0.75 1.5 µg/kg, i.e. 50–100 µg or 0.5–1.0 ml of 1:10 000, 5–10 ml of 1:100 000 slowly i.v. for a 70-kg patient (see p. 102).

(v)   *Extradural haemorrhage*

(a)   This may follow even trivial trauma. Look for a local bruise on the scalp, for instance in the temporoparietal area over the middle meningeal artery territory.

(b)   Watch for further deterioration in the level of consciousness, ultimately with the development of Cheyne–Stokes breathing and a unilateral fixed, dilated pupil.

(c)   Call an airway skilled doctor to pass a cuffed endotracheal tube if not already in place.

(d)   Refer the patient immediately to the neurosurgical team, before the latter signs develop. Arrange an urgent head CT scan.

(8)   The most common causes of an unconscious patient are:

(i)   poisoning (accidental or deliberate, including alcohol)

(ii)   hypoglycaemia

(iii) postictal state

(iv) stroke

(v)   head injury

(vi) subarachnoid haemorrhage

(vii) respiratory failure

(viii) hypotension, including cardiac arrhythmia or myocardial infarction.

(9) Less common causes of an unconscious patient are:

     (i)   meningitis or encephalitis

     (ii)   hepatic or renal failure

     (iii) septicaemia

     (iv) subdural haematoma

     (v)   hyperglycaemia

     (vi) hypothermia.

(10) Rare causes of an unconscious patient are:

     (i)   cerebral space occupying lesion

     (ii)   Addison's disease

     (iii) myxoedema

     (iv) hypertensive encephalopathy

     (v)   hyponatraemia or hypercalcaemia.

(11) Finally, in those who have recently been abroad, consider:

     (i)   cerebral malaria

     (ii)   typhus, yellow fever, trypanosomiasis and typhoid.

These four lists may seem daunting, but aim to build up a picture of the events as follows:

(12) History:

     (i)   Any clues from relatives, passers-by or ambulance crew?

     (ii)   Any prior medical or surgical conditions?

     (iii) Any known drug therapy or abuse?

     (iv) Any witnessed fit, trauma, alcohol or drug ingestion?

     (v)   Any recent travel abroad?

(13) Further examination:

     (i)   Search the clothing for a diabetic card, steroid card or outpatient card.

     (ii)   Look particularly for signs of trauma, needle puncture marks, or petechiae on the skin.

(iii) Reassess the vital signs, including the temperature.

(iv) Examine the front of the chest, feel the abdomen and examine the back, inspect the perineum and perform a rectal examination.

(v) Reassess the neurological state, including the level of consciousness using the Glasgow coma scale (GCS) score (see p. 168), the pupil responses, eye movements and fundi. Exclude any neck stiffness, and assess the muscle power, tone and reflexes including the plantar responses.

(14) Perform:

(i) CXR, ECG and urinalysis;

(ii) lateral cervical spine X-ray and pelvic X-ray in trauma cases;

(iii) head CT scan if intracranial pathology is suspected or cannot be excluded.

Having treated any urgent conditions and built up a list of the likely causes of unconsciousness, refer the patient to the medical (or surgical) team, or intensive care unit if they are not already involved.

ACUTE NEUROLOGICAL CONDITIONS

The following neurological conditions frequently present to the emergency department:

(1) syncope (faints)

(2) fits

(3) status epilepticus

(4) transient ischaemic attacks

(5) strokes.

Headache is covered separately in the next section.

SYNCOPE

Syncope or a faint is the transient loss of consciousness due to cerebral ischaemia from reduced perfusion, usually with a rapid onset associated with blurred vision, dizziness and sweating. A brief tonic–clonic fit may follow if perfusion remains impaired. Faints may be difficult to distinguish from fits or acute vertigo, so an eye-witness account is vital. Always interview ambulance crew or accompanying adults.

DIAGNOSIS

Causes include:
(1) Vasovagal – 'simple' faint, triggered by heat, pain or emotion.
(2) Hypoglycaemia.
(3) Cardiac:
    (i)   arrhythmia, Stokes–Adams attack
    (ii)   myocardial infarction
    (iii)   stenotic valve lesion (especially aortic stenosis)
    (iv)   hypertrophic cardiomyopathy.
(4) Vascular:
    (i)   carotid sinus hypersensitivity
    (ii)   pulmonary embolism.
(5) Haemorrhage:
    (i)   haematemesis
    (ii)   melaena
    (iii)   concealed (aortic aneurysm or ectopic pregnancy).
(6) Neurological:
    (i)   subarachnoid haemorrhage
    (ii)   vertebrobasilar insufficiency.
(7) Cough or micturition syncope.
(8) Postural hypotension:
    (i)   diabetes, hypoadrenalism
    (ii)   Parkinson's disease
    (iii)   drugs:
        (a) phenothiazines
        (b) tricyclic antidepressants
        (c) anti-hypertensives, e.g. ACE inhibitors, prazosin
        (d) diuretics
        (e) nitrates
        (f) levodopa.

MANAGEMENT

This is aimed at excluding the more serious of the conditions above, e.g. cardiac disease or haemorrhage.

(1) Examine carefully all patients, looking for hypotension (postural), a cardiac lesion, an abdominal mass or tenderness, and focal neurological signs.

(2) Check the Glucostix for hypoglycaemia, ECG and other investigations as indicated (FBC, U&E, LFTs, pregnancy test, G&S and CXR).

(3) Refer the patient to the medical or surgical team as appropriate, or for outpatient follow-up if no immediately life-threatening cause is found. A 24-h ambulatory ECG (Holter monitor) may help, particularly in unexplained recurrent syncope.

(4) Inform the GP by telephone or letter if the patient is discharged.

FITS

DIAGNOSIS

(1) An eye-witness account is crucial to establish the diagnosis. Helpful indicators of a true epileptic seizure having occurred are:
  (i)   bitten tongue, urinary incontinence;
  (ii) preceding aura or proceeding drowsiness;
  (iii) known epilepsy.

(2) In known epileptics, the commonest causes of fits are:
  (i)   not taking their medication;
  (ii) alcohol abuse (withdrawal or excess);
  (iii) intercurrent infection (remember meningitis);
  (iv) head injury;
  (v)   hypoglycaemia.

(3) In non-epileptic patients presenting with a first fit or a sporadic fit, never diagnose new-onset epilepsy until the following are excluded:
  (i)   hypoglycaemia
  (ii) head injury
  (iii) hypoxia
  (iv) infection – especially meningitis and encephalitis (or a febrile fit in a child), HIV
  (v)   acute poisoning, e.g. alcohol, theophylline, cocaine, amphetamine, tricyclics and isoniazid

(vi)   drug withdrawal, e.g. alcohol, benzodiazepine, narcotics, cocaine
(vii) intracranial pathology:
       (a) space-occupying lesion
       (b) cerebral ischaemia
       (c) subarachnoid or intracerebral haemorrhage
(viii) hyponatraemia, hypocalcaemia, uraemia and eclampsia.

Note: the above acute symptomatic causes of grand mal fits must also be excluded in status epilepticus (see p. 57).

MANAGEMENT

(1) Check a Glucostix. If it is low, take blood for a laboratory glucose estimation and give 50 ml of 50% dextrose i.v. (or glucagon 1 mg i.m. if venous access is impossible).
(2) If the patient is fitting, or if the fit recurs, give lorazepam 0.07 mg/kg (up to 4 mg) i.v. or diazepam (Diazemuls) 0.2 mg/kg i.v. and oxygen via a face mask, to maintain the oxygen saturation above 94%.
(3) Do not attempt to wedge the mouth open. Make sure the head is protected from harm and turn the patient semi-prone.
(4) Proceed to FBC, U&E, LFTs, drug screen, blood culture, blood gases, CXR, ECG and CT scan as indicated clinically, and send urgent anticonvulsant levels if the patient is on treatment.
(5) Refer the following patients to the medical team:
    (i)   a suspected underlying cause such as meningitis, tumour, etc.;
    (ii) a fit exceeding 5 min, or recurrent fits, especially if there is no full recovery between them;
    (iii) residual focal CNS signs;
    (iv) a fit following a head injury (refer to the surgeons).
(6) A previously known epileptic may be discharged home if:
    (i)   a rapid, full recovery is made;
    (ii) the fit lasted less than 5 min and was not associated with trauma either before or during the fit;

(iii) there are no residual focal CNS signs and the level of consciousness is normal;

(iv) their usual medication is adequate and being taken;

(v) there is an adult to accompany the patient.

(7) A patient under 40 years with a non-focal first fit, with no serious underlying cause (see point (3) on page 55), and who makes a full recovery without focal neurology, may also be discharged.

(a) Discuss this with the senior A&E doctor.

(b) Perform a CT head scan immediately or within days.

(c) Organise an outpatient EEG and medical clinic review.

(d) Advise the patient not to drive, operate machinery, etc. until seen by the specialist.

(8) Always inform the GP by telephone or letter on discharging a patient, and if the patient is referred to the medical or neurology clinic for follow-up.

STATUS EPILEPTICUS

Two or more seizures without full recovery of consciousness in between, or recurrent epileptic seizures for more than 30 min.

MANAGEMENT

(1) Give the patient oxygen via a face mask, attach a cardiac monitor and pulse oximeter, and aim for an oxygen saturation above 94%.

(2) Check the blood sugar:

(i) If it is low, give 50 ml of 50% dextrose i.v.

(ii) If chronic alcoholism or malnutrition is likely, give thiamine 100 mg i.v. in addition, to avoid precipitating Wernicke's encephalopathy.

(3) Give lorazepam 0.07 mg/kg (up to 4 mg) i.v. or diazepam (Diazemuls) 0.2 mg/kg i.v., but beware causing respiratory depression, bradycardia and hypotension, especially in the elderly.

(4) If the patient is still fitting, get senior A&E doctor help.
    (i)   Repeat the lorazepam or diazepam (Diazemuls) i.v.
    (ii)   Give phenytoin 15 mg/kg i.v. no faster than 50 mg/min by slow bolus or as an infusion in 250 ml normal saline over 30 min (never in dextrose).

(5) Other drugs that may be used include phenobarbitone 10–20 mg/kg i.v. no faster than 100 mg/min, and clonazepam 0.5–2 mg i.v.

(6) Occasionally, if i.v. access is impossible give:
    (i)   rectal diazepam, especially in children, using parenteral diazepam solution (Valium) 0.5 mg/kg given through a small syringe (see p. 300);
    (ii)   paraldehyde 0.4 ml/kg rectally diluted 1 : 1 with olive oil or normal saline if fitting persists.

TRANSIENT ISCHAEMIC ATTACKS

Transient ischaemic attacks (TIAs) are episodes of sudden transient focal neurological deficit, lasting for less than 24 h (often less than 10 min). They may recur and are important in that they may herald a major stroke or other serious vascular event (10% per year).

DIAGNOSIS

(1) The causes may be considered in three groups.
    (i)   Embolic:
        (a)   cardiac – post-myocardial infarction, atrial fibrillation, mitral stenosis, valve prostheses;
        (b)   extracranial vessels – carotid stenosis, narrowed vertebral artery.
    (ii)   Reduced cerebral perfusion:
        (a)   hypotension from hypovolaemia, drugs or a cardiac arrhythmia;
        (b)   hypertension (especially in hypertensive encephalopathy);
        (c)   polycythaemia, paraproteinaemia, antiphospholipid antibodies

(d) vasculitis, e.g. temporal arteritis, systemic lupus erythematosus, polyarteritis nodosa or syphilis.

(iii) Lack of nutrients:

(a) anaemia

(b) hypoglycaemia.

(2) TIAs present clinically as:

(i) carotid territory dysfunction causing hemiparesis, hemianaesthesia, hemianopia, dysphasia, dysarthria and amaurosis fugax (transitory monocular blindness);

(ii) vertebrobasilar territory dysfunction causing combinations of tetraparesis, crossed sensory symptoms, diplopia, nystagmus, ataxia, vertigo and cortical blindness.

(3) Examination must therefore include checking the pulse rhythm, heart sounds, BP (in both arms and postural), listening for carotid bruits and a full neurological assessment.

MANAGEMENT

(1) Perform FBC, erythrocyte sedimentation rate (ESR), coagulation profile, blood sugar, U&E, LFTs, lipids, CXR and ECG.

(2) Arrange an urgent CT brain scan to differentiate haemorrhage from infarction and to look for structural lesions. Organise a duplex carotid ultrasound for a suspected carotid territory ischaemic event[5].

(3) Refer the patient for medical admission if:

(i) an embolic source is suspected;

(ii) carotid stenosis is suspected;

(iii) the patient is hypertensive with a diastolic blood pressure over 110 mm Hg;

(iv) a significant systemic disorder is suspected;

(v) TIAs are recurring over a period of hours, or are of progressive severity and intensity;

(vi) a severe transient neurological deficit occurred or there are residual neurological findings.

(4) Otherwise, if complete recovery has occurred and there is well-documented hypertension, consider starting a beta blocker or diuretic. Refer to medical outpatients and inform the GP.

(5) In the remainder of cases, commence low-dose aspirin 75–150 mg once daily and refer to medical outpatients. Again, inform the GP.

Note: remember that patients can present with the consequences of their TIA, e.g. a head injury, Colles' fracture, or fracture of the neck of femur.

STROKES

These are due to a vascular disturbance producing a focal neurological deficit for over 24 h.

DIAGNOSIS

(1) The causes include:
    (i)   Cerebral ischaemia (80%):
        (a) cerebral thrombosis from atherosclerosis, hypertension or rarely arteritis, etc.;
        (b) cerebral embolism from atrial fibrillation, mitral stenosis, post-myocardial infarction or from atheromatous plaques in a neck vessel.
    (ii)   Cerebral haemorrhage (20%):
        (a) intracerebral haemorrhage associated with hypertension or rarely intracranial tumour and bleeding disorders including anticoagulation;
        (b) subarachnoid haemorrhage from ruptured berry aneurysm or arteriovenous malformation.

(2) Presentation may give a clue to aetiology.
    (i)   Cerebral thrombosis is often preceded by a TIA and the neurological deficit usually progresses gradually. Headache and loss of consciousness are uncommon.
    (ii)   Cerebral embolism causes a sudden, complete neurological deficit.

(iii) Intracerebral haemorrhage causes sudden onset of headache, vomiting, stupor or coma with a rapidly progressive neurological deficit.

(iv) Subarachnoid haemorrhage is heralded by:
  (a) sudden severe headache often after exertion, associated with meningism, i.e. stiff neck, photophobia, vomiting and Kernig's sign (see p. 63);
  (b) confusion or lethargy, which are common, or focal neurological deficit and coma, which are rare and serious.

(3) Record the vital signs, including the temperature, pulse, blood pressure and respiratory rate.

(4) Perform a careful neurological examination, recording any progression of symptoms and signs.

MANAGEMENT

This is essentially supportive.

(1) If the patient is unconscious:
  (i) open the airway by tilting the head and lifting the chin, insert an oropharyngeal airway, give oxygen and pass a nasogastric tube (NGT);
  (ii) place the patient in the left lateral position. Get senior A&E help, and consider endotracheal intubation if there is respiratory depression, deteriorating neurological status and/or signs of raised intracranial pressure.

(2) Otherwise, commence oxygen, and attach a cardiac monitor and pulse oximeter to the patient. Aim for oxygen saturation above 94%.

(3) Gain i.v. access and send blood for FBC, ESR, coagulation profile, U&E, LFTs and blood sugar. Give 50 ml of 50% dextrose i.v. if the Glucostix is low. Catheterise the bladder.

(4) Obtain an ECG and CXR, and arrange an urgent CT head scan.

(5) Refer the patient to the medical team for admission and definitive diagnosis.

(i)   Avoid the temptation to treat acutely raised blood pressure unless hypertensive encephalopathy (see p. 65) or aortic dissection (see p. 21) are suspected.

(ii)   Seek an urgent neurosurgical opinion for a cerebellar stroke presenting with headache, dizziness, vertigo, truncal or limb ataxia, and gaze palsy.

HEADACHE

DIFFERENTIAL DIAGNOSIS

Consider the serious or life-threatening diagnoses first:
(1) meningitis
(2) subarachnoid haemorrhage
(3) space-occupying lesion
(4) hypertensive encephalopathy
(5) temporal arteritis.
The majority, however, will be due to:
(6) migraine
(7) tension headache
(8) post-traumatic headache
(9) disease in other cranial structures.
The history is vital as physical signs may be lacking, even in the serious group. A new headache or a change in quality of a usual one must be evaluated carefully.

MENINGITIS

DIAGNOSIS

(1) Prodromal malaise, followed by generalised headache, fever, vomiting and drowsiness occur, progressing to confusion or coma.
(2) Pyrexia, photophobia and neck stiffness are found. Localised cranial nerve palsies or fits may occur.
(3) Eliciting signs of meningeal irritation are rarely positive (<10%).

(i)   Kernig's sign: pain and spasm in the hamstrings on attempted knee extension, with a flexed hip.
(ii) Brudzinski's sign: involuntary flexion of both hips and knees on passive neck flexion.
(4) A petechial rash suggests meningococcal septicaemia.
(5) Always consider meningitis in the confused elderly, sick neonate, status epilepticus and coma of unknown cause.

MANAGEMENT

(1) Give the patient oxygen and gain i.v. access. Send blood for FBC, coagulation profile, U&E, LFTs, blood sugar, viral studies and blood culture.
(2) Commence a normal saline infusion and perform a CXR.
(3) Seek immediate senior A&E doctor help.
    (i)   Give cefotaxime 2 g i.v. and benzylpenicillin 2.4 g i.v. as soon as the diagnosis is suspected.
    (ii) Perform a CT scan, especially if there are focal neurological signs, papilloedema or mental obtundation. Even if this scan is normal, a lumbar puncture (LP) should be delayed until the signs improve.
    (iii) Otherwise, consider LP without CT if there are no focal neurological signs and the patient has a normal mental state.
(4) Admit the patient under the medical team.

SUBARACHNOID HAEMORRHAGE

DIAGNOSIS

(1) A family history, hypertension, polycystic kidneys and coarctation of the aorta are associated with berry aneurysm, which cause the majority of cases on rupturing.
(2) Prodromal episodes of headache or diplopia due to 'warning leaks' may precede a sudden, severe, 'worst headache ever', often following exertion.

(3) Lethargy, nausea, vomiting and meningism with photo-phobia and neck stiffness occur, although fever is usually absent. A III nerve oculomotor palsy suggests bleeding from a posterior communicating artery aneurysm.

(4) Presentation may also be with acute confusion, transient loss of consciousness or coma, when a stiff neck and subhyaloid (preretinal) haemorrhages are useful diagnostic pointers.

MANAGEMENT

(1) Give the patient oxygen and nurse head upwards. Aim for an oxygen saturation above 94%.

(2) Gain i.v. access and send blood for FBC, coagulation profile, U&E and blood sugar, and perform an ECG and CXR.

(3) Give lorazepam 4 mg or diazepam (Diazemuls) 5 mg i.v. for fits or severe agitation. Give paracetamol 500 mg and codeine phosphate 8 mg (co-codamol 8/500) two tablets orally or occasionally morphine 2.5–5 mg i.v. for pain relief, with an antiemetic such as metoclopramide 10 mg i.v.

(4) Refer the patient to the medical team or neurosurgical unit.

   (i)   Arrange a CT head scan urgently to confirm the diagnosis.

   (ii) Perform a lumbar puncture if the CT scan is negative or unavailable, providing there are no focal neurological signs or papilloedema. Always request xanthochromia studies by spectrophotometry of the CSF to differentiate a traumatic tap (absent) from a true subarachnoid haemorrhage (positive).

   (iii) Consider a nimodipine infusion at 1 mg/h, increased to 2 mg/h after 2 h if the blood pressure is stable, or nimodipine 60 mg orally 4-hourly when the diagnosis is confirmed, after specialist consultation.

SPACE-OCCUPYING LESION

DIAGNOSIS

(1) Causes include an intracranial haematoma, cerebral tumour or cerebral abscess.
(2) The headaches become progressively more frequent and severe, worse in the mornings and exacerbated by coughing, bending or straining.
(3) Vomiting without nausea occurs, and focal neurological signs develop, ranging from subtle personality changes, ataxia, and visual problems to cranial nerve palsies, hemiparesis and seizures.
(4) Papilloedema is seen with loss of venous pulsation and blurring of the disc margin with filling in of the optic cup as the earliest signs on fundoscopy.

MANAGEMENT

(1) Give oxygen, and treat seizures with lorazepam 4 mg i.v. or diazepam (Diazemuls) 5 mg i.v.
(2) Perform a CXR to look for a primary tumour and arrange an immediate CT head scan. Only if this is not readily available, consider a skull X-ray to look for a fracture, shift of the pineal, bony erosion or sclerosis and eroded posterior clinoids or pituitary fossa floor.
(3) Refer any patient with a possible extradural or subdural haematoma to the neurosurgical team.
(4) Otherwise refer the patient to the medical team for full investigation.

HYPERTENSIVE ENCEPHALOPATHY

DIAGNOSIS

(1) An acute hypertensive crisis causing severe hypertension (diastolic over 140 mm Hg), headache, confusion, vomiting, deteriorating vision, and retinal haemorrhages, exudates or papilloedema.
(2) Focal neurological signs, fits and coma develop later.

MANAGEMENT

(1) Give the patient oxygen, attach a cardiac monitor and pulse oximeter, and aim for an oxygen saturation above 94%.
(2) Gain intravenous access and send blood for FBC, U&E, LFTs and blood sugar.
(3) Request a CXR and perform an ECG.
(4) Get senior A&E doctor help.
　　(i)　Aim to initially reduce mean arterial pressure (MAP) by 25% or for a diastolic BP of 100–110 mm Hg.
　　(ii)　Give sodium nitroprusside (SNP) 0.25–10 μg/kg/min i.v. with intra-arterial BP monitoring.
　　(iii)　Or use nifedipine 5–10 mg orally or sublingually.
(5) Refer the patient to the medical team for blood pressure control and to observe for the complications of heart failure, aortic dissection, intracranial haemorrhage and renal impairment.

TEMPORAL ARTERITIS

DIAGNOSIS

(1) Severe, bitemporal headache often associated with a history of malaise, weight loss and myalgia occurring in a patient over 50 years old is typical.
(2) Localised scalp tenderness, hyperaesthesia and decreased temporal arterial pulsation are seen, occasionally with pain on chewing (jaw claudication).
(3) The immediate danger is sudden visual loss due to ophthalmic artery involvement, which may affect both eyes if treatment is delayed.

MANAGEMENT

(1) Send blood for an urgent ESR.
(2) Commence prednisolone 60 mg orally.
(3) Refer the patient to the medical or ophthalmology team for admission for temporal artery biopsy and high-dose steroid therapy.

MIGRAINE

DIAGNOSIS

(1) Classic migraine attacks begin before the age of 40 years with a positive family history in up to 70%.

    (i) A visual prodrome with flashing lights, fortification spectra, teichopsia (zigzag lines of light) and a central scotoma is usual (i.e. migraine with aura).

    (ii) Hemianopia, hemisensory, dysphasic or hemiplegic aura is less common.

    (iii) Headache is unilateral, throbbing or pulsating, recurrent and periodic, lasting from 4 h to 3 days.

    (iv) Nausea, vomiting, photophobia and phonophobia are associated.

(2) Common migraine is more usual in females. It resembles classic migraine, but may be bilateral and lacks the typical prodrome (i.e. migraine without aura).

(3) Rare variants include hemiplegic, ophthalmoplegic and vertebrobasilar migraine.

MANAGEMENT

(1) Nurse the patient in a darkened room, give oxygen by face mask and an analgesic such as aspirin 400 mg and codeine phosphate 8 mg (co-codaprin 8/400) two tablets orally.

(2) Give an antiemetic with anti-dopaminergic effects, such as prochlorperazine (Stemetil) 12.5 mg i.v. If this fails, give chlorpromazine 0.2 mg/kg i.v. with a fluid bolus of normal saline 10 ml/kg[6].

(3) Give sumatriptan 6 mg s.c. only for resistant headache:

    (i) Side effects of tingling, heat and flushing may occur, or rarely chest pain and tightness.

    (ii) Sumatriptan is contraindicated in known coronary artery disease, previous myocardial infarction, and in patients with possible unrecognised coronary artery disease, e.g. post-menopausal women or men over 40 years with risk factors.

    (iii) Sumatriptan is also contraindicated within 24 h of ergotamine-containing therapy.

(4) Discharge the patient back to the GP, having discussed precipitating factors such as chocolate, cheese, alcohol, hunger, etc. that could then be avoided.

TENSION HEADACHE

DIAGNOSIS

(1) Women are more commonly affected with headaches associated with stress but lacking any prodrome.
(2) The pain comes on gradually, and is bilateral, dull, constant and band-like.
(3) Mild nausea, phonophobia and photophobia can occur, but vomiting is rare. Headaches often become chronic.

MANAGEMENT

(1) Give the patient an analgesic such as paracetamol 500 mg and codeine phosphate 8 mg (co-codamol 8/500) two tablets orally.
(2) Reassure the patient and discharge back to the care of the GP.

POST-TRAUMATIC HEADACHE

DIAGNOSIS

(1) Headache following head injury may begin immediately or after a few days, and is present in up to 30% of patients at 6 weeks after mild concussion.
(2) Inability to concentrate, dizziness, insomnia, irritability and even depression may develop, known as the 'post-concussion syndrome'.

MANAGEMENT

(1) Persistent worsening of headache, clouding of consciousness or focal neurological signs require urgent CT scan and referral to the neurosurgical team to exclude a subdural haematoma.

(2) Otherwise treatment is supportive, including analgesics, rest and reassurance that complete recovery is the rule.

(3) Refer the patient back to the GP, as symptoms may persist for up to 1 year.

DISEASE IN OTHER CRANIAL STRUCTURES

DIAGNOSIS AND MANAGEMENT

(1) Glaucoma (see p. 336), iritis (see p. 335), otitis media (see p. 310), sinusitis or dental caries may all present with headache.

(2) Treatment is aimed at the underlying condition.

ACUTE POISONING

Most cases will be acts of deliberate self-harm in the adult, whereas in children they are usually accidental. Initially, all cases are managed as medical emergencies, including resuscitation, substance identification and elimination, specific and nonspecific treatment, and a period of observation. Thereafter, cases will require psychiatric assessment. Remember that an apparently trivial act of self-harm may still indicate serious suicidal intent (see p. 372).

DIAGNOSIS

(1) Consider acute poisoning in any unconscious patient or patient exhibiting bizarre behaviour, or in unexplained metabolic, respiratory or cardiovascular problems.

(2) Obtain information from any witnesses to the circumstances of the poisoning. Ask if tablets were found, and the approximate time of their ingestion.

(3) Corroborate the history with the patient, although he or she may be unable to remember exactly what was taken and when, or may deliberately mislead.

(4) Remember that two or more drugs are taken in 30% of cases, and that alcohol is a common adjunct.

MANAGEMENT

This will depend on whether the patient is unconscious or conscious.

(1) If the patient is unconscious or collapsed:

  (i) Clear the airway by extending the head, remove dentures, vomit or blood by a quick sweep round the mouth with a Yankauer sucker, and give oxygen via a face mask.

  (ii) If the patient is not breathing or the gag reflex is reduced, insert an oropharyngeal (Guedel) airway and use an Ambu or Laerdal bag and face mask to ventilate the patient. Call an airway skilled doctor urgently to pass a cuffed endotracheal tube.

  (iii) Record the pulse, blood pressure, respiratory rate and temperature (beware of hypothermia), and attach a cardiac monitor and pulse oximeter to the patient. Aim for an oxygen saturation above 94%.

  (iv) Gain venous access. Take blood for glucose, U&E, LFTs, and a drug screen for salicylate and paracetamol, and give:

    (a) 50 ml of 50% dextrose i.v. if the Glucostix is low;

    (b) naloxone 0.8–2 mg i.v. if the pupils are pinpoint.

  (v) Maintain the circulation with an infusion of normal saline unless the hypotension is secondary to an arrhythmia or myocardial depression, in which case specific drug therapy and inotropic support with dopamine or dobutamine are indicated.

  (vi) Check the arterial blood gases, CXR and ECG: metabolic acidosis occurs with salicylate, methanol, ethanol, iron and ethylene glycol poisoning.

  (vii) If the patient is cardiovascularly stable, and only if the airway is protected by a cuffed endotracheal tube, perform gastric lavage.

    (a) This must not be done if there is known ingestion of a corrosive substance, oil or petrol, or if this is suspected from scalding of the lips and mouth or a characteristic fetor.

(b) Pass activated charcoal 50 g in 100–200 ml water down the lavage tube prior to removal (see p. 72).

(viii) Get senior A&E doctor help and consult ITU.

(2) If the patient is conscious, do not be misled, as serious poisoning may still have occurred and the effects may be delayed.

    (i) Obtain a history of the substances taken, the time of ingestion, associated alcohol consumption, current medical conditions, and any toxic effects experienced from the poisoning.

    (ii) Examine for clues to the substance taken:

        (a) dilated pupils – tricyclics, amphetamine, cocaine, antihistamines, anticholinergics

        (b) pinpoint pupils – opiates (remember Lomotil), organophosphates

        (c) nystagmus – alcohol, benzodiazepines, phenytoin

        (d) nasal bleeding or perioral sores – solvent abuse

        (e) hyperventilation – salicylate.

    (iii) Check the vital signs and examine the chest for signs of aspiration.

    (iv) Send blood routinely for a paracetamol level.

        (a) This drug may have been taken, and the patient may be seriously poisoned with no overt signs initially. Ask the laboratory staff to save a sample of serum.

        (b) Other drug levels are only indicated in specific cases according to the history and physical findings.

        (c) Send additional blood for U&E, blood sugar and osmolarity as appropriate and obtain an ECG and CXR.

(3) Perform gastrointestinal decontamination. This is no longer routine, and should be considered only in significant poisonings after appropriate supportive care.

    (i) *Gastric lavage*

        (a) Perform gastric lavage in the rare patient who presents early within 1 h of ingestion, who has taken a potentially lethal amount of drug that is not adsorbed by charcoal, such as iron or lithium, or is unconscious.

(b) If the patient has a reduced cough or gag reflex, the airway must first be protected by a cuffed endotracheal tube.

(c) Position the patient head down in the left lateral position, and use 200–300 ml of warm tap water for each lavage cycle.

(d) Corrosive, caustic or petroleum derivative ingestion are absolute contraindications to lavage.

(e) Pass activated charcoal 50 g down the lavage tube before removal (see below).

(ii) *Induced emesis*

(a) This is rarely used, except in children with a potentially lethal ingestion who present within 1 h and will not take charcoal or if the drug is not adsorbed by charcoal.

(b) Give syrup of ipecacuanha 15 ml with water, repeated once after 20 min if necessary.

(c) Never use ipecacuanha if it is known that corrosive material, oil or petrol were ingested, or if the substance taken could induce seizures or drowsiness before the emesis has occurred, as the patient may then aspirate vomitus.

(iii) *Activated charcoal*

(a) This is now considered a first-line measure to reduce the absorption of many drugs, ideally administered within 1–2 h of ingestion.

(b) The dose is 50 g for adults (1 g/kg body weight in children) in 100–200 ml water as a slurry given orally or down a nasogastric tube.

(c) Give repeated 25–50 g doses every 4 h in salicylate, theophylline, digoxin, carbamazepine, quinine, phenytoin, phenobarbitone and dapsone poisoning.

(d) Warn the patient that charcoal is somewhat unpalatable and will turn the stools black.

(e) Avoid if an oral antidote such as methionine is to be given.

(f) Remember that charcoal is not effective for poisoning by cyanide, alcohols, iron, lithium, acid, alkali, petroleum or pesticides.
(4) Admit the patient to the A&E observation ward once relevant drug levels are known and the clinical severity of the poisoning is apparent, or to the medical team or ITU.

SPECIFIC POISONS

Advice on the management of all types of poisoning may be obtained from the Poisons Information Centres:
(1) Telephone the UK National Poisons Information Service (24 h) contact number 0870 600 6266, which directs the caller to the relevant local centre for specialised information.
(2) Individual centres may still be contacted directly on the following numbers:
   (i) Belfast: (028) 9024 0503
   (ii) Birmingham: (0121) 507 5588/9
   (iii) Cardiff: (029) 2070 9901
   (iv) Dublin: (01) 837 9964/6
   (v) Edinburgh: (0131) 536 2300
   (vi) London: (020) 7635 9191
   (vii) Newcastle: (0191) 282 0300
(3) TOXBASE provides information about routine diagnosis, treatment and management of patients exposed to drugs, household products and industrial and agricultural chemicals.
   (i) It is available on the Internet: www.spib.axl.co.uk.
   (ii) Contact (0131) 536 2298 for further information.
(4) TICTAC is a computer-aided tablet and capsule identification system. Contact a Poisons Information Centre to use.

SALICYLATES

DIAGNOSIS

(1) The patient is restless, flushed, sweating and hyperventilating, and may complain of nausea, vomiting, tinnitus or deafness.

(2) Confusion, coma, fits or cardiac arrest are rare and signify severe poisoning.
(3) Complicated metabolic effects occur, including:
   (i)   hypokalaemic alkalosis (vomiting);
   (ii)   respiratory alkalosis (hyperventilation);
   (iii)   metabolic acidosis (several causes);
   (iv)   dehydration and hyperpyrexia;
   (v)   hypoglycaemia or hyperglycaemia;
   (vi)   bleeding tendency (low prothrombin and platelet effect);
   (vii)   pulmonary oedema (hypersensitivity).

MANAGEMENT

(1) Perform gastrointestinal decontamination (see p. 71), including repeat doses of activated charcoal 4-hourly.
(2) Check levels early. In adults, symptoms occur at 350 mg/l (2.5 mmol/l), and toxicity is serious over 500 mg/l (3.6 mmol/l). Repeat the level at least once to monitor for further drug absorption.
(3) Check FBC, U&E, blood sugar, PTI and blood gases if the salicylate level is high or rising, or the patient is symptomatic.
(4) Give i.v. normal saline or 1.26% sodium bicarbonate with potassium to maintain a high urine output. Refer all serious cases with levels over 500 mg/l (3.6 mmol/l) or markedly symptomatic to the medical team. Otherwise observe in the A&E overnight ward.
(5) Haemodialysis may be considered for severe poisoning with metabolic acidosis or a level over 700 mg/l (5.1 mmol/l).

PARACETAMOL

DIAGNOSIS

(1) The initial symptom may be nausea alone, but the danger is delayed fulminant hepatic failure causing abdominal pain, vomiting, hypoglycaemia, tender hepatomegaly, jaundice, encephalopathy and death.

(2) Patients who regularly take enzyme-inducing drugs, such as phenytoin, carbamazepine, phenobarbitone or rifampicin, or alcohol are at increased risk of hepato-toxicity. Starvation and debilitating illness such as AIDS may also increase the risk.

(3) A potentially fatal paracetamol dose is 12 g (150 mg/kg), although in patients on enzyme-inducing drugs it may be as low as 7.5 g (15 tablets).

(4) N-acetylcysteine (Parvolex) is a highly effective antidote, provided it is commenced within 8 h of poisoning. Figure 4 shows a treatment nomogram indicating when to use N-acetylcysteine.

MANAGEMENT

(1) Perform gastrointestinal decontamination (see p. 71).

(2) Check the blood level a minimum of 4 h after ingestion and determine whether the specific antidote is indicated according to the treatment nomogram (see Fig. 4).

(3) Commence N-acetylcysteine i.v. immediately if the blood level is in the toxic range, and send blood for baseline blood sugar, U&E, PTI and LFTs.

    (i) However, if the result of the paracetamol level will not be available within an estimated 8 h of the original ingestion, commence N-acetylcysteine anyway in a patient with a potentially fatal over-dose (see definition above) while awaiting the level.

    (ii) If the level is then found not to be in the toxic range, cease the infusion.

    (iii) In addition, give N-acetylcysteine to every patient who presents 15 h or longer after significant poi-soning, and send blood for serum creatinine, PTI and a paracetamol level. Discuss the further man-agement of these patients presenting late with a Poisons Information Centre clinical toxicologist.

(4) Give i.v. N-acetylcysteine (Parvolex) 150 mg/kg in 200 ml 5% dextrose over 15 min, followed by 50 mg/kg in 500 ml 5% dextrose over 4 h, then 100 mg/kg in 1000 ml 5% dextrose over 16 h.

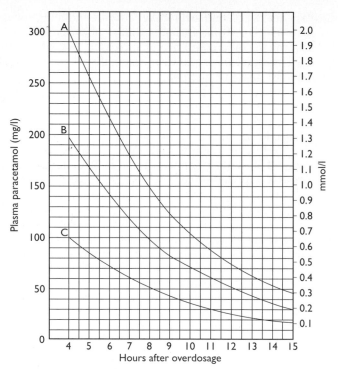

Fig. 4. Treatment nomogram for paracetamol poisoning. Line B: specific treatment is indicated above this line. Line C: specific treatment is indicated above this line in patients who regularly take enzyme-inducing drugs, such as phenytoin, carbamazepine, phenobarbitone and rifampicin, or alcohol. Line A: 90% of untreated patients will develop alanine transaminase (ALT) levels over 1000 u/l, and most fatal cases will be above this line (reproduced with permission from Proudfoot A.T. (1993). *Acute Poisoning Diagnosis and Management*, 2nd edn. Oxford: Butterworth-Heinemann).

    (i)   Side effects include flushing, urticaria, wheeze and hypotension. Stop the infusion and give promethazine 25 mg i.v. and hydrocortisone 200 mg i.v.

    (ii)   Once the adverse effects have settled, restart the N-acetylcysteine infusion cautiously at the lowest rate, e.g. 100 mg/kg over 16 h.

TRICYCLIC ANTIDEPRESSANTS

DIAGNOSIS

These cause drowsiness, dilated pupils, dry mouth, tachycardia and urinary retention, progressing to fits, coma, respiratory depression, hypotension, cardiac arrhythmias and cardiac arrest.

MANAGEMENT

(1) Perform gastrointestinal decontamination (see p. 71).
(2) Request a 12-lead ECG to look for a prolonged PR or QT interval, QRS widening or any arrhythmia.
   (i) Give 8.4% sodium bicarbonate 1–2 ml/kg (1–2 mmol/kg), providing respirations are adequate, which may dramatically improve cardiac arrhythmias even in the absence of acidosis.
   (ii) Avoid giving an antiarrhythmic drug if possible.
(3) Call for senior A&E doctor help to intubate the patient if the conscious level is reduced, respirations are inadequate, convulsions occur, or there are cardiac arrhythmias.
   (i) Hyperventilation also improves cardiac arrhythmias, similarly to sodium bicarbonate.
   (ii) Aim for pH of 7.50–7.55.
(4) Refer the patient to ITU or coronary care unit for ECG monitoring and supportive care. Patients with drowsiness and mild non-progressive or absent ECG changes may be observed in the A&E overnight ward.

BENZODIAZEPINES

DIAGNOSIS

(1) These are comparatively safe taken alone, causing drowsiness, ataxia, dysarthria and nystagmus.
(2) Coma is unusual unless combined with other sedatives or alcohol, or in the elderly.

MANAGEMENT

(1) Gastrointestinal decontamination is rarely necessary unless there was co-ingestion or the patient is unconscious, in

which case airway protection with endotracheal intubation is required first.

(2) Otherwise, give oxygen and place in the left lateral position to prevent aspiration.

(3) Flumazenil, a specific benzodiazepine antagonist, may avoid the need for intubation in severe cases, and clarify the extent of benzodiazepine involvement in coma of unknown aetiology. It is rarely if ever indicated, and must be discussed with the senior A&E doctor.

   (i) Perform an ECG first to exclude additional tricyclic antidepressant poisoning suggested by:
       (a) rate over 100 beats/min
       (b) QRS width over 0.1 s
       (c) corrected QT interval over 0.42 s.
   (ii) If the ECG is abnormal as above, suggesting tricyclic poisoning, or if the patient is epileptic on long-term benzodiazepines, then flumazenil must not be used.
   (iii) Otherwise, give flumazenil 200 μg over 15 s followed by 100 μg/min up to 1 mg total.

(4) Admit the patient to the A&E overnight ward or medical team.

OPIATES

DIAGNOSIS

Opiates cause respiratory depression, pinpoint pupils and hypotension. Vomiting, convulsions and pulmonary oedema may also occur.

MANAGEMENT

(1) Commence supportive care with oxygen and assisted ventilation, and check the blood glucose.

(2) Give naloxone 0.8–2 mg i.v. titrated carefully to response, to avoid precipitating an acute agitated withdrawal.

   (i) Repeat at intervals of 2–3 min to a maximum of 10 mg.
   (ii) Naloxone has a short half-life, and further doses or an infusion may be required.

(3) Refer all patients for overnight admission, as they may relapse as the naloxone wears off.

Note: naloxone may be given intramuscularly or through the endotracheal tube, if venous access is difficult. Remember also to give naloxone in Lomotil and co-proxamol overdoses, and in any case of coma or respiratory depression with pin-point pupils.

IRON

DIAGNOSIS

(1) Iron tablets are often mistaken for sweets by children.
(2) Iron tablets cause initial haemorrhagic gastroenteritis with vomiting and bloody diarrhoea, followed by hypotension, fits, coma, metabolic acidosis, acute liver and renal failure.
(3) A plain abdominal X-ray may show residual whole tablets or a concretion.

MANAGEMENT

(1) Perform gastric lavage, providing the airway is protected, or whole bowel lavage if there are significant numbers of tablets beyond the pylorus.
(2) Give desferrioxamine 2 g i.m. for potentially serious poisoning (>60 mg elemental iron/kg body weight ingested) while awaiting an iron level.
(3) Send blood for FBC, coagulation profile, U&E, LFTs, G&S and an iron level. An iron level in adults of over 50 μmol/l is significant and over 90 μmol/l is serious.
(4) Refer all cases to the medical team. Admission to intensive care and i.v. desferrioxamine 15 mg/kg/h are required for severe cases.

DIGOXIN

DIAGNOSIS

(1) Toxicity occurs from acute overdose or in long-term therapy, particularly in the elderly, associated with

      hypokalaemia, renal impairment, hypercalcaemia and drugs such as amiodarone and quinidine, which increase plasma digoxin concentration.

(2) Foxglove and oleander ingestion will also cause acute cardiac glycoside poisoning.

(3) Fatigue, anorexia, nausea, vomiting, diarrhoea, visual disturbances and altered mental status occur.

(4) Any cardiac arrhythmia may be seen, although brady-cardia, heart block, paroxysmal atrial tachycardia with block, ventricular ectopics and ventricular tachycardia are characteristic.

MANAGEMENT

(1) Perform gastrointestinal decontamination (see p. 71).

(2) Give oxygen and monitor the ECG.

(3) Send blood for U&E and a digoxin level. Toxicity occurs with levels over 2 ng/ml, although the level should be repeated after 4 h in acute poisoning.

(4) In chronic toxicity, correct hypokalaemia with 20 mmol potassium i.v. per hour (1.5 g KCl), but note that in severe acute poisoning hyperkalaemia may occur.

(5) Refer the patient to the medical team for ECG monitoring. Digoxin-specific antibody fragments (Digibind) are indicated for haemodynamically unstable arrhythmias or hyperkalaemia, i.e. serum potassium over 5 mmol/l in severe acute poisoning.

LITHIUM

DIAGNOSIS

(1) Lithium causes nausea, vomiting, diarrhoea, tremor, hypertonia and hyper-reflexia, slurred speech and ataxia, progressing to fits and coma.

(2) Toxicity may be precipitated inadvertently by dehydration or the use of diuretics or nonsteroidal anti-inflammatory drugs, as the therapeutic (0.7–1.3 mmol/l) and toxic (1.5 mmol/l or over) ranges of lithium are close.

MANAGEMENT

(1) Check the lithium level, U&E, blood sugar and ECG.
(2) Perform gastric lavage within 1–2 h of serious poisoning, but do not give activated charcoal (ineffective).
(3) Commence i.v. normal saline, or 5% dextrose if there is hypernatraemia.
(4) Refer all cases to the medical team. The patient may require peritoneal or haemodialysis if the level is over 3.5 mmol/l.

THEOPHYLLINE

DIAGNOSIS

(1) Nausea, intractable vomiting, abdominal pain, agitation, hyperventilation and tachycardia occur, progressing to gastrointestinal bleeding, convulsions, coma and cardiac arrhythmias such as ventricular tachycardia.
(2) Severe hypokalaemia, hypomagnesaemia and hyperglycaemia are seen.
(3) Delayed toxicity occurs with sustained-release preparations.

MANAGEMENT

(1) Perform gastrointestinal decontamination (see p. 71), including repeat doses of activated charcoal 4-hourly.
(2) Give high-dose metoclopramide 10–40 mg i.v. for intractable vomiting. If this fails, consider ondansetron 4 mg i.v.
(3) Monitor the ECG and send blood for U&E, blood sugar, arterial blood gases and theophylline level.
   (i)   Toxic symptoms occur with theophylline levels over 25 mg/l.
   (ii) In acute poisoning, levels over 40 mg/l are dangerous and over 60 mg/l potentially fatal.
   (iii) In chronic toxicity, levels over 20 mg/l cause symptoms and over 40 mg/l are life threatening.
(4) Give lorazepam 4 mg i.v. or diazepam (Diazemuls) 5–10 mg i.v. for convulsions, although endotracheal intubation may then be required.

(5) Correct fluid depletion and hypokalaemia with normal saline and potassium under ECG control.

(6) In non-asthmatic patients, hypokalaemia, hyperglycaemia and tachycardia respond to propranolol 1 mg i.v. over 1 min repeated up to a maximum of 10 mg.

(7) Refer all patients to the medical team for ECG monitoring, intensive care and possibly charcoal haemoperfusion.

BETA BLOCKERS

DIAGNOSIS

Beta blockers may cause bradycardia, hypotension, coma, convulsions and cardiogenic shock.

MANAGEMENT

(1) Perform gastrointestinal decontamination (see p. 71).

(2) Give oxygen, and check U&E and blood sugar.

(3) Give atropine 0.6–1.2 mg i.v. for bradycardia, up to a maximum of 0.04 mg/kg.

(4) Give glucagon 50–150 μg/kg i.v. bolus followed by an infusion at 2–5 mg/h.

(5) In resistant cases, an adrenaline/isoprenaline infusion and cardiac pacing may be necessary.

(6) Admit all cases to coronary care unit (CCU) or ITU.

CALCIUM-CHANNEL-BLOCKING DRUGS

DIAGNOSIS

(1) Nausea, vomiting, lethargy, confusion, coma, bradycardia, hypotension and heart block occur, with hyperglycaemia and lactic acidosis.

(2) The elderly and sustained-release tablet ingestion are the greatest risk.

MANAGEMENT

(1) Perform gastrointestinal decontamination (see p. 71).

(2) Give oxygen, and check U&E, LFTs, ABG and ECG.

(3) Give 10% calcium chloride 5–10 ml i.v. repeated as necessary, with a fluid challenge.
(4) If this fails, give glucagon 5 mg i.v. followed by an infusion at 1–5 mg/h.
(5) Admit the patient to CCU or ITU.

CARBON MONOXIDE

DIAGNOSIS

(1) Carbon monoxide poisoning is usually caused by a car exhaust or the combustion of fuel with an inadequate flue, e.g. a blocked domestic heater.
(2) It causes impaired consciousness, vomiting, headache, neurological signs, hypotension and arrhythmias.
(3) It should be suspected if there are several members of one household who present in a similar fashion.

MANAGEMENT

(1) Give 100% oxygen by tight-fitting mask with reservoir bag, and monitor the ECG.
   (i)   Remember a pulse oximeter will record a misleadingly normal oxygen saturation.
   (ii)   Likewise, the partial pressure of oxygen and calculated oxygen saturation will be normal on arterial blood gases. However, there may be a metabolic acidosis due to tissue hypoxia.
(2) Check the carboxyhaemoglobin level and blood gases, and beta human chorionic gonadotrophin (HCG) pregnancy test in females.
   (i)   A carboxyhaemoglobin level up to 9% is seen in smokers. Higher than this indicates toxic exposure, although there is no absolute correlation between the initial level and eventual outcome.
   (ii)   A carboxyhaemoglobin level over 60% is likely to be associated with severe poisoning and the risk of death.
(3) Comatose patients require endotracheal intubation plus mannitol for cerebral oedema, acid–base correction

and general measures such as i.v. fluid and inotrope support.

(4) If the patient was found unconscious or has neurological symptoms other than headache, cardiac complications, a carboxyhaemoglobin level of 20% or is pregnant, refer to a hyperbaric medicine unit (see p. 127).

    (i)   The best results are achieved if hyperbaric treatment is started within 2 h of the patient being found.

    (ii)   Efficacy is now challenged, so practices may vary.

ORGANOPHOSPHATES

DIAGNOSIS

These are widely available as insecticides.

(1) Absorption is through the skin or bronchi, or orally.

(2) Agitation, headache, sweating, pinpoint pupils, salivation, lachrymation, bronchorrhoea, bronchospasm, abdominal pain and diarrhoea occur.

(3) Weakness, muscle paralysis, bradycardia or tachycardia, coma, convulsions and asystole occur in severe cases.

MANAGEMENT

(1) Remove soiled clothing and wash the skin wearing gloves, give oxygen, and call an airway skilled doctor to pass an endotracheal tube for respiratory failure and severe bronchorrhoea.

(2) Perform gastrointestinal decontamination for oral poisoning (see p. 71).

(3) Monitor the ECG and give atropine 2 mg i.v. repeated until the skin becomes dry, and bronchial secretions are minimal. Massive doses may be necessary, although pupillary dilatation and tachycardia should not be relied on as end points.

(4) Give pralidoxime 1–2 g i.v. over 10 min in all significant cases, although not for carbamate insecticide poisoning.

(5) Admit the patient to ITU.

PARAQUAT

DIAGNOSIS

(1) As little as 10–15 ml of 20% liquid paraquat is fatal.
(2) It causes oral and pharyngeal ulceration, nausea, vomiting and diarrhoea, myocarditis, hepatic and renal damage, and life-threatening pulmonary oedema or progressive pulmonary fibrosis.

MANAGEMENT

(1) Gastric lavage should be performed if the patient presents under 2 h (a rare exception to the rule concerning corrosive materials).
(2) Instil up to 1000 ml of 15% aqueous suspension of Fuller's earth into the stomach via the gastric lavage tube, and give 20% mannitol 200 ml as a cathartic. Use activated charcoal 50–100 g if Fuller's earth is unavailable.
(3) Check the blood gases, but do not give oxygen initially unless the S_aO_2 is under 90%, as this enhances the pulmonary toxicity.
(4) Refer the patient immediately for admission to ITU.

CHLOROQUINE

DIAGNOSIS

(1) This causes nausea, vomiting and drowsiness, followed by dyspnoea, convulsions and coma.
(2) Cardiac effects include hypotension, QRS and QT prolongation, and ventricular arrhythmias.
(3) As little as 2.5–5 g may be rapidly fatal.

MANAGEMENT

(1) Perform gastrointestinal decontamination (see p. 71).
(2) Check the U&E and arterial blood gases, and monitor the ECG.
(3) Give high-dose diazepam 1–2 mg/kg i.v. for severe cardiotoxicity, after an airway skilled doctor has intubated

the patient first. Inotropic support with adrenaline will also be necessary.

(4) Refer the patient to ITU.

CYANIDE

See under smoke inhalation (p. 177).

DISEASES IMPORTED FROM ABROAD

Patients who have been travelling outside the UK should be asked specifically about the time, place and type of travel. They should also be asked how much time they spent in each foreign country and how long they have been back in the UK.

Enquire about malaria prophylaxis and whether it was taken for 4 weeks after leaving the malarial zone, and about immunisations before going abroad.

Advice is always available from:

(1) Departments of tropical medicine or infectious diseases:
- (i) London (Hospital for Tropical Diseases): (020) 7387 4411
- (ii) Liverpool (School of Tropical Medicine): (0151) 708 9393
- (iii) Oxford (John Radcliffe Hospital): (01865) 741 166
- (iv) Birmingham (Heartland Hospital): (0121) 766 6611
- (v) Glasgow (Ruchill Hospital): (0141) 946 7120.

(2) The Internet: this is now the most current source of regional variation in the incidence of various international infections. The US Centers for Disease Control and Prevention at www.cdc.gov/travel/travel.html includes a summary of health information for international travel, and lists of recent disease outbreaks.

(3) Communicable Disease Surveillance Centre Travel Unit: (020) 8200 6868.

COMMON IMPORTED DISEASES OF TRAVELLERS

Some of these diseases are endemic in the UK but more frequently are contracted abroad. They are considered under the following headings:
  (1) Human immunodeficiency virus (HIV) infection
  (2) Gastrointestinal tract infections:
      (i)   *Escherichia coli* gastroenteritis
      (ii) *Salmonella* and *Shigella* gastroenteritis
      (iii) *Campylobacter* enteritis
      (iv) giardiasis
      (v)   amoebiasis
  (3) Helminth infections:
      (i)   schistosomiasis
      (ii) roundworm infection
      (iii) tapeworm infection
  (4) Malaria
  (5) Typhoid
  (6) Dengue
  (7) Meningococcaemia, pneumonia, pyelonephritis
  (8) Viral hepatitis:
      (i)   hepatitis A
      (ii) hepatitis B
      (iii) hepatitis C, D, E and G.

HUMAN IMMUNODEFICIENCY VIRUS INFECTION

DIAGNOSIS

  (1) Casual sexual intercourse, i.v. drug use and blood transfusion in countries with high carrier rates of HIV will expose the patient to infection.
  (2) Assessment and diagnosis require a thorough clinical and laboratory appraisal. HIV testing in the A&E department is inappropriate as skilled counselling and follow-up are not available.
  (3) Moreover, relying on a single serum test for HIV to exclude infection is unwise as:
      (i)   occasional false positives occur;

(ii)   false negatives occur in those infected due to:
    (a)   early infection
    (b)   lack of seroconversion in the first 4 months.

MANAGEMENT

(1) All patients should be referred to the appropriate hospital outpatient clinic that provides a specialist screening service for HIV (see p. 113 on acquired immune deficiency syndrome).

(2) If acute HIV illness is possible, it may then be preferable to perform nucleic acid amplification (NAA) using the polymerase chain reaction (PCR) testing for HIV, or the p 24 antigen.

GASTROINTESTINAL TRACT INFECTION

DIAGNOSIS

(1) 'Traveller's diarrhoea' is most often due to enterotoxigenic *E. coli*, which is usually self-limiting over 2–5 days, causing watery stools and occasionally vomiting. Fever is not a feature.

(2) *Salmonella* and *Shigella* infections tend to cause fever, diarrhoea (which may be blood-stained), vomiting and abdominal pain.

(3) *Campylobacter* infection presents with colicky abdominal pain, which may precede the onset of diarrhoea, which is watery and offensive and sometimes blood-stained.

(4) Giardiasis causes acute watery diarrhoea, which often persists beyond 10 days. Chronic infection may eventually cause malabsorption with steatorrhoea.

(5) Amoebiasis may also cause a chronic, recurrent diarrhoea, with stools containing blood and mucus.

(6) The most important feature in all cases is to assess the patient for dehydration. Dehydration causes thirst, lassitude, dry lax skin, tachycardia and postural hypotension, leading to oliguria, confusion and coma.

MANAGEMENT

(1) In all dehydrated and febrile or toxic patients, send blood for FBC, U&E and blood culture, and commence an i.v. infusion of normal saline. Admit the patient for observation.

(2) Other patients may be allowed home and encouraged to drink plenty of fluid. Alternatively, give the patient an oral glucose and electrolyte solution such as Dioralyte or Rehidrat, or simply advise the patient to drink a mixture of half a teaspoon of salt and six teaspoons of sugar added to a litre of water.

(3) If symptoms persist, ask the patient to return within 24–48 h:

    (i)   Send stools for microscopy and culture then.

    (ii)   Give an antimotility agent such as loperamide 4 mg initially, followed by 2 mg after each loose stool to a maximum of 16 mg/day.

    (iii)   Give empirical treatment for moderate to severe bloody diarrhoea or for associated rigors with ciprofloxacin 500 mg orally b.d. for 3 days (not in children).

    (iv)   If giardia is suspected, give tinidazole 2 g orally once.

    (v)   Arrange follow-up in medical outpatients or by the local GP.

HELMINTH INFECTION

DIAGNOSIS

(1) Schistosomiasis rarely presents acutely, but it should be suspected in cases from endemic areas presenting with fever and diarrhoea associated with eosinophilia, or in cases with painless terminal haematuria or obstructive uropathy.

(2) Roundworm infection is discovered when the adult worm is passed in the stool, although occasionally allergic pneumonitis, abdominal pain or urticaria occur.

(3) Tapeworm infection usually presents with lassitude, weight loss and anaemia.

MALARIA

DIAGNOSIS

(1) The patient usually presents within 4 weeks of returning from a malarious area with fever, rigors, nausea, vomiting, diarrhoea and headache. Hepatosplenomegaly is common.

(2) However, symptoms may occur months or even years later due to release of parasites from the exoerythrocytic phase in the liver (this does not occur in falciparum malaria).

(3) Falciparum malaria is the most dangerous form and may prove rapidly fatal. Most cases are imported from sub-Saharan Africa, South East Asia, Papua New Guinea, the western Pacific, the Amazon basin and Oceania.

   (i)   Large numbers of destroyed red cells affect the capillary circulation, leading to damage to the brain, kidneys, liver, heart, gastrointestinal tract and lungs.

   (ii)   Abrupt onset of encephalopathy with headache, confusion, fits and coma may occur, known as cerebral malaria.

   (iii) Other presentations include an influenza-like illness, diarrhoea and vomiting, jaundice, acute renal failure, acute respiratory distress, arthralgia, postural hypotension or shock, progressive anaemia and thrombocytopenia.

   (iv)   The patient may not appear ill in the first few days, but non-immune patients may then deteriorate rapidly over a few hours and die.

MANAGEMENT

(1) Send a thick and thin film for malarial parasites for every patient returning from abroad with fever and any of the above symptoms or signs. Also send blood for a FBC, U&E and blood culture.

(2) Falciparum malaria is a medical emergency requiring prompt treatment with oral or i.v. quinine therapy. Immediate i.v. treatment is essential if there is altered conscious level, vomiting, jaundice, oliguria, severe

anaemia, over 2% red cells parasitised, hypoglycaemia or acidosis.

(3) Other types of malaria should also be referred to the medical team, although some cases will be treated as outpatients.

(4) Ask patients with negative films but a suggestive history to return for repeat blood films if symptoms persist. Inform the GP of the possibility of malaria by telephone and letter.

(5) If falciparum malaria is likely, admit the patient immediately and begin treatment, if necessary before the blood results are available.

TYPHOID

DIAGNOSIS

(1) The incubation period is up to 3 weeks, with initial symptoms of malaise, headache, fever, anorexia, dry cough and constipation in the first week.

(2) The illness may progress to abdominal distension and pain associated with diarrhoea, splenomegaly, bronchitis, confusion or coma, and rarely a characteristic crop of fine rose-pink macules on the trunk.

(3) In the first week, blood cultures are positive in up to 90%, whereas in the second week stool culture becomes positive in 75% and urine culture in 25%.

MANAGEMENT

(1) Always send blood for a blood culture in all suspected cases and a FBC that may show a leucopenia with a relative lymphocytosis.

(2) Refer all suspected cases to the medical team for ciprofloxacin 500 mg b.d. orally or 200 mg i.v.

(3) Late cases should also have stool and urine cultures sent.

DENGUE

DIAGNOSIS

(1) Dengue occurs after a short 1-week incubation period from infection by one of four serotypes of mosquito-borne

flavivirus, particularly in Central or South America and South East Asia.

(2) There is abrupt fever, chills, retro-orbital or frontal headache, myalgia, back pain, lymphadenopathy and rash.

    (i)   The initial rash is transient, blanching and macular.

    (ii)   Secondary rash on days 3–6 is maculopapular.

(3) Dengue haemorrhagic fever (DHF) and dengue shock syndrome occur in second infections with a different serotype.

MANAGEMENT

(1) Send blood for FBC, coagulation profile, U&E, LFTs, blood culture and serology.

(2) Admit the patient for supportive care, including ITU for DHF.

MENINGOCOCCAEMIA, PNEUMONIA AND PYELONEPHRITIS

DIAGNOSIS AND MANAGEMENT

These important causes of fever and malaise following travel are covered on p. 63 (meningococcaemia), p. 24 (pneumonia) and p. 202 (pyelonephritis).

VIRAL HEPATITIS

See p. 197.

ACUTE MONOARTHROPATHY

DIFFERENTIAL DIAGNOSIS

It is important to distinguish between:
(1) trauma
(2) septic arthritis
(3) gout or pseudogout

and occasionally

(4) rheumatoid arthritis
(5) osteoarthritis.

TRAUMATIC ARTHRITIS

DIAGNOSIS

(1) Severe joint pain is usually associated with obvious trauma, although occasionally the trauma is mild or even forgotten. Haemarthroses may also occur spontaneously in haemophilia A, haemophilia B (Christmas disease) or severe von Willebrand disease.
(2) X-rays are required although may not always demonstrate an obvious fracture (e.g. scaphoid or radial head), but may show only a joint effusion or periosteal elevation as supporting evidence of the fracture.
(3) If septic arthritis cannot be excluded, joint aspiration should be performed by a senior A&E doctor, which generally yields a haemorrhagic effusion, with fat globules in cases of intra-articular fracture.

MANAGEMENT

(1) Refer the patient to the orthopaedic team. Management varies according to the joint involved (see Section IV, Orthopaedic emergencies).
(2) Give Factor VIII to a patient with known haemophilia A or von Willebrand's, and factor IX to a known haemophilia B patient. This should be organised as rapidly as possible in consultation with the haematology team.

SEPTIC ARTHRITIS

DIAGNOSIS

(1) This may occur with penetrating trauma, which may be trivial such as a rose thorn or following arthrocentesis.

(2) Most cases develop from haematogenous spread, predisposed to in patients with rheumatoid arthritis, i.v. drug abuse, debility, immunosuppression, disseminated meningococcal or gonococcal infection, and sickle cell disease.

(3) There is localised pain, warmth and severely restricted movement with a less precipitate onset than with gout.

(4) X-rays will initially be normal, but subsequently will show destruction of bone with loss of the joint space.

(5) Ultrasound is more helpful in demonstrating an effusion, particularly in infection of the hip (see p. 303).

MANAGEMENT

(1) Check the temperature, pulse and BP. Send blood for blood culture, FBC, ESR and C-reactive protein.

(2) Refer the patient immediately to the orthopaedic team for joint aspiration under sterile conditions, rest, i.v. antibiotics and repeated drainage.

GOUTY ARTHRITIS

DIAGNOSIS

(1) Gout is predisposed to by thiazide diuretic therapy, myeloproliferative disease (especially following treatment), and dietary excess, alcohol and trauma.

(2) It is commonest in the metatarsophalangeal joint of the great toe or knee, sometimes with a precipitate onset waking the patient from sleep.

(3) Chronic cases may be associated with gouty tophi on the ear and around the joints, and recurrent acute attacks.

(4) The patient may be mildly pyrexial with a leucocytosis.

(5) The uric acid level is raised (over 0.4 mmol/l), but can be normal in an acute attack.

(6) Definitive diagnosis is by joint aspiration and polarising light microscopy showing strongly negative birefringent crystals.

MANAGEMENT

(1) In a known relapsing case, or if there is strong clinical suspicion of gout, give the patient diclofenac (Voltarol) 50 mg orally t.d.s. for 24 h, then 25 mg orally t.d.s. until the attack settles. Alternatively, use naproxen (Naprosyn) 500 mg orally, followed by 250 mg orally t.d.s.

(2) Refer the patient back to the GP or to medical outpatients.

(3) If septic arthritis cannot be excluded, refer the patient immediately to the orthopaedic team for joint aspiration.

PSEUDOGOUT

(1) This is much less common than gout, typically affecting the knee or wrist, and is associated with diabetes, osteoarthritis, hyperparathyroidism, haemochromatosis and many other rare conditions.

(2) X-ray may show chondrocalcinosis, and joint aspiration shows weakly positive birefringent crystals under polarising light microscopy.

(3) Treatment is as for acute gout, with referral back to the GP or to medical outpatients for follow-up.

RHEUMATOID ARTHRITIS

DIAGNOSIS

(1) This occasionally presents as a monoarthritis, though generally it causes a symmetrical polyarthritis affecting the metacarpophalangeal and proximal interphalangeal joints in particular.

(2) Other joints affected include the knees, elbows and hips.

(3) X-rays initially show soft-tissue swelling only.

(4) Systemic involvement with malaise, weight loss, fever, pleurisy and pericarditis may occur.

MANAGEMENT

(1) If the patient is systemically unwell, refer to the medical team.

(2) If septic arthritis cannot be excluded, refer the patient to the orthopaedic team, remembering that rheumatoid arthritis actually predisposes to septic arthritis.

(3) Otherwise, check FBC, ESR, rheumatoid factor, ANF and DNA antibodies, and refer the patient to medical outpatients or the GP.

(4) Commence a nonsteroidal anti-inflammatory agent such as diclofenac 50 mg orally t.d.s. or naproxen 500 mg orally b.d.

OSTEOARTHRITIS

DIAGNOSIS

(1) This usually presents as a polyarthritis of insidious onset, typically affecting the distal interphalangeal joints.

(2) However, an acute monoarthritis with minimal systemic symptoms may be seen associated with marked joint crepitus.

(3) X-ray shows loss of joint space, osteophyte formation and bony cysts.

MANAGEMENT

(1) Refer the patient to the orthopaedic team if septic arthritis cannot be excluded.

(2) Otherwise, give the patient diclofenac 50 mg orally t.d.s. or naproxen 500 mg orally b.d. and return to the care of the GP.

ACUTE POLYARTHROPATHY

DIAGNOSIS

(1) There are many causes, including:
    (i)   rheumatoid arthritis
    (ii)   systemic lupus erythematosus
    (iii) osteoarthritis

(iv)   psoriatic arthritis
(v)   ankylosing spondylitis
(vi)   Reiter's syndrome
(vii) viral illness, e.g. hepatitis B, rubella, parvovirus B_{19}, HIV
(viii) serum sickness
(ix)   ulcerative colitis, Crohn's disease, Behçet's disease, etc.

MANAGEMENT

(1) Send blood for FBC, ESR, U&E, LFTs, uric acid, rheumatoid factor, ANF and DNA antibodies.
(2) If the patient is systemically unwell, refer to the medical team for bed rest, drug treatment and definitive diagnosis.
(3) Otherwise, commence a nonsteroidal anti-inflammatory agent such as diclofenac (Voltarol) 50 mg orally t.d.s. or naproxen 500 mg orally b.d., and refer the patient to medical or rheumatology outpatients.

NON-ARTICULAR RHEUMATISM

(1) Joint pain, swelling and tenderness mimicking arthritis can be due to inflammation of periarticular structures.
(2) Most patients may be treated with nonsteroidal anti-inflammatory analgesics such as diclofenac 50 mg orally t.d.s. or naproxen 500 mg orally b.d., and then referred to outpatients or their GP.
(3) Joint aspiration and steroid injection are best left to the experts, as complications such as septic arthritis and joint destruction could occur.
(4) Conditions in this category include:
   (i)   torticollis
   (ii)   frozen shoulder
   (iii) supraspinatus tendinitis
   (iv)   subacromial bursitis
   (v)   tennis and golfer's elbow
   (vi)   olecranon bursitis

(vii)   de Quervain's stenosing tenosynovitis
(viii) housemaid's knee.

TORTICOLLIS (WRY NECK)

DIAGNOSIS AND MANAGEMENT

(1) Ask the patient about recent trauma, particularly in the elderly. Look specifically for local sepsis, including tonsillitis, quinsy or a submandibular abscess, and for sensory or motor signs suggesting a cervical disc prolapse.

(2) Exclude drug-induced dystonia due to metoclopramide, phenothiazines or haloperidol. Oculogyric crisis may also occur. Give benzatropine (Cogentin) 1–2 mg i.v. followed by 2 mg orally once daily for 3 days if dystonia is likely.

(3) In the absence of the causes in points (1) and (2) above, manipulate the neck into the neutral position and immobilise in a soft collar.

(4) Give an analgesic such as paracetamol 500 mg and codeine phosphate 8 mg (co-codamol 8/500), and return the patient to their GP.

FROZEN SHOULDER

DIAGNOSIS AND MANAGEMENT

(1) This occurs spontaneously, or following local trauma, or following disuse of the arm after a fracture, CVA, myocardial infarction or even shingles. It is more common in the elderly.

(2) There is pain and loss of all movement from an adhesive capsulitis.

(3) Encourage active shoulder movements following the conditions above to prevent the capsulitis in the first place. Otherwise prescribe an anti-inflammatory analgesic and return the patient to their GP.

(4) Physiotherapy may help, but although the pain subsides, the loss of movement tends to persist for months or even years.

SUPRASPINATUS TENDINITIS

DIAGNOSIS AND MANAGEMENT

(1) This is one of the causes of the 'painful arc' between 60 and 120 degrees of shoulder abduction.
(2) X-ray may show calcification in the supraspinatus tendon.
(3) Give an anti-inflammatory analgesic, and consider referral to the orthopaedic clinic for aspiration and local steroid injection (or to the rheumatology clinic or GP).

SUBACROMIAL BURSITIS

DIAGNOSIS AND MANAGEMENT

(1) This may be due to rupture of calcific material into the subacromial bursa, again causing a 'painful arc' or constant severe pain.
(2) Treat as for supraspinatus tendinitis above.

TENNIS AND GOLFER'S ELBOW

DIAGNOSIS AND MANAGEMENT

(1) Tennis elbow causes pain over the lateral epicondyle of the humerus from a partial tear of the extensor origin of the forearm muscles used in repetitive movements (e.g. using a screwdriver or playing tennis).
(2) Advise the patient to avoid the activity causing the pain, and to rest the arm. Give an anti-inflammatory analgesic.
(3) If the pain is persistent, refer for local steroid injection.
(4) Golfer's elbow is a similar condition affecting the medial epicondyle and the flexor origin.

OLECRANON BURSITIS

DIAGNOSIS AND MANAGEMENT

(1) Painful swelling of this bursa is due to trauma, gout or infection, usually with *Staphylococcus aureus*.
(2) Aspirate under sterile conditions and send fluid for culture and polarising light microscopy if the latter two conditions are likely.

(3) The patient may require immediate referral for drainage of the bursa under anaesthesia if infection is confirmed. Otherwise, refer the patient to orthopaedic outpatients for removal of the bursal sac.

DE QUERVAIN'S STENOSING TENOSYNOVITIS

DIAGNOSIS AND MANAGEMENT

(1) This causes tenderness over the radial styloid, a palpable nodule from thickening of the fibrous sheaths of the abductor pollicis longus and extensor pollicis brevis tendons, and pain on moving the thumb.
(2) Treat by resting the thumb in a splint and by using an anti-inflammatory analgesic.
(3) This condition may require surgical release of the tendon sheaths if local injection of steroid fails.

HOUSEMAID'S KNEE

DIAGNOSIS AND MANAGEMENT

(1) This is a prepatellar bursitis due to friction or occasionally infection.
(2) Treat by giving an anti-inflammatory analgesic, avoiding further trauma and, if necessary, by aspiration and steroid injection by the GP or outpatient clinic (orthopaedic or rheumatology).
(3) If infection is suspected, refer the patient to the orthopaedic team.

ALLERGIC OR IMMUNOLOGICAL CONDITIONS

The following conditions may present, ranging from socially inconvenient to imminently life threatening:
(1) urticaria (hives)
(2) angioedema
(3) anaphylaxis.

URTICARIA (HIVES)

DIAGNOSIS

(1) Itchy, oedematous, transient skin swellings are seen, which may occur in crops lasting several hours.
(2) There are many causes, including:
    (i)   foods – shellfish, eggs, nuts, strawberries, chocolate;
    (ii)   drugs – penicillin, sulphonamide, aspirin, NSAIDs, codeine, morphine;
    (iii) insect stings, animals, parasitic infections (children);
    (iv) physical – cold, heat, sun, pressure, exercise;
    (v)   systemic illness – neoplasm, vasculitis, viral;
    (vi) idiopathic (over 90% of chronic cases).

MANAGEMENT

(1) Give the patient an H_1 antagonist such as loratadine (Claratyn) 10 mg orally b.d. This is not sedating, unlike chlorpheniramine (Piriton). Refractory cases may respond to the addition of an H_2 antagonist such as ranitidine 150 mg orally b.d.
(2) Attempt to identify the likely cause from the recent history. Most reactions occur within minutes but may be delayed for up to 24 h.
(3) Observe for any multisystem involvement suggesting progression to anaphylaxis (see later).

ANGIOEDEMA

DIAGNOSIS

(1) An urticarial reaction involving the deep tissues of the face, eyelids, lips, tongue and occasionally the larynx, often without pruritus.
(2) The causes are as for urticaria, especially ACE inhibitors, aspirin or a bee sting.
(3) It may cause facial, lip and tongue swelling, progressing to laryngeal oedema with hoarseness, dysphagia and stridor.

(4) A rare autosomal dominant hereditary form is due to C1 esterase inhibitor deficiency. A family history of attacks often following minor trauma and recurrent abdominal pain are suggestive.

MANAGEMENT

(1) Commence high-dose oxygen, and attach a cardiac monitor and pulse oximeter to the patient. Aim for an oxygen saturation above 94%.

(2) Give 1:1000 adrenaline 0.3–0.5 ml (0.3–0.5 mg) i.m. repeated as necessary.

    (i)   Change to 1:10 000 or 1:100 000 adrenaline 0.75–1.5 µg/kg i.v., i.e. 50–100 µg or 0.5–1.0 ml of 1:10 000 or 5–10 ml of 1:100 000 over 5 min if rapid deterioration occurs.[7] The ECG must be monitored.

    (ii)   Give 1:1000 adrenaline 1–2 mg (1–2 ml) nebulised whilst preparing the i.v. adrenaline.

(3) If airway obstruction persists, call the senior A&E doctor urgently and be prepared to intubate.

(4) Give H_1 and H_2 blockers and steroids only when cardiorespiratory stability has been achieved (see below).

(5) Hereditary angioedema responds poorly to adrenaline and requires urgent fresh frozen plasma or C1 esterase inhibitor i.v.

(6) Admit the patient when stable for 6–8 h observation, as late deterioration may occur in up to 5%.

ANAPHYLAXIS

DIAGNOSIS

(1) An immunologically mediated systemic illness that may rapidly follow drug ingestion, particularly parenteral penicillin, a bee or wasp sting, and food such as nuts and shellfish. An anaphylactoid reaction is a clinically identical syndrome most commonly following radio-contrast media or aspirin or NSAID exposure, which is not triggered by IgE antibody and therefore does not necessarily require previous exposure.[7]

(2) Respiratory manifestations:
    (i)   rhinitis
    (ii)   cough and bronchospasm
    (iii)   laryngeal oedema, hoarseness and stridor.
(3) Cardiovascular manifestations:
    (i)   tachycardia
    (ii)   hypotension
    (iii)   circulatory collapse.
(4) Other manifestations:
    (i)   erythema, pruritus
    (ii)   local or widespread urticaria
    (iii)   angioedema
    (iv)   headache
    (v)   nausea, vomiting or diarrhoea
    (vi)   joint pains and back pain.

MANAGEMENT

(1) Give high dose oxygen via a face mask, and attach a cardiac monitor and pulse oximeter to the patient. Aim for an oxygen saturation above 94%.
(2) *Laryngeal oedema and wheeze*
    (i)   Give 0.3–0.5 ml of 1:1000 adrenaline i.m. immediately.
    (ii)   Change to 1:10 000 or 1:100 000 adrenaline 0.75–1.5 µg/kg i.v., i.e. 50–100 µg or 0.5–1.0 ml of 1:10 000 or 5–10 ml of 1:100 000 over 5 min if rapid deterioration occurs. The ECG must be monitored.
    (iii) Give 1:1000 adrenaline 1–2 mg (1–2 ml) nebulised while preparing the i.v. adrenaline.
    (iv) Give hydrocortisone 200 mg i.v. Consider aminophylline 5 mg/kg i.v. over 20 min for persistent wheeze (providing the patient is not already taking oral theophylline).
(3) *Shock and circulatory collapse*
    (i)   Give 0.3–0.5 ml of 1:1000 adrenaline (0.3–0.5 mg) i.m. immediately, repeated every 5–10 min until improvement occurs.
    (ii)   Give a bolus of polygeline (Haemaccel) 10–20 ml/kg i.v.

     (iii)   Change to 1:10 000 or 1:100 000 adrenaline 0.75–1.5 μg/kg i.v., i.e. 50–100 μg or 0.5–1.0 ml of 1:10 000 or 5–10 ml of 1:100 000 over 5 min if rapid deterioration occurs. The ECG must be monitored.

(4) Second-line measures after achieving cardiorespiratory stability include:

     (i)   promethazine 12.5–25 mg i.v. plus ranitidine 50 mg i.v.;

     (ii)   hydrocortisone 200 mg i.v. (if not given already);

     (iii)   glucagon 1 mg i.v. repeated as necessary, for patients on beta blockers resistant to the above treatment.

(5) Admit all patients receiving adrenaline for 6–8 h observation as late deterioration may occur in up to 5%.

     (i)   Discharge home on prednisolone 50 mg o.d., promethazine 10 mg t.d.s. and ranitidine 150 mg b.d. all orally for 3 days.

     (ii)   Inform the GP by telephone or letter.

     (iii)   Refer to the allergy clinic all significant or recurrent attacks, especially if the cause is unavoidable or unknown.[7]

SKIN DISORDERS

The vast majority of skin disorders are managed by GPs and the dermatology department, although some patients may present as emergencies with blistering, itching or purpuric conditions. Malignant melanoma may also be seen.

BLISTERING CONDITIONS

DIAGNOSIS

(1) Common causes:

     (i)   viral:

          (a)   herpes zoster

          (b)   herpes simplex

- (ii) impetigo
- (iii) scabies
- (iv) insect bites and papular urticaria
- (v) bullous eczema and pompholyx
- (vi) drugs – sulphonamides, penicillin, barbiturates.
- (2) Less common causes:
  - (i) erythema multiforme and Stevens–Johnson syndrome:
    - (a) drugs such as sulphonamides, salicylates and penicillins
    - (b) mycoplasma pneumonia
    - (c) herpes simplex
  - (ii) toxic epidermal necrolysis
  - (iii) dermatitis herpetiformis
  - (iv) pemphigus and pemphigoid
  - (v) porphyria cutanca tarda.
- (3) Rare causes: congenital – epidermolysis bullosa.

MANAGEMENT

- (1) Refer patients with widespread or potentially life-threatening blistering immediately to the dermatology team or medical team. This should include patients with erythema multiforme, toxic epidermal necrolysis, pemphigus and pemphigoid.
- (2) Otherwise give symptomatic treatment including:
  - (i) antihistamine such as chlorpheniramine 4 mg orally q.d.s. if there is associated pruritus, with a warning about drowsiness;
  - (ii) antibiotics such as flucloxacillin 500 mg orally q.d.s. for secondary staphylococcal infection in herpes zoster, impetigo, insect bites and eczema, or erythromycin 500 mg orally q.d.s. for patients allergic to penicillin;
  - (iii) parasiticidal preparation for scabies (see p. 107);
  - (iv) antiviral agent such as aciclovir 200 mg orally five times a day for 5 days for severe herpes simplex or 800 mg orally five times a day, or famciclovir 250 mg orally t.d.s. for 7 days for severe herpes zoster;

       (v)   topical steroid antiseptic such as 0.1% betamethasone with 3% clioquinol (Betnovate-C) cream three times daily for papular urticaria and bullous eczema.

(3) Return the patient to the care of their GP.

PRURITUS (ITCHING CONDITIONS)

DIAGNOSIS

(1) Causes of pruritus with skin disease:
   - (i)   scabies, pediculosis, insect bites, parasites (roundworm)
   - (ii)   eczema
   - (iii)   contact dermatitis
   - (iv)   urticaria
   - (v)   lichen planus
   - (vi)   pityriasis rosea
   - (vii) dermatitis herpetiformis
   - (viii) drugs.

(2) Causes of pruritus without skin disease:
   - (i)   hepatic or biliary – jaundice, including primary biliary cirrhosis
   - (ii)   chronic renal failure
   - (iii)   haematological:
       - (a) lymphoma
       - (b) polycythaemia rubra vera
   - (iv)   endocrine:
       - (a) myxoedema
       - (b) thyrotoxicosis
   - (v)   carcinoma:
       - (a) lung
       - (b) stomach
   - (vi)   drugs.

MANAGEMENT

(1) Refer patients unable to sleep with intractable pruritus to the dermatology team or medical team.

(2) Otherwise give symptomatic treatment including:

- (i) Antipruritic drug:
  - (a) chlorpheniramine 4 mg orally q.d.s. with a warning about drowsiness;
  - (b) loratadine – although non-sedating, it does not cross the blood–brain barrier and is therefore ineffective for non-allergic pruritus.
- (ii) For scabies:
  - (a) Scabies is suggested by itch worse at night that does not involve the head, a close partner affected, and finding burrows (often excoriated) in interdigital webs around the genitalia or the nipples.
  - (b) Treat the patient and close contacts with 5% permethrin aqueous lotion over the whole body, excluding the head, washed off after 8–24 h. All clothes should also be washed.
  - (c) Explain to the patient that although itching may persist, it is no longer contagious.
  - (d) Advise the patient to attend a genitourinary medicine clinic to exclude an associated sexually transmitted disease if the scabies follows casual sex.
- (iii) For urticaria, see p. 101.
- (iv) Cease any recent drug therapy considered causal, including non-prescription drugs.
- (4) Return the patient to the care of their GP.

PURPURIC CONDITIONS

DIAGNOSIS

- (1) Petechiae and purpura are non-blanching, cutaneous bleeding that may be non-palpable or palpable.
- (2) Causes of non-palpable purpura include:
  - (i) thrombocytopenia with splenomegaly:
    - (a) normal marrow:
      - liver disease with portal hypertension
      - myeloproliferative disorders
      - lymphoproliferative disorders
      - hypersplenism

      (b) abnormal marrow:
- leukaemia
- lymphoma
- myeloid metaplasia

  (ii)   thrombocytopenia without splenomegaly:

      (a) normal marrow:
- immune: idiopathic thrombocytopoenic purpura (ITP), drugs, infections including HIV
- non-immune: vasculitis, sepsis, disseminated intravascular coagulation (DIC), haemolytic-uraemic syndrome

      (b) abnormal marrow:
- cytotoxics
- aplasia, fibrosis or infiltration
- alcohol, thiazides

  (iii) non-thrombocytopoenic:

      (a) cutaneous disorders:
- trauma, sun
- steroids, old age

      (b) systemic disorders:
- uraemia
- von Willebrand's disease
- scurvy, amyloid.

(3) Causes of palpable purpura include:

  (i)   vasculitis:

      (a) polyarteritis nodosa

      (b) leucocytoclastic (allergic), Henoch–Schönlein purpura

  (ii)   emboli:

      (a) meningococcaemia

      (b) gonococcaemia

      (c) other infections: staphylococcus, rickettsia.

(4) The history must include at least any drugs taken, systemic symptoms, bleeding tendency and alcohol use.

MANAGEMENT

(1) Check the temperature, pulse, BP, S_aO_2 and urinalysis, and examine for a spleen, liver and lymphadenopathy.

(2) Send blood for FBC and film, coagulation profile, U&E, LFTs and blood cultures according to the likely aetiology.

(3) Management is of the underlying cause.

MALIGNANT MELANOMA

The incidence of malignant melanoma has doubled in many countries over the last decade.

DIAGNOSIS AND MANAGEMENT

(1) Revised seven-point checklist for suspected malignant melanoma:
   (i) Major signs:
      (a) change in size, e.g. an increase in size of a new or pre-existing cutaneous lesion
      (b) change in shape, especially an irregular outline
      (c) change in colour.
   (ii) Minor signs:
      (a) inflammation
      (b) crusting or bleeding
      (c) sensory changes, including mild itch
      (d) diameter 7 mm or more.
(2) Refer a patient with a pigmented lesion with any major sign urgently to the dermatology team.
(3) A patient with a pigmented lesion and a minor sign should also be referred, although less than 50% will have a melanoma.
(4) Remember that the most common sites for melanoma are on the back and on the legs.

SEXUALLY TRANSMITTED DISEASES

DIAGNOSIS

(1) Urethral discharge, dysuria, penile ulceration, warts and balanitis may present in males.

(2) Vaginal discharge, vaginal pruritus, ulceration, warts, menstrual irregularities and abdominal pain may present in females.

MANAGEMENT

(1) All sexually transmitted diseases require expert diagnosis, treatment, follow-up and partner contact tracing readily available in the Special Clinic (genitourinary medicine clinic).

(2) As many patients are reluctant to attend these clinics, explain carefully the local appointment system, what to expect, and how to locate the clinic. Advise males not to empty the bladder for at least 4 h before attendance.

(3) Occasionally, the patient will require hospital admission for the acute manifestations of AIDS, secondary syphilis, acute Reiter's syndrome, disseminated gonococcal infection, severe primary genital herpes or acute salpingitis.

(4) Genital herpes simplex infection:
   (i)   Treatment started early will reduce pain and shorten the acute attack.
   (ii)   Give aciclovir 200 mg orally five times a day or famciclovir 125 mg orally b.d. for 5 days.
   (iii)   Neither of these influence the likelihood of later reactivation.

ACQUIRED IMMUNE DEFICIENCY SYNDROME (AIDS)

DIAGNOSIS

(1) This is caused by an RNA retrovirus called human immunodeficiency virus (HIV). It is transmitted by sexual contact, syringe sharing in i.v. drug abusers, blood transfusion and transplacentally.

(2) HIV risk groups include:
   (i)   homosexual and bisexual males

- (ii) i.v. drug abusers
- (iii) haemophiliacs and transfusion recipients in the early 1980s
- (iv) heterosexual partners of HIV patients
- (v) children of affected mothers.

(3) CDC classification of HIV infection (Centers for Disease Control and Prevention, Atlanta, Georgia USA) 1986:
- (i) Group 1: acute infection.
- (ii) Group 2: asymptomatic infection.
- (iii) Group 3: persistent generalised lymphadenopathy (PGL).
- (iv) Group 4: symptomatic infection:
  - (a) subgroup A: nonspecific constitutional disease
  - (b) subgroup B: neurological disease
  - (c) subgroup C: secondary infectious diseases categories C1 and C2
  - (d) subgroup D: secondary cancers
  - (e) subgroup E: other conditions.

(4) The revised classification system for HIV infection and an expanded surveillance case definition for AIDS among adolescents and adults were published by the CDC in 1992.[8]
- (i) These emphasised the clinical importance of the absolute CD4+ T-lymphocyte count or its percentage of the total lymphocyte count.
- (ii) A CD4 count under $200/\mu l$ may be used to define AIDS in the USA, and $<100/\mu l$ is associated with invasive infection, i.e. atypical mycobacteria.

(5) Presentation varies according to the disease group.
- (i) Group 1: acute infection
  - (a) 50–70% of patients infected with HIV develop an acute illness with lethargy, fever, pharyngitis, myalgia, rash and lymphadenopathy about 2 weeks after exposure. Acute meningitis or encephalitis are seen occasionally.
  - (b) Although the patient is infectious, serology for HIV antibodies at this early stage will be negative.
- (ii) Group 2: asymptomatic infection

(a) Acute infection symptoms usually resolve by 3 weeks.

(b) Infected patients seroconvert to HIV positive over the next 4 months, most within 2–12 weeks of exposure.

(c) 50% of these patients will have fully developed AIDS by 10 years, with a near 100% mortality within 3 years of its development.

(iii) Group 3: persistent generalised lymphadenopathy

(a) Enlarged nodes in two or more non-contiguous extra-inguinal sites for at least 3 months and not due to a disease other than HIV.

(b) The patient is otherwise relatively well.

(iv) Group 4: symptomatic infection

(a) Subgroup A: constitutional disease with persistent fever, unexplained weight loss of 10% body mass or diarrhoea for over 1 month.

(b) Subgroup B: neurological disease, including encephalopathy, myelopathy and peripheral neuropathy.

(c) Subgroup C: secondary infectious diseases due to opportunistic infections, including *Pneumocystis carinii* pneumonia, recurrent pneumonia, *Mycobacterium tuberculosis*, atypical mycobacteria, toxoplasmosis, cryptosporidiosis, strongyloidosis, cytomegalovirus, systemic candidiasis, cryptococcosis and many others.

(d) Subgroup D: secondary cancers including Kaposi's sarcoma, high-grade non-Hodgkin's lymphoma, primary lymphoma of the brain, and invasive cervical cancer.

(e) Subgroup E: other conditions such as the HIV wasting syndrome and chronic lymphoid interstitial pneumonitis.

(6) AIDS-defining illnesses in a HIV-positive patient are in Subgroups B–E, most commonly *Pneumocystis carinii* pneumonia and *Cryptococcus neoformans* meningitis.

(7) Patients encountered in the A&E department with HIV will range from the asymptomatic carrier state in the

majority, to nonspecific illness or acute problems as varied as collapse, respiratory failure, gastrointestinal bleeding, skin disorders, depression, dementia, stroke and coma.

MANAGEMENT

(1) Always maintain a high index of suspicion to identify the HIV-risk patient, if necessary by direct questioning.
(2) However, consider all patients to be potentially infected and adopt Universal Blood and Body Fluids Precautions with every patient to prevent any disease transmission.
   - (i) Hands should always be washed before and after contact with patients.
   - (ii) Gloves should always be worn when handling blood specimens and body fluids.
   - (iii) Disposable aprons should be worn if there is likely to be contamination of clothing (e.g. from bleeding), and face masks and goggles should be used if splashing is a possibility.
   - (iv) Great care should be taken in handling needles or scalpel blades, particularly on disposal.
   - (v) Blood spills must be cleaned immediately with a suitable chlorine-based disinfectant.
(3) If the patient is acutely ill, refer him or her to the medical team in the usual way. Otherwise refer the patient to the genitourinary medicine Special Clinic or to the appropriate medical outpatient clinic.

Note: HIV antibody testing should not be offered on demand unless the patient has been counselled fully on the use and implications of a positive or negative test, and follow-up is guaranteed.

INOCULATION ACCIDENTS

INOCULATION ACCIDENTS WITH HIV RISK

If accidental inoculation of blood or infectious material from a suspected HIV antibody-positive patient occurs:
(1) Use a skin antiseptic such as 0.5% chlorhexidine in 70% alcohol and encourage bleeding by local venous occlusion.

(2) Take 10 ml clotted blood with consent from the injured person, and if possible 10 ml with consent from the source. Send for HIV testing.

(3) If the source is known to be HIV positive and higher-risk exposure has occurred, e.g. deep needlestick or laceration with blood inoculated, and source is high viral load or late-stage disease:

  (i)   Commence immediate (within hours) triple anti-retroviral therapy with zidovudine 300 mg orally b.d., lamivudine 150 mg orally b.d. and nelfinavir 1.25 g orally b.d. or indinavir 800 mg orally t.d.s. all for 4 weeks. Check your local policy for regional variations.

  (ii) Side effects are complex and significant, including fatigue, headache, anorexia, nausea, vomiting and blood dyscrasias.

  (iii) Every case should be discussed with an infectious diseases expert.

(4) If the source is HIV positive with a low viral load and lower-risk exposure has occurred, e.g. superficial scratch or mucous membrane, commence zidovudine and lamivudine only as above, or according to local policy.

(5) Refer the injured person to Occupational Health for follow-up, advice and counselling. Report the incident to a senior member of the A&E department staff and infection control officer.

(6) The risk of seroconversion following a needlestick injury with HIV-positive blood is less than 1 in 300.

  (i)   However, the exposed person should be followed up for 6 months, should practise safe sex, should not donate blood and should avoid pregnancy.

  (ii) Confidentiality and sensitivity for all concerned must be assured.

(7) Consider the additional possibility of transmission of hepatitis B (see below) and the need for tetanus prophylaxis.

INOCULATION ACCIDENTS WITH HEPATITIS B RISK

(1) Wash the area with soap and water, dress the wound, and give tetanus prophylaxis.

Table 3. Hepatitis B prophylaxis following significant percutaneous, ocular or mucous membrane exposure

Source	Exposed person	
	Unvaccinated	Previously vaccinated with HB vaccine
HBsAg positive	(i) HBIG immediately (ii) Initiate HB vaccine series	(i) Test exposed person for anti-HBs (ii) If anti-HBs level inadequate, give HBIG immediately and booster HB vaccine
Known source; high risk of being HBsAg positive	(i) Initiate HB vaccine series (ii) Test source for HBsAg; if positive, give exposed person HBIG in addition	(i) Test exposed person for anti-HBs; if level inadequate, test source for HBsAg (ii) If source positive, treat as (ii) above
Known source; low risk of being HBsAg positive	Initiate HB vaccine series	No action required
Source unknown or untraceable	Initiate HB vaccine series	No action required

HBsAg, hepatitis B surface antigen; anti-HBs, antibody to HBsAg; HBIG, hepatitis B immunoglobulin; HB vaccine, hepatitis B vaccine.

HB vaccine series: three doses of 1 ml (20 µg) on day 1, at 1 month and at 6 months. For children (birth–12 years) give 0.5 ml (10 µg). Give i.m. into deltoid or anterolateral thigh, not the buttock (efficacy reduced).

(2) Use Table 3 for recommendations for hepatitis B prophylaxis following significant percutaneous, ocular or mucous membrane exposure.

(3) Refer the patient to Occupational Health for follow-up. Inform the senior A&E department doctor and infection control officer.

(4) The risk of seroconversion in a non-immunised person following a needlestick injury with HBV-positive blood is about 1 in 5.

THE ELDERLY PATIENT

(1) An increasing number of patients over the age of 65 years attend A&E departments and pose unique problems of their own.

(2) These problems begin in the waiting area, where old people may become frightened or confused due to their inability to see, hear or move easily and understand instructions.

(3) Particular factors must always be considered before discharging an elderly patient. Ask yourself the following questions:

    (i)   Can the patient walk safely with or without a stick?

    (ii)   Can the patient get home safely and easily?

    (iii)   Once home, can the patient cope with dressing, washing, using the toilet, shopping, cooking, cleaning or relaxing?

    (iv)   Can the patient understand new or existing medication?

    (v)   Can relatives or friends cope any more?

(4) If the answers to any of the above are 'no', do not discharge the patient until help has been sought from the following people. If necessary, keep the patient in overnight to facilitate arrangements:

    (i)   General practitioner:

        (a)   the key person to coordinate the care of the patient at home;

        (b)   always contact by telephone as well as by letter.

    (ii)   Social worker (hospital- or community-based), who can offer:

        (a)   home help

        (b)   'meals on wheels'

        (c)   lunch and recreational clubs

        (d)   voluntary visiting services

        (e)   laundry service

        (f)   chiropody service

        (g)   home adaptation service

        (h)   emergency accommodation.

(iii) District nursing service: this includes an evening and night nursing service.
(iv) Health visitor.
(v) Domiciliary physiotherapist or occupational therapist.

DISORDERED BEHAVIOUR IN THE ELDERLY

A breakdown in a patient's normal, socially acceptable behaviour can be classified into three broad categories:
(1) delirium (toxic confusional state)
(2) dementia (organic confusional state)
(3) depression (psychiatric confusional state).

DIAGNOSIS

(1) *Delirium or toxic confusional state*
    (i) This includes clouding of consciousness, inattention and failure of recent memory.
    (ii) It results in an acute or fluctuating confusional state with recent memory loss, associated with aggressive, restless behaviour and hallucinations, and is often worse at night.
    (iii) Causes are many, including:
        (a) infection – pneumonia, urinary tract infection (UTI), cholecystitis, septicaemia
        (b) hypoxia – respiratory disease, heart failure, anaemia
        (c) cerebral ischaemia – TIA, stroke
        (d) cerebral lesion – haematoma, tumour, infection
        (e) iatrogenic – many drugs (remember poisoning, both accidental and deliberate), alcohol
        (f) vitamin deficiency – poor diet
        (g) metabolic – including dehydration, electrolyte imbalance and hypoglycaemia or hyperglycaemia
        (h) pain, cold, urinary retention, faecal impaction.
(2) *Dementia or organic confusional state*
    (i) This includes disorientation in place, time and person, abnormal or antisocial behaviour, short-term memory loss, loss of intellect and loss of insight.

  (ii)   The causes are many, although a definitive new
         diagnosis is seldom made in the emergency
         department.
  (iii) However, if a known demented patient is brought
         into the A&E department with recent deterior-
         ation, the causes in listed in (1 iii) above should be
         sought.
(3) *Depression or psychiatric confusional state*
  (i)   This includes difficulty in sleeping, demanding or
         withdrawn behaviour, hypochondriasis, a loss of
         self-interest and a sense of futility.
  (ii)   Suicide is a risk, particularly if the patient lives
         alone and is physically incapacitated or has made
         previous attempts at suicide.

MANAGEMENT

(1) A toxic confusional state and decompensated dementia
    require hospital admission (do not simply sedate).
(2) Depression and a high suicide risk require urgent refer-
    ral to a psychiatrist and possible hospital admission.

FALLS IN THE ELDERLY

DIAGNOSIS

Two aspects must always be considered following a fall in the
elderly:
(1) The cause of the fall:
  (i)   Accidental:
         (a) obstacles in the home, such as a trailing flex,
             the edge of a carpet, poor lighting, or no
             handrails
         (b) inappropriate footwear.
  (ii)   Musculoskeletal:
         (a) arthritis
         (b) obesity
         (c) physical inactivity.
  (iii) Visual failure:
         (a) cataracts

    (b)   senile macular degeneration
    (c)   glaucoma.
(iv) Sedating drugs:
    (a)   benzodiazepines
    (b)   antihistamines
    (c)   psychotropics
    (d)   alcohol.
(v)   Postural hypotension:
    (a)   autonomic failure
    (b)   drug-induced
    (c)   occult bleeding.
(vi) Syncopal episode:
    (a)   vertebrobasilar insufficiency
    (b)   cardiac arrhythmia, infarction, heart block.
(vii) Cerebral disorder:
    (a)   Parkinson's disease
    (b)   seizure
    (c)   stroke.
(viii) Balance disorder:
    (a)   inner ear disease
    (b)   impaired proprioception.
(2) The result of the fall:
    (i)   Fracture:
        (a)   Colles'
        (b)   neck of femur or pelvis
        (c)   skull
        (d)   ribs.
    (ii) Hypothermia.
    (iii) Pressure sores, rhabdomyolysis.
    (iv) Hypostatic pneumonia.
    (v)   Loss of confidence and independence.

MANAGEMENT

(1) All falls in the elderly, particularly if recurrent, must be diagnosed and managed correctly, otherwise a fatal injury will eventually occur.
(2) Refer the patient to the medical or geriatric team for admission if acute care is needed or if there is any doubt about their ability to cope at home.

(3) Otherwise, refer to outpatients, physiotherapy, occupational therapy or social services and liaise closely with the GP.

REFERENCES

1   Advanced Life Support Working Group. European Resuscitation Council guidelines 2000 for adult advanced life support. *Resuscitation* 2001;48:211–21.
2   British Thoracic Society. Suspected acute pulmonary embolism. *Thorax* 1997;52:S1–24.
3   Chan SSW. Current opinions and practices in the treatment of spontaneous pneumothorax. *J Accid Emerg Med* 2000;17: 165–9.
4   British Thoracic Society. Guidelines for the management of asthma. *BMJ* 1993;306:776–82.
5   Hankey GJ. Transient ischaemic attacks and stroke. *Med J Aust* 2000;172:394–400.
6   Kelly A-M. Migraine: pharmacotherapy in the emergency department. *J Accid Emerg Med* 2000;17:241–5.
7   Brown AFT. Therapeutic controversies in the management of acute anaphylaxis. *J Accid Emerg Med* 1998;15:89–95.
8   CDC. 1993 revised classification system for HIV infection and expanded surveillance case definition for AIDS among adolescents and adults. *Morbidity and Mortality Weekly Report* 1992;41(RR-17):1–19.

ENVIRONMENTAL EMERGENCIES

HEAT, COLD AND NEAR-DROWNING

Heat illness, hypothermia and near-drowning are considered together here; sports diving accidents are considered in the next section.

HEAT ILLNESS

This is predisposed to by hot weather, exercise, obesity, lack of physical fitness or acclimatisation, fever, and recent alcohol intake or anticholinergic drug use.

DIAGNOSIS

(1) Mild to moderate heat illness with intact thermoregulatory mechanisms:
  (i) Heat cramps – pains develop in heavily exercising muscles in hot weather.
  (ii) Heat exhaustion:
    (a) thirst, cramps, headache, vertigo, anorexia, nausea and vomiting occur
    (b) the patient is flushed and sweating, with rectal temperature 38–39°C
    (c) tachycardia and orthostatic hypotension occur from dehydration.
(2) Severe heat illness with failure of thermoregulatory mechanisms – heat stroke:
  (i) hot dry skin, or profuse sweating in up to 50%, headache, vomiting and diarrhoea, progressing to aggressive or bizarre behaviour, collapse, seizures and coma;
  (ii) the rectal temperature is over 40°C;
  (iii) the patient is flushed, tachypnoeic, tachycardic and hypotense; muscle rigidity, transient hemiplegia, dilated pupils and disseminated intravascular coagulation all occur.

MANAGEMENT

(1) *Heat cramps*
   (i)   Rest in a cool environment, and replace fluid orally with added salt or give 1 l normal saline i.v.
   (ii) The patient is usually able to go home.
(2) *Heat exhaustion*
   (i)   Rest in a cool environment and give up to 3 l cooled normal saline i.v.
   (ii) Cool the patient with tepid sponging and fanning.
   (iii) Admit for observation, particularly when elderly or if orthostatic hypotension persists.
(3) *Heat stroke*
   (i)   Give oxygen and attach an ECG monitor and pulse oximeter. Aim for an oxygen saturation above 94%.
   (ii) Commence urgent cooling with tepid sponging, fans and cold packs to the groin and axillae until the temperature is less than 38.5°C.
   (iii) Gain i.v. access and send blood for FBC, coagulation profile, U&E, blood sugar, LFTs and creatine kinase (CK), and check the blood gases.
   (iv) Give 1 l cooled 4% dextrose 0.18% normal saline over 20 min, then according to the blood pressure, U&E and urine output following bladder catheterisation.
   (v)   Give lorazepam 4 mg i.v. or diazepam (Diazemuls) 5–10 mg i.v. for fits, and chlorpromazine 25 mg i.v. to suppress shivering if the rate of cooling is inadequate. Endotracheal intubation is usually necessary.
   (vi) Refer the patient to the medical team for admission to ITU.

HYPOTHERMIA

This is present when the core temperature drops to less than 35°C (95°F). Mild hypothermia is classified as 32–35°C, moderate hypothermia as 29–32°C, and severe hypothermia as less than 29°C.

DIAGNOSIS

(1) Hypothermia is predisposed to in the following:
   (i)   exposure to low air temperatures, particularly if there was associated wind and rain;
   (ii)   exposure in cold water;
   (iii)   unconscious patients, or patients who have taken sedative drugs, especially alcohol;
   (iv)   babies or the elderly, with intercurrent illness, e.g. stroke, pneumonia, diabetic ketoacidosis (DKA);
   (v)   endocrine disorders, such as myxoedema or hypopituitary coma (rare).
(2) Mild hypothermia causes lethargy, ataxia, shivering and tachypnoea. Moderate hypothermia causes bradycardia, hypotension, bradypnoea, confusion and absent shivering.
(3) In severe hypothermia, the patient is comatose and may appear dead with an undetectable pulse, absent reflexes and fixed pupils.
(4) ECG changes include low-voltage complexes, bradycardia, atrial fibrillation, prolonged QT interval, and a slurred notching of the terminal portion of the QRS complex – the J wave.

MANAGEMENT

(1) Record the core temperature rectally with a low-reading thermometer or using a tympanic membrane device.
(2) Give high-dose oxygen, which should be warmed and humidified if the core temperature is 32°C or less. Extreme care with endotracheal intubation is essential, as this may precipitate a cardiac arrhythmia.
(3) Cover the patient in warm woollen blankets and layers of polythene. Use a forced-air rewarming blanket, e.g. Bair Hugger, and minimise handling, aiming for a core temperature rise of at least 0.5°C/h in the elderly, and 1°C/h in younger patients.
(4) Take blood for FBC, coagulation profile, U&E, blood sugar and lipase/amylase, as rarely pancreatitis may be associated. Send ABG, and check ECG and CXR.

(5) Give i.v. fluids cautiously through a warming device. Pulmonary oedema may be precipitated by excessive fluid administration.

(6) If a cardiac arrest occurs in a hypothermic patient:

    (i)   Commence cardiac massage and deliver three DC shocks while a skilled doctor passes an endotracheal tube. Use warmed, humidified oxygen (see p. 8).

    (ii)   Drugs and DC shocks are usually ineffectual.

    (iii) Continue resuscitation attempts until the core temperature rises to at least 33°C or until a senior doctor advises to the contrary.

        (a) This may involve a prolonged period of time when aggressive measures must be resorted to.

        (b) Such measures include left pleural, gastric or peritoneal dialysis with warmed fluid.

        (c) Extracorporeal rewarming is the method of choice when available.[1]

Note: with elderly, debilitated or deprived patients, remember to determine the predisposing factors to hypothermia before considering their discharge home, to prevent recurrence.

NEAR-DROWNING

DIAGNOSIS

(1) The initial difference between sea water (hypertonic) and fresh water (hypotonic) near-drowning is of little clinical significance, as only small amounts of fluid may have been aspirated.

(2) Consider other more relevant factors:

    (i)   Preceding injury, especially to the cervical spine in diving accidents.

    (ii)   Sudden prior illness, such as a myocardial infarction, cerebrovascular accident or epileptic fit, that may have led to the drowning.

    (iii) Alcohol or drug use.

    (iv) Hypothermia.

(3) The presence of lung crackles indicates likely inhalation of water.

MANAGEMENT

(1) Commence cardiopulmonary resuscitation if the patient has no detectable cardiac output or is not breathing, taking due care for any possible neck injury. Prolonged resuscitation efforts may be successful, particularly if there was rapid associated hypothermia in cold water.

(2) Otherwise, give high-dose oxygen and measure the rectal temperature. Rewarm the patient if the core temperature is low (see p. 124). Attach a cardiac monitor and pulse oximeter to the patient. Aim for an oxygen saturation above 94%.

(3) Check U&E, blood sugar, blood gases, CXR and ECG.

(4) Call an airway skilled doctor to intubate the patient if they are unconscious or develop respiratory failure with a P_aO_2 of less than 10 kPa (75 mm Hg) on 50% oxygen, or a rising P_aCO_2 above 7.5 kPa (56 mm Hg).

(5) Refer all patients to the medical team for admission. Delayed adult respiratory distress syndrome may develop 6–48 h after submersion 'secondary drowning'.

SPORTS DIVING ACCIDENTS

Two main groups of sports (scuba) diving accidents were traditionally classified as decompression sickness and barotrauma, but may now be collectively termed decompression illness (DCI), further described by the acuity, evolution, organs involved and presence of barotrauma.[2]

DECOMPRESSION ILLNESS

When due largely to inert nitrogen gas absorbed under pressure through the lungs becoming liberated throughout the body, the following predominate:

DIAGNOSIS

(1) Symptoms occur from several min up to 48 h after diving.

(2) *Mild*
- (i)   Joint pain occurs, usually in a large joint such as the elbow or shoulder. Pain may migrate, and ranges from a dull ache to the crippling 'bends'. Unusual fatigue and malaise are common.
- (ii) Skin itching, marbling or scarlatiniform rashes.
- (iii) Painful lymphadenopathy and local oedema.

(3) *Serious*
- (i)   Central nervous system involvement causes:
  - (a) motor and sensory losses, personality disorder and seizures;
  - (b) labyrinthine damage, with deafness, tinnitus, nystagmus, vertigo and nausea – 'the staggers';
  - (c) hemiplegia, paraplegia and urinary retention.
- (ii) Cardiopulmonary involvement causes retrosternal or pleuritic pain, dyspnoea, cough and haemoptysis – 'the chokes'. This can progress to respiratory failure and hypotension.

MANAGEMENT

(1) Give the patient 100% oxygen by tight-fitting face mask with reservoir bag.

(2) Gain i.v. access and commence normal saline rehydration.

(3) Give lorazepam 4 mg i.v. or diazepam (Diazemuls) 5 mg i.v. for fits. This may also be used for severe labyrinthine disturbance after discussion with a hyperbaric medicine unit.

(4) Minimise strong analgesics, particularly opiates, as they mask symptoms.

(5) Refer every patient, however strange their symptoms, to a hyperbaric medicine unit:
- (i)   Provide information about any dive in the preceding 48 h, including the depth and duration, and time of symptoms.
- (ii) Advice on diagnosis and arrangements for treatment are available by telephoning the following hyperbaric medicine units:
  - (a) England
    - Royal Navy, Portsmouth: (023) 9281 8888

      – Diving Disease Research Centre: (01752)
      261 910
  (b) Scotland – Aberdeen Royal Hospitals:
      (01224) 681 818
  (c) Northern Ireland – Craigavan Hospital, Co.
      Armagh: (028) 3833 6711

DECOMPRESSION ILLNESS WITH BAROTRAUMA

DIAGNOSIS

(1) *Middle ear barotrauma*
   (i) Local pain, sometimes with bleeding from the ear,
   occurs associated with conductive deafness if the
   drum ruptures.
   (ii) The tympanic membrane appears reddened or
   may rupture.
(2) *Inner ear barotrauma.* Vertigo, tinnitus and sensorineural deafness occur due to a perilymph fistula,
which mimics labyrinthine CNS decompression illness
(see p. 127).
(3) *Sinus barotrauma.* Local pain occurs over the maxillary
and frontal sinus, sometimes associated with bleeding.
(4) *Dental barotrauma.* Pain occurs in or around fillings or
carious teeth.
(5) *Pulmonary barotrauma.* This is the most serious form of
barotrauma causing:
   (i) Surgical emphysema or pneumothorax associated
   with chest pain and dyspnoea.
   (ii) Arterial gas embolus affecting:
      (a) the coronary circulation, with cardiac pain,
      arrhythmia and cardiac arrest;
      (b) the cerebral circulation, with sudden onset of
      neurological symptoms just before or within
      5 min of surfacing (without the delay seen in
      CNS decompression illness);
      (c) any neurological symptom or sign may occur
      from confusion to fits or coma, and may
      fluctuate.

MANAGEMENT

(1) *Middle ear barotrauma*
  (i) Give an analgesic such as paracetamol 500 mg and codeine phosphate 8 mg (co-codamol 8/500) and an antibiotic such as amoxycillin 500 mg orally t.d.s. for 5 days.
  (ii) Refer the patient to the next ENT clinic and ban further diving until the drum is fully healed.
(2) *Inner ear barotrauma* should be discussed immediately with a hyperbaric medicine unit as labyrinthine CNS decompression illness is a possibility.
(3) *Sinus and dental barotrauma* require an analgesic such as paracetamol 500 mg and codeine phosphate 8 mg (co-codamol 8/500).
(4) *Pulmonary barotrauma*
  (i) Give oxygen and perform a CXR. Insert an intercostal drain if a significant pneumothorax is present (see p. 26).
  (ii) If arterial gas embolus is suspected:
    (a) keep the patient horizontal on their left side (not head down, as this raises intracranial pressure);
    (b) give 100% oxygen by tight-fitting face mask with reservoir bag;
    (c) gain i.v. access and commence normal saline rehydration;
    (d) give lorazepam 4 mg i.v. or diazepam (Diazemuls) 5 mg i.v. for fits;
    (e) refer the patient immediately to a hyperbaric medicine unit, even after apparent recovery, as delayed deterioration can occur (see p. 127 for telephone contact numbers).

VENOMOUS BITES AND STINGS

These are exceedingly rare in Britain, but may present following an altercation with an exotic pet, or in zoo handlers and herpetologists. Specialist advice is available from the

following centres:
  (1) National Poisons Information Service, London: (020) 7635 9191
  (2) Liverpool School of Tropical Medicine: (0151) 708 9393
  (3) John Radcliffe Hospital, Oxford: (01865) 741 166
  (4) Poisons Information Centres (see p. 73).

SNAKE BITES

DIAGNOSIS

  (1) The adder is the only naturally occurring venomous snake in the UK.
  (2) Immediate local pain, bruising or swelling within hours of the bite indicate envenomation. However, less than 50% of bites are associated with envenomation, and occasionally systemic poisoning may occur with no local reaction.
  (3) Systemic envenomation causes vomiting, abdominal pain and diarrhoea. Transient hypotension and coma may occur early, although hypotension may persist in severe cases. Spontaneous bleeding, coagulopathy and acute renal failure may follow.

MANAGEMENT

  (1) Reassure the patient, apply a firm bandage proximal to the bite, immobilise the dependent limb, and transport the patient rapidly to hospital.
  (2) Gain i.v. access, send blood for FBC, clotting screen, U&E and LFTs, and monitor the ECG. Give tetanus prophylaxis.
  (3) European viper venom antiserum is available for adder envenomation.
      (i)   Indications for antivenom:
            (a) hypotension
            (b) bleeding
            (c) ECG changes
            (d) leucocytosis over $20\,000/mm^3$
            (e) extending limb swelling within 4 h of the bite.

(ii) Add one 10-ml ampoule to normal saline 5 ml/kg diluent and infuse over 30 min.

(iii) Adrenaline must be available immediately for hypersensitivity reactions.

(4) Refer all patients to the medical team for admission, even in the absence of symptoms or signs initially.

MARINE ENVENOMATION

DIAGNOSIS

Several hazardous marine animals are found in UK coastal waters, including the following:

(1) Jellyfish:
   (i) sea nettle, compass, Portuguese man-of-war;
   (ii) these cause burning local pain and oedema, with occasional systemic symptoms.

(2) Poisonous fish:
   (i) sting ray, lesser weever;
   (ii) these cause extreme local pain and oedema, with various systemic effects, including diarrhoea, respiratory depression and hypotension.

(3) Sea urchins:
   (i) injury is caused by the many tiny spines that may break off and enter joint cavities, or the deep palmar or plantar spaces;
   (ii) there is excruciating local pain and oedema, with systemic effects, including cardiorespiratory failure.

MANAGEMENT

(1) Rinse jellyfish wounds with sea water, remove adherent tentacles, and prevent further nematocyst discharge with 5% acetic acid (vinegar).

(2) Use supportive measures, including oxygen, analgesics and fluid replacement.

(3) Poisonous fish and sea urchin wounds:
   (i) Relieve pain by immersion in hot water or by using a local anaesthetic block, followed by exploration, irrigation and debridement as necessary.

(ii)   Give tetanus prophylaxis and an antibiotic such as co-trimoxazole two tablets orally b.d. if there is extensive tissue damage.

BEE AND WASP STINGS

DIAGNOSIS

(1) There are more deaths in Britain and the USA from anaphylaxis following a bee or wasp sting than from all the other venomous bites and stings put together.
(2) Local pain predominates and may be followed by a severe anaphylactic reaction causing angioedema, laryngeal oedema, difficulty in breathing, hypotension and collapse.

MANAGEMENT

(1) Remove a bee sting by scraping out the sting with a knife without squeezing.
(2) Treat anaphylaxis with 0.3–0.5 ml of 1:1000 adrenaline i.m. or 1:10 000 adrenaline 0.75–1.5 µg/kg, i.e. 50–100 µg or 0.5–1.0 ml for a 70-kg patient given slowly i.v. if circulatory collapse supervenes (see p. 102).
(3) Other measures include oxygen, airway management, hydrocortisone, promethazine and ranitidine.
(4) Patients prone to anaphylaxis from bee or wasp stings should carry a prefilled adrenaline syringe (Epipen) at all times.

REFERENCES

1   International Resuscitation Guidelines 2000 – A Consensus on Science. Part 8: Advanced Challenges in Resuscitation. Section 3: Special Challenges in ECC. 3A: Hypothermia. *Resuscitation* 2000;46:267–71.
2   Emerson GM. Dysbarism. In Cameron P, Jelinek G, Kelly A-M, Murray L, Heyworth J, Brown AFT. *Textbook of Adult Emergency Medicine*. Churchill Livingstone, Edinburgh; 2000: 615–22.

SURGICAL EMERGENCIES

MULTIPLE INJURIES

The management of the severely injured patient is best coordinated by adopting a standard routine for assessment as taught, for example, in advanced trauma life support (ATLS) courses. This involves a rapid primary survey, resuscitation of vital functions, a detailed secondary survey, and the initiation of definitive care.

(1) The primary survey identifies life-threatening conditions that are corrected immediately, as the respiratory and circulatory status are optimised in the resuscitation phase. Initial X-rays are taken, bloods sent, and procedures such as nasogastric tube and urinary catheterisation performed.

(2) The secondary survey commences after the primary survey is complete and the resuscitation phase well under way.
　　(i)　　A detailed head-to-toe examination is made.
　　(ii)　Special X-rays, CT scans and angiographic studies are performed.

(3) Definitive care is the management of all the injuries identified, including surgery, fracture stabilisation, hospital admission or the preparation for patient transfer, should this be necessary.

(4) Expect serious injuries in the following high-risk patients:
　　(i)　　high-speed impact, ejection or death of another vehicle occupant
　　(ii)　entrapment
　　(iii)　motorcyclist or pedestrian struck
　　(iv)　fall greater than 5 m (15 feet)
　　(v)　abnormal vital signs (systolic BP under 90 mm Hg, Glasgow Coma Scale (GCS) 12 or less, respiratory rate under 10/min or over 29/min).

(5) Call senior A&E department staff immediately for any multiple-injury patient, so that they may organise an integrated team response incorporating anaesthetic, surgical and orthopaedic colleagues.

(6) The time-honoured mnemonic for the initial sequence of care is:

A   Airway maintenance with cervical spine control.
B   Breathing and ventilation.
C   Circulation with haemorrhage control.
D   Disability: brief neurological evaluation.
E   Exposure/environmental control: completely undress
     the patient, but prevent hypothermia.

IMMEDIATE MANAGEMENT

(1) *Airway*
    (i)   Clear the airway by sucking out any debris,
          remove loose or broken dentures, and insert an
          oropharyngeal airway. Give 100% oxygen by
          tight-fitting mask with reservoir bag. Aim for an
          oxygen saturation above 94%.
    (ii) Intubation
          (a) If the gag reflex is absent or reduced, the
               patient requires intubating by an airway
               skilled doctor, e.g. emergency physician or
               anaesthetist.
          (b) Take great care to minimise neck movements
               in the unconscious head injury or suspected
               neck injury by in-line manual immobilisation.
          (c) Use capnography to measure the end tidal
               CO_2 to confirm correct endotracheal tube
               placement.
    (iii) Cricothyrotomy: if intubation is impossible due to
          laryngeal injury or severe maxillofacial injury,
          proceed directly to cricothyrotomy (see p. 34).
(2) *Maintain the integrity of the cervical spine*
    (i)   Place the unconscious head injury and the sus-
          pected neck injury in a semi-rigid collar.
    (ii) Head movements must be minimised. When the
          patient requires turning, the body should be 'log
          rolled', holding the head in the neutral position at
          all times.
(3) *Breathing and ventilation*
    (i)   Close a sucking chest wound with open pneumo-
          thorax using an occlusive dressing such as paraffin
          gauze under an adhesive film dressing (OpSite),

secured along three sides only, leaving the fourth open for air to escape. Proceed to formal intercostal tube drainage (see p. 26).

(ii) Tension pneumothorax

    (a) Suspect a tension pneumothorax if there are tachycardia, hypotension, distended neck veins, unequal chest expansion and absent or decreased breath sounds.

    (b) Insert a wide-bore needle or cannula into the second intercostal space in the mid-clavicular line. If this is followed by the rush of released air, proceed to formal intercostal tube drainage (see p. 26).

(iii) Flail chest

    (a) This will cause paradoxical movement of a part of the chest wall and may necessitate positive pressure ventilation.

    (b) An associated haemothorax or pneumothorax will require an intercostal tube drain to prevent the development of a tension pneumothorax when positive pressure ventilation is used.

(4) *Circulation with haemorrhage control*

(i) Apply a bulky sterile dressing to compress any external bleeding point (not a tourniquet, as this increases bleeding by venous congestion).

(ii) Establish an i.v. infusion.

    (a) Insert two large-bore (14 or 16 gauge) cannulae into the antecubital veins.

    (b) In mediastinal or neck injuries, one cannula should be below the diaphragm, e.g. in the femoral vein.

(iii) Monitor the pulse, blood pressure, ECG and pulse oximetry.

(iv) Take blood for haemoglobin, U&E, LFTs and blood sugar, and cross-match at least 4 units of blood according to the suspected injuries. Save serum for a drug screen in case alcohol or drug intoxication is subsequently suspected. Send arterial blood gases.

(v) Infusion fluid:
- (a) Infuse normal saline or a plasma expander such as polygeline (Haemaccel) to correct hypovolaemia.
- (b) Remember in healthy adults loss of up to 30% of the blood volume, e.g. 1.5 l, causes tachycardia with a narrowed pulse pressure only. Therefore, a consistent fall in systolic blood pressure indicates that at least 30% of the blood volume has already been lost.
- (c) Change to blood if 1.5 l of normal saline and 1 l of Haemaccel fail to reverse hypotension. A full cross-match takes 1.5 h and type-specific cross-match 10 min; and O rhesus-negative blood is available immediately.
- (d) Use a blood warmer and macropore blood filter for multiple transfusions. Fresh frozen plasma 5 units and platelets may be required after transfusing 10 units of blood. Discuss this with the haematologist.

(vi) Cardiac tamponade:
- (a) If there is persistent hypotension with distended neck veins that fill on inspiration (Kussmaul's sign), consider cardiac tamponade.
- (b) Call the surgical team for a decision on urgent thoracotomy and consider pericardiocentesis (see p. 9).

(vii) A CVP line is useful, but should be inserted only by a skilled operator to avoid inadvertent arterial puncture or causing a pneumothorax.

(5) *Disability: brief neurological evaluation*
- (i) Assess the level of consciousness using the GCS (see p. 168).
- (ii) Examine the pupil size, pupil reactions and eye movements.
- (iii) Assess for abnormal tone, weakness and gross sensory loss, or an asymmetric response to pain if the patient is unconscious. Check the limb reflexes, including the plantar responses.
- (iv) Examine the face and scalp for injuries (see p. 140).

(6) *Exposure: completely undress the patient*
- (i) Request a lateral cervical spine X-ray, CXR and pelvic X-ray, known as the 'trauma series'.
- (ii) These are performed in the resuscitation bay without interrupting patient care.

(7) (i) Examine the front of the abdomen, including the perineum, for evidence of penetrating trauma or blunt trauma, e.g. the imprint of clothing or a tyre mark on the skin. Cover any exposed abdominal viscera with saline-soaked packs.
- (ii) Examine the back for evidence of penetrating or blunt trauma. Palpate the spine for deformity and widened interspinous gaps.

(8) Assess the pelvis by springing to detect instability from major pelvic ring fracture, although this is an unreliable sign. Look for associated urethral injury.
- (i) Perform a rectal examination to assess the position of the prostate, integrity of the rectal wall, anal sphincter tone and to check for evidence of internal bleeding.
- (ii) If there is any bleeding from the urethral meatus, a scrotal haematoma or a high-riding prostate, suspect urethral transection. Do not attempt urethral catheterisation.
- (iii) Otherwise, insert a urethral catheter and measure the urine output, which should be over 50 ml/h in the adult, and 1 ml/kg/h in a child.

(9) Pass a large-bore nasogastric tube, or orogastric tube if a basal skull or midface fracture is present. This is particularly important in children, who commonly develop acute gastric dilation following trauma.

(10) (i) Splint major limb fractures, cover compound injuries with sterile dressings, and check the peripheral pulses.
- (ii) Administer increments of morphine 2.5–5 mg i.v. titrated to analgesic response.

The above procedures will save life and allow a decision on priorities in proceeding to definitive care. Make sure an ongoing record is kept of all clinical findings and vital signs, and keep re-examining the patient regularly.

Obtain as full a history as possible from ambulance crew, witnesses or relatives, as well as the patient. A useful mnemonic for the history is AMPLE:

A   Allergies
M   Medications
P   Past history, including alcohol and cigarette use
L   Last meal
E   Events/environment relating to the injury, including time, speed of impact, initial vital signs, and any change in condition.

FURTHER DIAGNOSIS AND MANAGEMENT OF MULTIPLE INJURIES: DEFINITIVE CARE

This is considered under the following headings:
(1) Head and facial injuries
   (i)   scalp
   (ii)   face
   (iii)   eyes
   (iv)   nose
   (v)   mouth
   (vi)   ears.
(2) Neck injuries
   (i)   cervical spine injury
   (ii)   neck sprain
   (iii)   airway injury
   (iv)   vascular injury
   (v)   nerve injury
   (vi)   oesophageal injury.
(3) Chest injuries
   (i)   pneumothorax
   (ii)   haemothorax
   (iii)   rib and sternum fractures
   (iv)   myocardial contusion
   (v)   aortic rupture
   (vi)   diaphragm rupture
   (vii)   oesophageal rupture
   (viii) penetrating chest injuries.
(4) Abdominal injuries
   (i)   blunt abdominal trauma

      (ii)   penetrating injury.
- (5) Pelvic and urethral injuries
    - (i)   bladder and urethral injury
    - (ii)   pelvic injury.
- (6) Back injuries
    - (i)   thoracic and lumbar spine injury
    - (ii)   blunt renal injuries
    - (iii)   penetrating renal injuries.
- (7) Limb injuries.

HEAD AND FACIAL INJURIES

(1) *Scalp*
- (i)   Look for lacerations, haematomas, penetrating wounds and foreign bodies, and palpate for evidence of deformity and fracture.
- (ii)   If a major head injury is suspected, assess the level of consciousness and manage as described on p. 166.

(2) *Face*
- (i)   Check the integrity of the airway again, and remember the possibility of an unsuspected neck injury.
- (ii)   Look for bruising, swelling or deformity suggesting orbital, nasal, malar or mandibular fractures (see p. 344–8).
- (iii)   Look for parotid and facial nerve damage in injuries to the face in the area in front of the ear.
- (iv)   Clean and inspect all the facial lacerations. They will require meticulous debridement and suture when the patient's condition is stable and all serious injuries have been dealt with.

(3) *Eyes*
- (i)   Inspect the eyes for evidence of penetrating or blunt injury, looking for iris prolapse, hyphaema, lens dislocation and traumatic mydriasis (see p. 328).
- (ii)   Check the visual acuity and eye movements.
- (iii)   Assess the pupil size and reactions, and examine the fundi for evidence of vitreous or retinal haemorrhage and retinal detachment.

(4) *Nose*

    (i)   Examine for evidence of blood or CSF leakage suggesting a basal skull fracture (see p. 170).

    (ii)   Palpate for deformity and nasal bone fracture (see p. 312).

    (iii) Look specifically for a septal haematoma, which, if large, will require incision and drainage to reduce the risk of subsequent cartilage necrosis (see p. 312).

(5) *Mouth*

    (i)   Examine for broken or missing teeth. They may have been inhaled (see p. 343).

    (ii)   Check for dental malocclusion, suggesting maxillary or mandibular fracture (see p. 344).

    (iii) Assess for nasopharyngeal bleeding, which may be profuse and associated with a basal skull fracture. Look for any tongue lacerations, although they rarely need repairing (see p. 342).

(6) *Ears*

    (i)   Examine for skin and cartilage damage, which will require drainage and suture later.

    (ii)   Consider perforation of the eardrum, although if frank bleeding is seen, do not examine with a speculum to avoid introducing infection. This bleeding will be associated with a basal skull fracture or damage to the external ear canal (see p. 308).

NECK INJURIES: CERVICAL SPINE INJURY

This should be considered in all patients with localised neck pain or stiffness following trauma. It should also be assumed in any unconscious head injury, multiply injured patient or with a local distracting injury.

DIAGNOSIS

    (1) If the patient is conscious, ask about local pain, tenderness on palpation and associated limb weakness or sensory deficit.

    (2) Palpate for areas of tenderness, swelling or deformity in the neck. Assess for limb tone, weakness, reflex loss and

sensory deficit, including loss of saddle area sensation and anal tone.

(3) A cervical or high thoracic cord lesion will cause respiratory difficulty, tachypnoea and abdominal breathing. Loss of sympathetic tone will cause bradycardia, hypotension and hypothermia from vasodilation if the ambient temperature is low.

(4) Motor weakness should be described by myotome and reflex abnormalities:

    (i)   Myotomes in the upper limb:

Root	Action
C5	Shoulder abduction
C6, C7	Shoulder adduction
C5, C6	Elbow flexion
C7	Elbow extension
C6	Pronation and supination
(C6), C7	Wrist flexion
C6, (C7)	Wrist extension
C8	Finger flexion
C7	Finger extension
T1	Intrinsic hand muscles

    (ii)   Use the Medical Research Council scale to grade muscle weakness:

Grade 0	Complete paralysis
Grade 1	A flicker of contraction only
Grade 2	Movement possible only if gravity is eliminated
Grade 3	Movement against gravity
Grade 4	Movement against gravity and resistance
Grade 5	Normal power

    (iii)   Reflexes in the upper limb:

Root	Reflex
C5, (C6)	Biceps
(C5), C6	Supinator
(C6), C7, C8	Triceps

    (iv)   Use reinforcement (the Jendrassik manoeuvre) before concluding that a reflex is absent, e.g. ask the patient to clench the teeth hard or hold the knees together.

(5) Assess sensation by testing pain fibres using pinprick (spinothalamic tracts), and examine fine touch or joint position sense (posterior columns). Describe any changes by dermatome abnormalities:

    (i) Dermatomes in the upper limb:

Root	Distribution
C5	Outer, upper arm
C6	Outer forearm
C7	Middle finger
C8	Inner forearm
T1	Inner, upper arm

    (ii) C4 and T2 dermatomes are adjacent on the front of the chest at the level of the first and second ribs (C5–T1 supply the upper limb).

(6) The myotomes, reflexes and dermatomes in the leg are described on p. 267.

MANAGEMENT

(1) Always apply a semi-rigid collar in any suspected neck injury, minimise head movements, and use laterally placed sandbags taped to the forehead to prevent head rotation.

(2) Urgent airway control with orotracheal or nasotracheal intubation may be required for hypoventilation. An airway skilled doctor should perform this with manual in-line stabilisation provided.

(3) Restore the circulatory volume if the patient is hypotensive. First look for sources of blood loss before concluding that the hypotension is due to vasodilation with bradycardia from loss of sympathetic tone in a cervical cord injury (i.e. neurogenic shock).

(4) X-ray the neck:

    (i) Lateral cervical spine: make sure all seven cervical vertebrae and the C7/T1 junction are seen. Look for signs of displacement, wedge fracture, teardrop fracture, odontoid peg fracture and an increase in the soft-tissue shadow in front of the vertebral bodies (see Fig. 5).

        (a) The retropharyngeal space should be less than 4 mm at the level of C3.

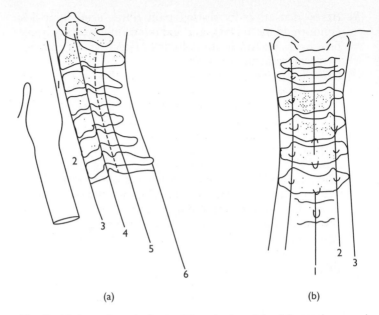

(a)　　　　　　　　　　　　　　　　(b)

Fig. 5. (a) Lateral cervical spine X-ray in the adult. I Retropharyngeal space (<4 mm); 2 retrotracheal space (less than the width of one vertebral body); 3 anterior longitudinal ligament line; 4 posterior longitudinal ligament line; 5 spinolaminar line; 6 posterior spinal line. Lines 3–6 should all be parallel, following the normal gentle lordotic curve of the cervical spine. The spinal cord runs between lines 4 and 5. (b) Anteroposterior cervical spine X-ray. I Interspinous line; 2 foramen transversarium line; 3 transverse processes line. Lines I–3 should be straight in the normal neck.

      (b)　The retrotracheal space should be less than the width of one vertebral body in adults.
  (ii)　Open-mouth view for odontoid peg fracture.
 (iii)　Anteroposterior view: look for rotation of the vertebrae, loss of joint space and transverse process fracture.
(5)　However, severe ligamentous damage may occur, leaving the neck unstable yet with an apparently normal X-ray.

(i)   This is more likely in children, in whom 50% of serious spinal injuries have normal X-rays (SCIWORA – spinal cord injury without radiological abnormality).

(ii) In elderly patients with cervical spondylosis, neck hyperextension may cause predominant weakness of the arms without any associated fracture or dislocation (central cord syndrome).

(6) Refer all suspected cervical spine injuries to the orthopaedic or surgical team and begin pressure area nursing.

(7) The value of high-dose methylprednisolone to improve neurological outcome in patients with complete or incomplete spinal cord damage is unconvincing and controversial.[1]

(i)   Start treatment within 8 h of injury, guided by the advice of the regional Spinal Injuries Unit.

(ii) Infuse methylprednisolone 30 mg/kg over 15 min, followed 45 min later by 5.4 mg/kg/h for 23 h.

NECK INJURIES: NECK SPRAIN

DIAGNOSIS

(1) Hyperextension injury due to sudden deceleration in a motor vehicle accident is commonly termed 'whiplash injury'.

(i)   In practice, neck sprain occurs with other directions of impact, including hyperflexion.

(ii) All result in neck pain and stiffness that typically occur 12–24 h after the injury, sometimes associated with headache.

(2) The pain may radiate to the shoulders and arms, causing paraesthesiae, but neurological examination does not show any objective deficit.

(3) Neck movements are restricted by pain.

(4) Unfortunately, symptoms may continue for months, and may be exacerbated by further minor injuries.

MANAGEMENT

(1) Request a cervical spine X-ray, which may show loss of the normal anterior curvature due to muscle spasm.

(2) Treat the patient with a nonsteroidal anti-inflammatory analgesic such as diclofenac 50 mg oraiiy t.d.s., and encourage early mobilisation.

(3) If the pain fails to settle, refer the patient to the physiotherapy department for heat treatment, etc.

(4) Refer the patient to the orthopaedic clinic in the event that the above measures are unsuccessful.

NECK INJURIES: AIRWAY INJURY

DIAGNOSIS

(1) Airway injuries may be penetrating or blunt, isolated or associated with multiple injury.

(2) They cause stridor, hoarseness, cough, haemoptysis and pain, with the development of local swelling, subcutaneous emphysema, pneumothorax or haemothorax.

(3) An anteroposterior and lateral cervical spine X-ray and CXR should be performed. The patient must not be left unattended at any stage.

MANAGEMENT

(1) Call for urgent senior A&E doctor help.

(2) Perform endotracheal intubation or cricothyrotomy, or insert an endotracheal tube directly into a gaping wound in the trachea to maintain patency of the airway.

(3) Refer the patient immediately to the surgical team for admission.

NECK INJURIES: VASCULAR INJURY

DIAGNOSIS AND MANAGEMENT

(1) Vascular injury causes obvious external haemorrhage or internal bleeding, with rapid haematoma formation, which may compromise the airway.

(2) (i) Do not attempt to probe or explore any penetrating wounds in the A&E department. Leave all penetrating objects in situ.

(ii) Refer the patient immediately to the surgical team for admission. The patient will require angiography and panendoscopy with urgent surgical exploration in theatre.

NECK INJURIES: NERVE INJURY

DIAGNOSIS AND MANAGEMENT

(1) Damage to the following nerves causes:
   (i) Recurrent laryngeal branch of the vagus: hoarseness and vocal cord paralysis.
   (ii) Accessory nerve: loss of function of trapezius and sternomastoid.
   (iii) Phrenic nerve: loss of diaphragmatic movement.
   (iv) Hypoglossal nerve: deviation of the tongue to the affected side.
   (v) Cervical sympathetic cord: Horner's syndrome, with partial ptosis, a constricted pupil, and decreased sweating on the same side of the face.
(2) Refer any of these injuries to the surgical team.

NECK INJURIES: OESOPHAGEAL INJURY

DIAGNOSIS AND MANAGEMENT

(1) Oesophageal injury causes dysphagia, drooling and localised pain, with the development of surgical emphysema.
(2) Refer this rare condition to the surgical team for immediate admission.

PNEUMOTHORAX

DIAGNOSIS

(1) *Tension pneumothorax*
   (i) This causes severe respiratory distress, tachypnoea and hypotension. There is tracheal deviation away

from the affected side, distended neck veins, loss of chest expansion on the affected side, a hyper-resonant percussion note, and diminished or absent breath sounds.

(ii)   It requires immediate decompression. Use a large-bore i.v. cannula inserted into the second intercostal space in the mid-clavicular line, followed by the insertion of an intercostal drain (see p. 9).

(2) *Simple pneumothorax*

(i)   This is surprisingly easy to miss. Examine for sub-cutaneous emphysema, decreased chest expansion, and quiet breath sounds.

(ii)   It is caused by blunt or penetrating chest trauma, and penetrating abdominal trauma breaching the diaphragm.

(iii)   An erect CXR, taken on expiration to highlight a small apical pneumothorax, confirms the diagnosis. A supine CXR may, however, appear normal and miss a small pneumothorax lying anteriorly.

MANAGEMENT

(1) Insert an intercostal drain into the fifth or sixth inter-costal space in the mid-axillary line (see p. 26).

(2) Virtually all cases of traumatic pneumothorax require a chest drain to avoid the subsequent development of tension, especially if positive pressure ventilation is necessary.

HAEMOTHORAX

DIAGNOSIS

(1) This results from chest wall damage, penetrating or blunt lung injury and great vessel damage.

(2) It causes hypotension, respiratory difficulty with reduced chest expansion, quiet breath sounds, and a dull percussion note at the base of the lung.

(3) An erect or semi-erect CXR is necessary to identify a fluid level.

(4) If only a supine CXR is possible, look for diffuse ground-glass haziness over one hemithorax, which is easily missed. Alternatively, a lateral decubitus CXR may be taken.

MANAGEMENT

(1) Give high-dose oxygen and commence i.v. fluid, including blood.

(2) Insert a large-bore 32 or 36 French gauge intercostal drain in the fifth or sixth intercostal space in the mid-axillary line, using blunt dissection down to and through the pleura (see p. 26).

(3) Autotransfusion devices are available to collect and return the intrathoracic blood to the circulation, providing contamination from gastrointestinal injury is excluded.

(4) Otherwise, if bleeding is severe and persists, a thoracotomy may be required (see p. 155).

CHEST INJURIES: RIB AND STERNUM FRACTURES

DIAGNOSIS

(1) These cause localised pain and tenderness, worse on breathing or springing the chest wall, following direct trauma.

(2) A CXR is indicated to look for the complications of a pneumothorax, haemothorax and a widened mediastinum, not simply to visualise the fractures.

(3) A lateral sternal X-ray is indicated for a suspected sternal fracture, and an ECG to exclude myocardial contusion (see p. 151).

(4) Associated injury may occur with fractures in the following areas:

    (i) Clavicle, first and second ribs: damage to the subclavian vessels, aorta, trachea, main bronchus, and spinal cord or brachial plexus.

    (ii)   Sternum: damage to the myocardium, great vessels and upper thoracic spine.

    (iii)   Right lower ribs: damage to the liver and right kidney.

    (iv)   Left lower ribs: damage to the spleen and left kidney.

(5) A flail segment with paradoxical chest wall movement from multiple rib fractures in two sites causes hypoxia, mainly from underlying pulmonary contusion.

MANAGEMENT

(1) (i)   Give the patient oxygen, check the blood gases, titrate morphine 2.5–5 mg i.v. and refer to the surgical team for ongoing pain relief, possibly by thoracic epidural.

    (ii)   Positive pressure ventilation may be required for deteriorating respiratory function, after insertion of an intercostal drain for any pneumothorax, however small.

(2) Refer the following patients also to the surgical team for admission after resuscitation, insertion of an intercostal drain if indicated, and adequate non-sedating analgesia such as diclofenac 75 mg i.m.:

    (i)   pneumothorax, haemothorax

    (ii)   fractured sternum with severe pain or ECG abnormalities

    (iii)   complications listed in point (4) above

    (iv)   pre-existing lung disease with poor respiratory reserve

    (v)   rib fractures with significant pain.

(3) Remaining patients with uncomplicated rib fractures or an isolated sternal fracture with a normal ECG and CXR may be discharged.

    (i)   Provide an analgesic such as paracetamol 500 mg and codeine phosphate 8 mg (co-codamol 8/500) two tablets orally q.d.s.

    (ii)   Recommend regular deep breathing exercises to prevent atelectasis.

    (iii)   Contact the GP by telephone or letter.

MYOCARDIAL CONTUSION

DIAGNOSIS

(1) This is due to blunt deceleration injury and is associated with rib fractures, sternal fracture and chest wall contusion. It is difficult to diagnose.

(2) It may be asymptomatic, cause chest pain or rarely cause transient right ventricular dysfunction with distended neck veins and hypotension.

(3) ECG abnormalities range from sinus tachycardia, atrial fibrillation, bundle branch block and ventricular extrasystoles to nonspecific ST- and T-wave abnormalities or ST elevation.

(4) Cardiac enzyme changes, including creatine phosphokinase (CK) and CK-MB isoenzymes, are unreliable. They may, however, incidentally diagnose antecedent myocardial infarction.

(5) Echocardiography may show wall motion abnormalities, but is most useful to exclude cardiac tamponade or acute valvular rupture.

MANAGEMENT

(1) Give the patient high-dose oxygen and attach a cardiac monitor. Gain i.v. access, send blood for FBC, cardiac enzymes and G&S, and give a fluid challenge if there is hypotension.

(2) Give morphine 2.5–5 mg i.v. with an antiemetic such as metoclopramide 10 mg i.v. for pain.

(3) Perform a 12-lead ECG.

    (i) Refer the patient for cardiac monitoring if there are any ECG abnormalities.

    (ii) Obtain an urgent echocardiogram if hypotension persists or cardiac tamponade cannot be excluded.

AORTIC RUPTURE

DIAGNOSIS

(1) This occurs from a high-speed deceleration injury, when the aorta is torn just distal to the left subclavian artery.

(2) Only 10–15% of patients with rupture of the thoracic aorta survive to reach hospital. Always consider this diagnosis in any deceleration injury over 45 miles/h or a fall from over 15 feet.

(3) Look for chest or interscapular pain, unequal blood pressure in each arm, or a different femoral and brachial pulse volume. In contained aortic rupture, initial hypotension responds to modest fluid replacement.

(4) Perform a CXR to look for signs of aortic rupture:

    (i)   Widened mediastinum (8 cm or more in a 1-m supine anteroposterior X-ray):

        (a) about 10% of angiograms for a widened mediastinum will subsequently show contained aortic rupture;

        (b) other causes of a widened mediastinum include sternal fracture and lower cervical or thoracic spine fracture with mediastinal haematoma.

    (ii) Blurred aortic outline with obliteration of the aortic knuckle.

    (iii) Left apical cap of fluid in the pleural space and a left haemothorax.

    (iv) Depressed left main stem bronchus.

    (v) Displacement of the trachea to the right.

    (vi) Displacement of a nasogastric tube in the oesophagus to the right.

MANAGEMENT

(1) Insert two large-bore i.v. cannulae, cross-match at least 10 units of blood, and give fluid cautiously. Avoid over-transfusion or hypertension from poorly controlled pain, etc.

(2) Look for a cervical, thoracic or sternal fracture clinically and by X-ray, although exclusion of aortic rupture is still necessary irrespective of these if the CXR is suggestive.

(3) Perform a high-speed, helical CT chest scan to look for blood contiguous with the aorta, or an abnormal aortic wall indicative of rupture.

(4) If the CT scan is positive or unavailable and suspicion is high, refer the patient to the surgical team for immediate aortography or transoesophageal echo. Urgent thoracotomy and repair are needed if either of these is positive.

DIAPHRAGM RUPTURE

DIAGNOSIS

(1) This may occur from blunt or penetrating chest or abdominal trauma, including crush fracture of the pelvis. It causes difficulty in breathing, and occasionally bowel sounds are audible in the chest.
(2) Left-sided lesions are more common and allow eventration of the stomach or intestine into the chest.
(3) The diagnosis is often missed as the CXR appears normal in up to 25% of cases.
(4) Look for a haemothorax, pneumothorax, elevated hemidiaphragm and coils of bowel or a nasogastric tube curled up in the left lower chest.

MANAGEMENT

(1) Carefully insert an intercostal drain for any associated haemothorax or pneumothorax, using blunt dissection down to and through the parietal pleura (see p. 26). Never use the trocar introducer to insert the drain.
(2) Decompress the stomach with a nasogastric tube.
(3) Refer the patient to the surgical team.

OESOPHAGEAL RUPTURE

DIAGNOSIS

(1) This rare injury is most commonly from penetrating trauma or blunt trauma from a blow to the upper abdomen. Other causes include instrumentation, swallowing a sharp object, and spontaneous rupture from vomiting (Boerhaave's syndrome).

(2) There is retrosternal pain and difficulty in swallowing, sometimes with haematemesis and subcutaneous emphysema.
(3) CXR shows a widened mediastinum with mediastinal air, a left pneumothorax, pleural effusion or haemothorax. These findings in the absence of rib fracture should suggest the possibility of rupture.

MANAGEMENT

(1) Give the patient oxygen, establish venous access with a large-bore i.v. cannula, and replace fluids. Give morphine 2.5–5 mg i.v. for pain with an antiemetic.
(2) Carefully insert an intercostal drain. Particulate matter in the intercostal tube drainage would confirm the diagnosis.
(3) If rupture is considered likely, commence broad-spectrum antibiotics such as ampicillin 1 g i.v., gentamicin 5 mg/kg i.v. and metronidazole 500 mg i.v.
(4) Refer the patient to the surgical team for a gastrografin swallow and/or oesophagoscopy, followed by surgical repair if feasible.

PENETRATING CHEST INJURIES

DIAGNOSIS

(1) These injuries present with difficulty in breathing due to pain, pneumothorax, haemothorax or tension pneumothorax. However, some patients are surprisingly undistressed.
(2) Hypotension occurs due to blood loss, cardiac tamponade or the development of tension.
(3) A CXR may show some of the above complications, although airway management, needle thoracocentesis and fluid resuscitation must be performed first when indicated.
(4) Remember that penetrating wounds:
   (i)   medial to the nipple line or tips of the scapulae posteriorly are at high risk of heart or great vessel injury;

(ii) below the fourth intercostal space may also injure the abdominal contents;

(iii) above the umbilicus may injure the lungs, heart or great vessels.

MANAGEMENT

(1) 80% of penetrating chest injuries are managed conservatively by insertion of an intercostal drain (see p. 26).

(2) Injuries involving the heart and great vessels will require thoracotomy.

    (i) *Indications for immediate emergency department thoracotomy*[2]

        (a) Traumatic cardiac arrest, or near cardiac arrest, with vital signs (palpable pulse and spontaneous respirations) observed at the scene of the accident and a short pre-hospital transit time (up to 10 min, particularly when intubated).

        (b) Cardiac arrest from penetrating thoracic trauma due to a stab wound or a low-velocity bullet, as opposed to blunt chest trauma or a high-velocity bullet. The latter two are virtually always fatal if cardiac arrest occurs.

        (c) Absence of major brain injury.

    (ii) *Indications for urgent thoracotomy in theatre*

        (a) Cardiac tamponade following trauma that recurs after pericardiocentesis.

        (b) Massive haemothorax with greater than 1500 ml initial drainage or over 200 ml/h for 2–4 h.

        (c) Penetrating cardiac injuries.

        (d) Persistent large air leak suggesting tracheobronchial injury.

BLUNT ABDOMINAL TRAUMA

DIAGNOSIS

(1) This should be suspected following a road traffic accident or a fall from a height, particularly if there is evidence of

chest, pelvic or long-bone injury (e.g. injuries on either side of the abdomen). It must also be suspected when there is unexplained hypotension in the absence of obvious external bleeding or a thoracic injury.

(2) Look for the imprint of clothing or tyre marks as indicators of potential intra-abdominal injury. Bruising from a lap seat belt may overlie duodenal, pancreatic or small-bowel injury, and fracture/dislocation of the lumbar spine.

(3) Ask about referred shoulder-tip pain or localised pain suggesting lower rib, pelvic or thoracolumbar spine injury.

(4) Examine the chest, pelvis and back as well as the abdomen. Inspect the perineum and perform a rectal examination and a vaginal examination in the female.

(5) X-ray: an erect CXR, pelvic X-ray and lumbosacral spine X-ray are of most value. The plain abdominal film is rarely indicated.

  (i) Erect CXR: this may demonstrate a thoracic injury or free gas under the diaphragm. Look particularly for lower-rib fractures associated with liver, splenic and renal injury.

  (ii) Pelvic X-ray: a fractured pelvis may be associated with major abdominal injuries, which must be recognised.

  (iii) Plain abdominal film: look for loss of the psoas shadow, transverse process fracture, abnormal renal outlines and free gas within the peritoneal cavity on a lateral decubitus view.

MANAGEMENT

(1) Give oxygen and send blood for FBC, U&E, LFTs, blood sugar, amylase or lipase, and cross-match at least 4 units of whole blood.

(2) Insert two large-bore i.v. cannulae. Transfuse initially with crystalloid (e.g. normal saline) or colloid (e.g. polygeline (Haemaccel)), then whole blood when available.

(3) Insert a urethral catheter to measure the urine output and to look for haematuria.

(i) Omit this if a urethral injury is suspected from blood at the meatus, a scrotal haematoma or a high-riding prostate on rectal examination.

(ii) Pass a nasogastric tube to drain the stomach.

(4) Indications for immediate laparotomy include:
  (i) persistent shock
  (ii) rigid, silent abdomen
  (iii) radiological evidence of free gas or ruptured diaphragm.

(5) Commonly there are no immediate indications for laparotomy. Further investigation is needed:

  (i) *Ultrasound*
    (a) Focused abdominal sonogram for trauma (FAST). This is a rapid, bedside, repeatable, non-invasive, accurate test for free intra-peritoneal fluid.[3]
    (b) It is ideal for unstable patients. If positive, refer for laparotomy.
    (c) It demands expertise, and may miss hollow viscus, diaphragmatic and retroperitoneal injuries.

  (ii) *CT abdomen scan*
    (a) Provides anatomical information, allowing non-operative management. It also visualises the retroperitoneum, pelvis and lower chest.
    (b) Patients must be stable, as it takes time away from the resuscitation room.
    (c) It also may miss hollow viscus and diaphragmatic injuries.

  (iii) *Diagnostic peritoneal lavage (DPL)*
    (a) This may be used for unexplained hypotension in suspected abdominal injury or when abdominal examination is:
      – unreliable, due to coma, intoxication or spinal injury
      – equivocal, due to fractured lower ribs, pelvis or lumbar spine
      – impractical in planned extra-abdominal radiographic or surgical procedures.
    (b) It has largely been superseded by FAST and CT abdomen scan.

  (c) Insert a nasogastric and urethral catheter first.
  (d) The admitting surgical team should perform the lavage by a mini-laparotomy technique using local anaesthetic with adrenaline, then open dissection through all the layers of the abdominal wall.
  (e) The procedure is positive if:
       – 5–10 ml of frank blood or enteric contents are aspirated
       – peritoneal lavage fluid effluent exits via a chest tube or bladder catheter
       – laboratory analysis of lavage fluid shows over 100 000 red blood cells/mm^3.
  (f) It is highly sensitive for intraperitoneal bleeding, but may miss retroperitoneal injury to the duodenum, pancreas, kidney and pelvis or diaphragm rupture.
(6) Involve the admitting surgical team at all stages of investigation, as the decision on emergent laparotomy is theirs.

PENETRATING ABDOMINAL INJURIES

DIAGNOSIS

(1) An entry wound may be obvious, with evisceration of bowel, or may be difficult to find if it is hidden by a gluteal fold or in the perineum.
(2) Associated damage to the chest can occur with any wound above the umbilicus.
(3) The most important signs to look for are hypotension and shock. Local rigidity and guarding with reduced bowel sounds occur but are less common.
(4) The causes include:
   (i)   stabbing with a knife or hand-held sharp instrument;
   (ii)   industrial accidents, road accidents and explosions;
   (iii) gunshot wounds – these may be divided into three types:
          (a) *high-velocity wound:* the muzzle velocity of a bullet from a high-velocity rifle exceeds

1000 m/s, and a small entry wound is associated with gross internal tissue damage from cavitation and a large exit wound;

(b) *low-velocity wound*: the muzzle velocity from a handgun reaches 250 m/s, and the bullet causes local internal damage by perforation and laceration, often passing through several structures;

(c) *shotgun wound*: this causes massive superficial internal damage from close range (less than 7 m) and is usually fatal from a range of less than 3 m. If the shotgun is fired from more than 7 m, there is scattering of shot, perforating structures within the abdomen. A shot from over 40 m may not even penetrate the peritoneal cavity.

MANAGEMENT

(1) Cover any exposed bowel with saline-soaked pads.

(2) Give oxygen, send blood for FBC, cross-match, U&E, and amylase or lipase, and replace fluid initially with normal saline.

(3) Commence broad-spectrum antibiotics, e.g. ampicillin 1 g i.v., gentamicin 5 mg/kg i.v. and metronidazole 500 mg i.v. Give tetanus prophylaxis.

(4) Request a CXR to look for associated thoracic injury. An abdominal X-ray is indicated to assess for metallic foreign bodies.

(5) Test the urine for blood indicating a urological injury, although it is an unreliable sign.

(6) Refer all patients to the surgical team for urgent admission and laparotomy for all gunshot wounds and the majority of stab wounds.

PELVIC INJURIES

The major complication of a pelvic fracture is massive blood loss, with up to 3 l or more of concealed haemorrhage, which may continue despite resuscitation.

DIAGNOSIS

(1) Pelvic injuries may result from direct trauma in road, work or sports accidents, and from falls.

(2) There is local pain, tenderness and bruising. Bony instability demonstrated by distracting the iliac crests is an unreliable sign that may increase bleeding.

(3) Associated bladder, urethral, vaginal and rectal injuries occur, which account for further morbidity. A ruptured diaphragm must also be excluded (see p. 153).

(4) Pelvic X-ray should always be performed in all multiple-injury patients especially if there is unexplained hypotension. Pelvic fractures associated with the greatest risk of haemorrhage include:

    (i) quadripartite 'butterfly' fracture of all four pubic rami;

    (ii) open-book fracture with diastasis of the symphysis pubis over 2.5 cm;

    (iii) vertical shear fracture.

MANAGEMENT

(1) Give oxygen, send blood for FBC, U&E and blood sugar, cross-match at least 6 units of blood, and commence an i.v. infusion.

(2) Do not attempt to catheterise the bladder if urethral rupture is suspected, but await experienced surgical assistance.

(3) Call the surgical and orthopaedic team immediately.

    (i) Exclude intraperitoneal bleeding with bedside ultrasound (FAST) or supra-umbilical, open diagnostic peritoneal lavage (DPL).

    (ii) External fixation of fractures, arterial embolisation and laparotomy may be required for severe bleeding, intraperitoneal or urological injury.

(4) If hypotension persists with bony pelvic ring disruption, consider the temporary use of a pneumatic antishock garment such as MAST (military antishock trousers) while definitive care is being organised:

(i) These have three independent compartments, reducing the circulation through the pelvis and legs, thus supporting the blood pressure and splinting any fractures.

(ii) The garment must never be deflated until rapid fluid replacement therapy and immediate laparotomy are available.

(iii) Alternatively, a pelvic sling may be fashioned from a sheet secured tightly around the front of the pelvis.

BLADDER AND URETHRAL INJURIES

DIAGNOSIS

(1) These injuries may occur particularly with major pelvic fractures or from a direct blow to the lower abdomen.

(2) *Bladder rupture*. This may be intraperitoneal, causing shock and peritonism, or extraperitoneal, causing urine extravasation, local bruising and frank haematuria.

(3) *Urethral rupture*
   (i) Membranous urethra:
      (a) membranous urethral rupture causes difficulty voiding urine and urethral bleeding, which mimics extraperitoneal rupture of the bladder;
      (b) rectal examination reveals a high-riding prostate, often with an underlying boggy haematoma.
   (ii) Bulbous urethra: bulbous urethral rupture is caused by a fall astride an object, resulting in local perineal bruising, pain and meatal bleeding.

MANAGEMENT

(1) Do not attempt to catheterise the patient with a bladder or urethral injury.

(2) Treat the patient for pain and shock, and give antibiotics such as ampicillin 1 g i.v. and gentamicin 5 mg/kg i.v.

(3) Refer to the surgical team for an i.v. urogram, cystogram or ascending urethrogram as indicated.

BACK INJURIES

Always examine the back in multiple-injury patients, carefully log-rolling patients with suspected spinal injury.

THORACIC AND LUMBAR SPINE INJURY

DIAGNOSIS

(1) This type of injury is caused by blunt trauma from a fall, a direct blow or in a traffic accident. A fractured sternum may accompany a hyperflexion wedge fracture of the upper thoracic spine.

(2) Look for bruising, deformity and evidence of any penetrating injury.

(3) Palpate for localised tenderness and swelling around the vertebral column or an abnormal gap between the spinous processes suggesting a fracture, or overlying the renal areas suggesting a kidney injury (see p. 163).

(4) Perform a careful neurological examination, assessing for sensory deficit and a sensory level, loss of perianal sensation, and for motor and reflex loss in the legs (see p. 267).

(5) The spinal cord ends at the level of the first lumbar vertebra, so any injury distal to this involves the cauda equina only.

(6) Thoracolumbar spine X-rays are indicated in the following high-risk patients[4]:
   (i)   fall from 3 m (10 f)
   (ii) high-speed accident over 80 kph (50 mph)
   (iii) ejection from motor vehicle or motor cycle
   (iv) GCS score of 8 or less
   (v)   neurological deficit
   (vi) back pain or tenderness (may be absent).

(7) These X-rays may show a wedge fracture, dislocation (particularly between T12 and L1, and L4 and L5) or a transverse process fracture.

MANAGEMENT

(1) Treat associated thoracic and abdominal injuries as a priority, log-rolling the patient and minimising unnecessary

movements, as thoracolumbar fractures are commonly unstable.
(2) Commence i.v. fluids, send blood for FBC, U&E and blood sugar, and cross-match if there is hypotension from local or retroperitoneal bleeding or loss of sympathetic tone in high thoracic cord injury.
(3) Refer the patient to the orthopaedic team and organise:
    (i)   CT scan for significant or potentially unstable fractures;
    (ii) methylprednisolone for spinal cord damage within 8 h of injury, only on recommendation from the regional Spinal Injuries Unit (see p. 145).

BLUNT RENAL INJURIES

These may be associated with injury to the vertebral column, lower ribs, ureters, aorta, inferior vena cava and the abdominal contents.

DIAGNOSIS

(1) Loin pain and tenderness occur, which in association with haematuria suggest renal trauma.
(2) Hypotension is due to retroperitoneal bleeding or an associated paralytic ileus. A flank mass may be felt.
(3) Request a plain abdominal film and look for 11th and 12th rib fracture, loss of the psoas shadow, or an abnormal soft-tissue outline indicating retroperitoneal bleeding.
(4) Intravenous urography is performed for suspected renal injury, although CT scanning may be preferred. Indications for radiology of the kidney and ureters include:
    (i)   macroscopic haematuria
    (ii)   microscopic haematuria with shock (systolic BP 90 mm Hg or less) at any time
    (iii) significant deceleration with the risk of renal pedicle injury
    (iv)   local physical signs
    (v)   penetrating proximity trauma (see below).

MANAGEMENT

(1) Resuscitate the patient with i.v. fluids and send blood for FBC, U&E and blood sugar, and cross-match 2–6 units of blood.
(2) Exclude associated intra-abdominal injuries with ultrasound (FAST), CT or DPL.
(3) Refer the patient to the surgical team. Over 85% of blunt renal injuries settle on conservative management with bedrest and analgesia.

PENETRATING RENAL INJURIES

These are rare and usually involve injury to the abdominal contents, ureter or vertebral column. They may be multiple or associated with penetrating injury at the front of the trunk.

DIAGNOSIS

(1) There is usually haematuria, localised pain and tenderness, although significant renal or ureteric injury may be present without haematuria.
(2) Ureteric colic may occur from the passage of blood clots.

MANAGEMENT

(1) Resuscitate the patient with i.v. fluids, send blood for FBC and U&E, and cross-match.
(2) Give tetanus prophylaxis as indicated.
(3) Refer the patient to the surgical team for i.v. urography or contrast CT scan. These will not only demonstrate the nature of the renal injury but also confirm the presence and normal function of the other kidney. CT scan gives additional information on intra- or retroperitoneal injury.

LIMB INJURIES

The management of limb injuries does not take precedence over head, thoracic, abdominal or pelvic injuries in the multiply injured patient, even though they may appear more dramatic and attract instant attention. Limb injuries are covered in detail in Section IV Orthopaedic emergencies.

DIAGNOSIS

(1) Look for obvious deformity, swelling, tenderness, abnormal movement or crepitus (if the patient is unconscious).

(2) Check the distal pulses, particularly in a supracondylar humeral fracture or a dislocated knee.

(3) Remember that closed fractures bleed extensively with little external evidence, and open fractures bleed even more:

Site of closed fracture	Predicted blood loss
Pelvic ring	Up to 6 units or more
Femoral shaft	2–4 units
Tibial shaft	1–3 units

(4) Note any neurological deficit, e.g. radial nerve damage in a humeral shaft fracture or sciatic nerve damage in posterior hip dislocation.

MANAGEMENT

(1) Restore any deformity to a normal anatomical alignment. This is particularly important in a dislocated ankle to prevent ischaemic pressure necrosis of the skin overlying the malleolus (see p. 253).

(2) Cover compound fractures with a sterile dressing. Give flucloxacillin 2 g i.v. or cefuroxime 750 mg i.v. and tetanus prophylaxis.

(3) Give increments of morphine 2.5–5 mg i.v. for pain with an antiemetic such as metoclopramide 10 mg i.v.

(4) Immobilise the fracture using a plaster of Paris backslab, or a specially designed splint such as the Donway traction splint for femoral shaft fractures. Splinting reduces pain, making handling easier; it also reduces blood loss and the risk of neurovascular injury.

(5) Obtain urgent orthopaedic assistance if distal ischaemia is present. Otherwise refer the patient when the other major injuries have been stabilised.

(6) Traumatic amputation:
    (i) Control haemorrhage by direct pressure and elevation of the stump.
    (ii) Consider the possibility of replantation, especially in a clean, sliced wound without crushing.

(a) Preserve the amputated part by wrapping in a sterile dressing soaked in saline.

(b) Seal the wrapped part in a sterile, dry plastic bag, and immerse in a container of crushed ice and water.

(c) Give i.v. antibiotics and tetanus prophylaxis as for a compound fracture.

(d) X-ray the limb and severed part.

(e) Refer the patient to the orthopaedic or plastic surgery team for consideration of microvascular surgery ideally performed within 6 h of injury.

HEAD INJURY

The diagnosis and management of head injuries will be considered in two groups:

(1) The seriously injured or unconscious major head injury.

(2) The conscious head injury.

THE SERIOUSLY INJURED OR UNCONSCIOUS MAJOR HEAD INJURY

DIAGNOSIS

(1) The head injury may be obvious from the history or on immediate examination.

(2) The possibility of a head injury must also be considered in every instance of coma or abnormal behaviour, in at-risk groups such as drunks and epileptics, non-accidental injury in children, and in falls in the elderly.

MANAGEMENT

(1) Clear the airway by sucking out any secretions, remove loose or broken dentures, and insert an oropharyngeal airway. Give 100% oxygen by tight-fitting mask with reservoir bag.

(2) Immobilise the cervical spine by applying a semi-rigid collar, as up to 10% of patients with blunt head trauma have a concomitant neck injury. In addition, use sandbags on either side of the head taped to the forehead, unless the patient is excessively restless.

(3) If the gag reflex is reduced or absent, the patient must be intubated to protect and maintain the airway:

    (i) Call an airway skilled doctor immediately to pass a cuffed endotracheal tube.

    (ii) Take great care to minimise neck movements by an assistant providing in-line manual immobilisation of the neck throughout.

(4) If the respirations are rapid or ineffectual, consider whether a tension pneumothorax (see p. 136), open pneumothorax (see p. 135), massive haemothorax (see p. 148) or flail chest (see p. 136) is responsible.

(5) Record the temperature, pulse, blood pressure and respirations, and attach an ECG monitor and pulse oximeter to the patient. Aim for an oxygen saturation above 94%.

(6) (i) Gain i.v. access, send blood for FBC, coagulation profile, glucose, U&E, group and hold blood and save serum for a drug screen in case alcohol or drug intoxication is subsequently suspected.

    (ii) Send arterial blood gases, recording the percentage of inspired oxygen being given at the time.

    (iii) Avoid excessive fluid administration if the patient is normotensive, as this may contribute to cerebral oedema.

(7) However, if the patient is hypotensive:

    (i) Search for associated injuries, including chest, abdominal or pelvic bleeding, long-bone fracture and cardiac tamponade.

    (ii) Occasionally, brisk scalp bleeding alone is found to be responsible, usually in children.

    (iii) Alternatively, a cervical or high thoracic spinal cord injury with loss of sympathetic vascular tone may be the cause.

    (iv) Commence i.v. fluid administration to restore normotension using a plasma expander such as polygeline (Haemaccel) or a crystalloid such as normal saline.

(8) Record the level of consciousness using the Glasgow coma scale (GCS) score (see Table 4).

  (i)   A patient in coma has a score of 8 or less.

  (ii) A decrease in score of 2 or more points indicates significant deterioration.

  (iii) Repeated neurological examination, including the GCS, is essential for detecting and managing secondary brain damage.

(9) Treat the following complications immediately, as they worsen existing cerebral damage:

  (i)   *Hypoglycaemia*

    (a) Check a Glucostix; if it is low, send a blood glucose to the laboratory and give 50 ml of 50% dextrose i.v.

    (b) Remember this especially if the patient has been drinking alcohol.

  (ii) *Hypoxia*

    (a) A P_aO_2 of less than 9 kPa (70 mm Hg) breathing air or 13 kPa (100 mm Hg) on supplemental

Table 4. The Glasgow Coma Scale

		Score
Eye opening	Spontaneously	4
	To speech	3
	To pain	2
	None	1
Verbal response	Oriented	5
	Confused	4
	Inappropriate	3
	Incomprehensible	2
	None	1
Motor response	Obeys commands	6
	Localises pain	5
	Withdraws (pain)	4
	Flexion (pain)	3
	Extension (pain)	2
	None	1

The maximum score is 15. Any reduction in the score indicates a deterioration in the level of consciousness.

oxygen and hypercarbia with P_aCO_2 over 6 kPa (45 mm Hg) in the spontaneously breathing patient require rapid management.
- (b) Call an airway skilled doctor to intubate urgently.
- (iii) *Seizures.* Give i.v. lorazepam 4 mg or diazepam (Diazemuls) 5–10 mg in adults, followed by phenytoin 15 mg/kg i.v. (see p. 57).
- (iv) *Pinpoint pupils*
    - (a) Give naloxone 0.8–2 mg i.v.
    - (b) If there is no response, this may indicate pontine or cerebellar damage.
- (v) *Restless or aggressive behaviour*
    - (a) Check that the airway is still patent and high-dose oxygen is being delivered.
    - (b) Repeat the BP to look for hypotension.
    - (c) Catheterise the bladder, and exclude a constricting bandage or tight cast.
- (vi) *Gastric distension.* Pass a large-bore nasogastric tube, or orogastric tube if a basal skull or midface fracture is present.
(10) Perform a neurological examination, including:
- (i) conscious level: repeat the GCS record and look for any deterioration (decrease in score);
- (ii) pupil size and reactions: look in particular for an unequal or dilating pupil, indicating rising intracranial pressure;
- (iii) eye movements and fundoscopy:
    - (a) intact eye movements are one indicator of brainstem function
    - (b) fundoscopy may reveal papilloedema, subhyaloid haemorrhage or retinal detachment
- (iv) the other cranial nerves: include examination of the corneal reflex, facial movements and the cough and gag reflexes;
- (v) limb movements:
    - (a) assess for abnormal tone, weakness or loss of movement, or an asymmetric response to pain if the patient is unconscious;
    - (b) check the limb reflexes, including the plantar responses.

(11) In the patient with a deteriorating level of consciousness or focal neurological signs, particularly a dilating pupil associated with bradycardia and hypertension:

    (i)   Call an airway skilled doctor urgently to pass an endotracheal tube if not already positioned. Aim for a mildly lowered P_aCO_2 of 4.0–4.7 kPa (30–35 mm Hg) in consultation with the neurosurgical team.

    (ii) Give 20% mannitol 0.5–1 g/kg (2.5–5 ml/kg) as an osmotic diuretic, providing adequate circulatory volume resuscitation has occurred.

(12) Examine the scalp for bruising, lacerations and haematomas, and palpate for a deformity indicating a depressed fracture.

(13) Examine the face and mouth for signs of facial fracture or basal skull fracture.

    (i)   Basal skull fracture is indicated by:

        (a) periorbital and subconjunctival haemorrhage;

        (b) haemotympanum, external bleeding, or CSF leak from the ear;

        (c) mastoid bruising (Battle's sign), which may not appear for many hours;

        (d) haemorrhage or CSF leakage from the nose;

        (e) nasopharyngeal haemorrhage, which may be profuse.

(14) Perform a head-to-toe assessment for other injuries of the neck, chest, back, limbs, abdomen and perineum, including a rectal examination (loss of anal tone may indicate spinal cord damage).

(15) Request radiological examinations as follows:

    (i)   Lateral cervical spine:

        (a) This should always be performed in any unconscious head injury or in a suspected neck injury, combined with an anteroposterior and open-mouth view (for odontoid peg fracture) as well.

        (b) Make sure C1–C7/T1 are visualised, if necessary by traction on the shoulders.

    (ii) CXR and pelvic X-ray in all multiply injured patients.

(iii) Skull X-rays: these are of minimal value in the early management of a major head injury if there is ready access to CT scanning, but may indicate a radio-opaque foreign body or depressed skull fracture.

(iv) Do not request facial views or base-of-skull views at this stage.

(16) Confirm that a history from the ambulance crew, police or any witnesses as to the circumstances and nature of the injury, observed loss of consciousness or subsequent seizures has been completed.

(17) Obtain any other medical details, if a relative or friend is available, of current medical or surgical conditions, drug therapy, allergies and previous head injury or epilepsy.

(18) If a penetrating or compound skull fracture or intracranial air is found, give flucloxacillin 1 g i.v. or cefuroxime 750 mg i.v. and tetanus prophylaxis.

(19) Refer all patients to the care of the surgical team. Obtain immediate neurosurgical advice and arrange a CT scan.

(20) *Guidelines for CT head scan*[5]:

(i) GCS <9 after resuscitation

(ii) neurological deterioration, i.e. 2 points or more on the GCS, hemiparesis, squint

(iii) drowsiness or confusion (GCS 9–13 persisting for more than 2 h)

(iv) persistent headache, vomiting

(v) focal neurological signs

(vi) fracture known or suspected, including base of skull

(vii) penetrating injury known or suspected

(viii) age over 50 years

(ix) postoperative assessment.

(21) *Criteria for neurosurgical consultation*[5]:

(i) coma continues after resuscitation (GCS <9)

(ii) deterioration in neurological status, e.g. worsening in conscious state (2 or more points decrease in GCS), fits, increasing headache, new CNS signs

(iii) suspected base-of-skull fracture (see p. 170)

(iv) suspected or known penetrating injury

(v) compound depressed skull fracture

(vi)   skull fracture with confusion, decreased level of consciousness, epilepsy, focal neurological signs, and any other neurological symptoms or signs

(vii)   confusion or other neurological disturbance (GCS 9–13) for more than 2 h, no fracture

(viii) abnormality on CT head scan.

(22) It is essential that the patient's condition is stable and any associated injuries have been dealt with before transferring the patient, if this is required[6]. The transport team should be suitably experienced and carry appropriate monitoring equipment (see p. 397).

THE CONSCIOUS HEAD INJURY

The aim is to differentiate patients requiring admission from those who could be allowed home.

DIAGNOSIS

(1) *History*. Enquire about:
    (i)   the nature and speed of impact;
    (ii)   subsequent loss of consciousness, drowsiness, vomiting or fits;
    (iii) the length of post-traumatic amnesia (PTA) from the time of injury to the time of the return of memory for consecutive events. This is often underestimated. Over 10 min PTA is significant;
    (iv)   associated alcohol or drug intoxication;
    (v)   relevant medical conditions and drug therapy, including warfarin.

(2) *Examination*
    (i)   Examine the scalp for bruising, lacerations or palpable fractures and haematomas.
    (ii)   Assess the higher mental functions, including the level of consciousness using the GCS (see p. 168).
    (iii) Check the pupil size and reactions, eye movements, cranial nerves and the limbs for lateralising neurological signs.

(iv)   Record the temperature, pulse, blood pressure and respirations.

(v)   Exclude associated neck or other injuries.

(3) Skull X-ray.

   (i)   Patients with the following conditions should have a skull X-ray where a CT scan is not available or readily accessible[5]:

      (a)   any loss of consciousness or significant PTA; history unknown or unreliable (e.g. under the influence of alcohol or drugs);

      (b)   high-speed injury, injury from a sharp or heavy object, or a suspected penetrating injury;

      (c)   deep scalp laceration, large haematoma, or fracture suspected on palpation;

      (d)   focal neurological signs or impaired consciousness;

      (e)   repeated vomiting or headache;

      (f)   cerebrospinal fluid or blood loss from the nose or ear;

      (g)   difficulty assessing the patient, e.g. children, elderly, epileptic.

   (ii)   Look for a linear fracture, the double shadow of a depressed fracture, suture diastasis, an air-fluid level in a sinus, a traumatic aerocoele, shift of the pineal or a foreign body.

MANAGEMENT

(1) Scalp lacerations should be cleaned thoroughly, the edges trimmed and any foreign bodies removed. They are then sutured in layers using a monofilament synthetic material such as polyamide (Ethilon) to skin.

(2) Give tetanus prophylaxis according to the patient's immune status.

(3) *Admission*

   (i)   Refer any of the following for admission under the surgical team or A&E observation ward[5]:

      (a)   confusion or any other decreased level of consciousness

          (b)   neurological symptoms or signs, including persistent headache, vomiting

          (c)   difficulty assessing, e.g. alcohol, drugs, epilepsy

          (d)   other medical conditions, e.g. warfarin, coagulation defects

          (e)   skull fracture

          (f)   abnormal CT head scan

          (g)   age under 5 or over 50 years

          (h)   no responsible observation available outside hospital

          (i)   significant associated injuries.

    (ii)   All of the above should have had radiology, ideally a CT head scan, and many should then be discussed with the neurosurgical team.

(4) *Discharge*

    (i)   The following patients may be sent home, providing there is someone with them and home circumstances are suitable:

          (a)   fully conscious and oriented

          (b)   normal CT head scan

          (c)   normal skull X-ray (if CT unavailable)

          (d)   no other significant injuries

          (e)   no fits or focal neurological signs

          (f)   no persistent headache or vomiting.

    (ii)   Each patient must be given a standard head injury warning card advising him or her to return if any complications develop within the next 24 h, such as confusion, drowsiness, seizure, visual disturbance, vomiting or persistent headache.

(5) *The remainder*. This leaves the following patients, who should all be admitted to the short-stay ward for regular neurological observations:

    (i)   no one to accompany them

    (ii)   poor home circumstances

    (iii)   other significant injuries to the face or nose, etc.

    (iv)   an unreliable history, particularly if under the influence of alcohol or drugs.

(6) *Always remember:*

    (i)   In the elderly, the cause of the original fall may have been a TIA, Stokes–Adams attack or other

·   syncopal episode that requires diagnosis and management in its own right, in addition to the resultant head injury.

(ii)   In children, a head injury may be due to non-accidental injury (see p. 283).

BURNS

These are considered in the following categories:
(1) major burns
(2) minor burns and scalds
(3) electrocution and electrical burns
(4) chemical burns
(5) bitumen burns.

MAJOR BURNS

DIAGNOSIS

(1) History
    (i)   Ascertain the nature of the fire, how it started, whether there was any explosion, and how much delay there was in reaching hospital.
    (ii)   Ask if the patient was in an enclosed place, if so for how long, and whether smoke or fumes were present, which predispose to carbon monoxide and cyanide poisoning.
    (iii)   Ask about previous respiratory or cardiac problems, present drug therapy, known allergies, and tetanus status.
(2) Examine for signs of a respiratory burn.
    (i)   Look for burns around the face and neck, burnt nasal hairs, and soot particles in the nose and mouth.
    (ii)   Look for signs of tachypnoea, hoarseness, stridor or wheezing.
    (iii)   Assess for headache and confusion suggesting carbon monoxide poisoning.

(3) Check for associated injuries and circulatory collapse.
(4) Determine the extent of the burn.
    (i)   In adults, use Wallace's 'rule of nines', ignoring areas of mere erythema (see Fig. 6).
    (ii)   In children, the head is relatively larger (12–14%) and the legs relatively smaller (14%), so use comparison with the size of the child's palm (equal to 1% of body surface area) when estimating the extent of the burn.

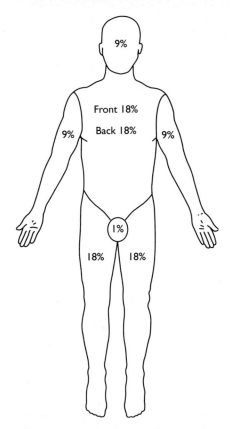

Fig. 6. Wallace's 'rule of nines' in adults to estimate the percentage of body surface area burned.

(5) Determine the depth of the burn.
   (i)   *Full-thickness*. The skin is white or brown, dry, leathery, and anaesthetic with no capillary refill. This will require skin grafting.
   (ii) *Partial-thickness*
         (a) Deep dermal. The skin is pink or white, feels thickened, does not blanch, and has reduced sensation. This should heal over in about 3 weeks, but some areas may require grafting to avoid leaving a scar.
         (b) Superficial. The skin is red and blistered, blanches and is painful. This should heal spontaneously in 10–14 days.
   (iii) *Superficial*. Erythema, blanching and pain occur, followed by peeling as in sunburn. This should heal rapidly in 5–7 days.

MANAGEMENT

(1) *Respiratory burn and smoke inhalation*
   (i)   Check the adequacy of the airway, give 100% oxygen by tight-fitting mask with reservoir bag, and nebulised salbutamol 5 mg for wheezing.
   (ii) Check the blood gases and carboxyhaemoglobin level, which will confirm exposure to carbon monoxide (see p. 83 for further management of carbon monoxide poisoning). Monitor the ECG and pulse oximetry.
   (iii) Request a CXR.
   (iv) Call an airway skilled doctor immediately to pass a cuffed endotracheal tube for burns of the face, tongue and pharynx, with stridor, hoarseness or a deteriorating level of consciousness.
   (v)   Consider the possibility of cyanide poisoning from burning plastics and fabrics, especially in patients with tachypnoea, coma, convulsions, cardiac arrhythmias, hypotension and severe metabolic acidosis with a raised anion gap and lactate.

(a) Act immediately on circumstantial evidence of cyanide poisoning, as no rapid measurement is available.

(b) Ventilate the patient with 100% oxygen.

(c) In patients seriously ill with coma and cardiorespiratory failure, and in whom the diagnosis is highly likely, give 1.5% dicobalt edetate (Kelocyanor) 20 ml i.v. immediately over 1 min followed by 50% dextrose 50 ml i.v.

(d) Repeat the dicobalt edetate if the response is inadequate, followed by a third dose after a further 5 min if necessary.

(e) Alternatively, a safer more reliable antidote is high-dose hydroxocobalamin (vitamin B_{12A}) at 70 mg/kg i.v. as a push or over 30 min, repeated up to a maximum of 15 g. Check with pharmacy on your local availability.

(f) Give 25% sodium thiosulphate 50 ml at 5 ml/min i.v. with the hydroxocobalamin[7].

(2) *Intravenous infusion*

(i) Commence i.v. fluids in any burn over 10% in a child or 15% in an adult, or for associated injuries causing hypovolaemia.

(ii) Insert a large-bore (14 or 16 gauge) cannula using an antecubital fossa vein or cut-down technique. Avoid central line insertion, as there is a high risk of sepsis from this procedure.

(iii) Send blood for Hb, PCV, U&E, blood sugar, CK, G&S and a drug screen if there is suspected alcohol or drug abuse.

(iv) (a) Give a volume of fluid according to the Muir and Barclay formula: (percentage area of burn × weight in kg)/2. This amount of fluid in millilitres should be given in each of three time periods: 0–4 h, 4–8 h and 8–12 h from the time the burn was sustained.

(b) Or use the Parkland formula at the rate of 4 ml/kg per percentage body surface area burned, 50% in the first 8 h and 50% in the remaining 16 h.

        (c)   More rapid fluid replacement may be required to catch up if there has been a delay in reaching hospital.

        (d)   Give additional maintenance fluid at 1.0–1.5 ml/kg/h of 4% dextrose 1/5 normal saline.

   (v)   Type of fluid:

        (a)   The quantity of fluid is more important than the type.

        (b)   Give polygeline (Haemaccel) initially in extensive, deep (e.g. electrical) burns, or when resuscitation is delayed, as it promotes a solute diuresis.

        (c)   Otherwise, use a crystalloid solution alone, such as compound sodium lactate (Hartmann's).

(3) Insert a urinary catheter to assess the adequacy of resuscitation, aiming for an hourly urine output of 50 ml in adults, or 1 ml/kg/h in children under 30 kg.

(4) Pass a nasogastric tube in patients with burns over 20%, who may develop gastric stasis.

(5) *Analgesia*

   (i)   Give morphine 0.1 mg/kg i.v. with an antiemetic such as metoclopramide 10 mg i.v.

   (ii)   Remember undertransfusion or hypoxia are more common causes of restlessness than pain.

(6) Give tetanus prophylaxis to all burn patients (see p. 261).

(7) *Escharotomy*

   (i)   Circumferential, leathery, full-thickness burns may cause difficulty in breathing by constricting chest wall movements, and distal ischaemia in a limb or digits by restricting the blood flow.

   (ii)   Request the surgical team to perform relieving incisions through the burn area. This is known as escharotomy; it does not require an anaesthetic, but will bleed.

(8) *Wound dressing*

   (i)   Leave any adherent clothing alone and do not break blisters in the burnt area.

(ii)   Cover the burn with a non-adherent, paraffin-impregnated gauze dressing or plastic cling wrap. Beware hypothermia in children if wet soaks were left on.

(iii) Avoid silver sulfadiazine (Flamazine) cream at this stage until the patient has been assessed by the surgical or burns unit team.

(9) *Admission*

(i)   All full-thickness burns over 1–2% body surface area require hospital admission by the surgical team.

(ii)   Refer patients to a specialist burns unit with:
   (a) burns over 10% in children and 15% in adults;
   (b) burns of important functional areas, such as the face, hands, feet, perineum and genitalia;
   (c) respiratory burns;
   (d) chemical burns and electrical burns, including lightning injury.

(iii) Serious burns must be assessed fully and resuscitated before departure, similar to the precautions taken when transferring serious head injuries to a neurosurgical unit.

(iv)   Avoid the risk of sudden respiratory obstruction during transit, by prior endotracheal intubation of any significant respiratory burn by an experienced airway doctor.

Note: burn injuries are always frightening and unexpected, and relatives (particularly parents of children) may feel guilty and angry. Special counselling and reassurance are needed from an early stage to help them come to terms with the injuries and to allay their anxieties, so they are useful as a support to the victim.

MINOR BURNS AND SCALDS

These include full-thickness burns under 1%, or partial-thickness burns under 15% body surface area in adults and under 10% in children. The aim is to manage them as outpatients, in distinction from patients with major burns who require admission (see above).

INITIAL MANAGEMENT

(1) Irrigate the wound immediately with copious running cold water until the pain is relieved.

(2) Assess the extent and depth of the burn (see p. 176). In general, superficial partial-thickness burns heal spontaneously, deep dermal partial-thickness burns heal slowly with scar formation, and full-thickness burns do not heal at all, unless under 1–2 cm in diameter when epithelium will cover the area from the edges. Otherwise grafting is required.

(3) Clean with saline or an antiseptic, e.g. chlorhexidine.

(4) Give an analgesic such as codeine phosphate 30–60 mg orally for adults, or paracetamol elixir 120–250 mg for children.

(5) Deroof large blisters that have broken, or aspirate the fluid if the blister is tense. Otherwise leave blisters intact to protect the healing epithelium.

(6) Apply silver sulfadiazine cream (Flamazine) and cover the burn with a non-adherent paraffin-impregnated gauze dressing.

(7) Then apply gauze and an absorbent layer consisting of a cotton-wool and gauze combine pad, overlapping the paraffin-impregnated gauze dressing by 3 cm either end.

(8) Finally, keep the absorbent layer in place with a firm crepe bandage, again overlapping each end by 3 cm and sealing with Elastoplast.

(9) Always elevate the limb using a high-arm sling for arm and hand burns.

(10) Give tetanus prophylaxis and analgesics to take home, such as codeine phosphate 30–60 mg orally q.d.s., or paracetamol 500 mg and codeine phosphate 8 mg (co-codamol 8/500) two tablets q.d.s.

(11) Remember that burns of the perineum, feet or hands in children may be due to non-accidental injury. Suspect this when there has been a delay in seeking treatment and the explanation is tenuous, or there is absence of any evidence of splashing. Refer the child to the paediatric team for admission if non-accidental injury is possible, however trivial the burn (see p. 283).

FOLLOW-UP MANAGEMENT

(1) Repeat the dressing after 2 days to check the area is pain free and clean, but omit the silver sulfadiazine.

(2) Thereafter, change the dressing every 5 days, unless the wound becomes painful, smells or the bandage becomes soaked ('strike through'), when the dressing should be renewed immediately.

  (i)   When changing the dressing, leave the paraffin-impregnated gauze in place if it has become adherent to the skin, to avoid destroying the delicate new epithelium forming underneath.

  (ii) Otherwise, replace the paraffin-impregnated gauze, the gauze and cotton-wool absorbent layer and the crepe bandage.

(3) When the wound is healing and has become epithelialised, it can be left exposed or covered with a dry, non-adherent dressing, e.g. Melolin.

(4) Refer burns that have not healed in 10–12 days to a plastic surgery unit for review and consideration for skin grafting.

(5) Warn the patient that healed burns will initially be both hypersensitive and photosensitive, will have dry, scaly skin and may be depigmented in dark-skinned races.

MINOR BURNS OF THE HAND

(1) These are difficult to dress. Cover the hand with silver sulfadiazine cream and place the hand inside a sterile polythene bag, bandaged over a gauze ring as a seal at the wrist.

(2) The hand is then elevated and the patient encouraged to move the fingers and use the hand.

(3) Give tetanus prophylaxis and analgesia.

(4) Replace the silver sulfadiazine cream and bag daily, as turbid fluid collects in the bag.

MINOR BURNS OF THE FACE

(1) These should be left alone and exposed to heal in 10 days. A proprietary moisturising lotion may be used.

(2) Exclude corneal damage by staining with fluorescein.
(3) Warn the patient that facial swelling may develop the following day.

ELECTROCUTION AND ELECTRICAL BURNS

These may be considered in three groups:
(1) electrical flash burns
(2) low-voltage electrocution
(3) high-voltage injuries.

ELECTRICAL FLASH BURNS

DIAGNOSIS

(1) These burns are caused by electrical arcing, which generates brief high temperatures that may ignite clothing.
(2) They are usually superficial partial-thickness burns, but may be deep dermal or even full-thickness.

MANAGEMENT

(1) Assess the depth and extent of the burn.
(2) Check the eyes for evidence of corneal injury using fluorescein.
(3) Dress the areas as for a thermal burn and treat accordingly (see p. 177).

LOW-VOLTAGE ELECTROCUTION

DIAGNOSIS

(1) Alternating current (AC) is more dangerous than direct current (DC), typically causing tetanic muscle spasm and cardiac arrhythmias.
(2) Injury usually occurs through carelessness or faulty electrical equipment, or to inquisitive children.
(3) The charge causes an entry wound that is often full-thickness, with potential underlying thermal tissue damage that may be extensive and include blood vessels and muscle. There is a similar exit (earthing) burn.

(4) If the charge crosses the heart or brain, arrhythmias including ventricular fibrillation and unconsciousness may occur.

MANAGEMENT

(1) Manage cardiac or respiratory arrest as for cardio-pulmonary resuscitation (see p. 2).
(2) Otherwise, give oxygen and attach a cardiac monitor and pulse oximeter to the patient. Aim for an oxygen saturation over 94%. Perform a 12-lead ECG.
(3) If there is no history of altered consciousness or cardiac arrhythmia, and the neurological state and ECG are normal, the patient may then be discharged, providing there is no significant thermal soft-tissue burn.
(4) All other patients require admission, with cardiac monitoring if the ECG is abnormal or there is a history of arrhythmias.
   (i)   Give i.v. normal saline for hypotension, aiming for a urine output of 100 ml/h if there is evidence of myoglobinuria (tea-coloured urine with a false-positive urine dipstick test for blood).
   (ii) Request a CT head scan if there is coma, confusion or focal neurological signs.

Note: remember that electrical burns look deceptively innocent. A white blister or small area of broken skin may cover extensive deep-tissue damage.

HIGH-VOLTAGE INJURIES

DIAGNOSIS

(1) These injuries occur from electric shocks greater than 1000 V, such as from lightning, pylons, electric train cables, etc. They are very serious injuries, and are often fatal.
(2) The victim's clothes may ignite or explode as the current arcs over the skin, particularly in lightning strike.

(3) Tetanic muscle spasm occurs, causing:
   (i)   direct long-bone fracture, vertebral crush fracture and muscle tears;
   (ii) indirect injury from falling;
   (iii) asphyxia from respiratory paralysis.
(4) The charge itself causes entry and exit wounds, which may be multiple if the charge jumps along the skin. The resultant tissue damage is deep and extensive, often requiring limb amputation.
(5) According to the pathway the charge follows, other effects include:
   (i)   Heart: cardiac arrest or arrhythmia.
   (ii) Brain: confusion, coma, cerebral haemorrhage, spinal cord damage and peripheral nerve damage.
   (iii) Eyes and ears: dilated pupils, uveitis, vitreous haemorrhage, ruptured ear drum, deafness and the late development of cataracts.
   (iv) Visceral and connective tissue: immediate damage to nerves, muscles and bone from heat and vascular thrombosis or later secondary haemorrhage.

MANAGEMENT

(1) Assess the airway, give oxygen, and commence cardio-pulmonary resuscitation if there is no pulse or absent respirations.
(2) Otherwise, attach an ECG monitor and pulse oximeter to the patient, examine for major injuries, and send blood for FBC, U&E, blood sugar, CK, G&S and blood gases.
(3) Commence an i.v. infusion guided by the blood pressure and urine output. Fluid requirements are higher than they appear from assessment of the burnt areas alone. Aim for a urine output of 100 ml/h if there is myo-globinuria from rhabdomyolysis.
(4) Request a cervical spine X-ray, CXR and pelvic or limb X-rays, according to the suspected injuries.
(5) Refer patients to the surgical team for admission or referral to a specialist burns unit. Escharotomy,

fasciotomy, surgical debridement and limb amputation may all be necessary.

CHEMICAL BURNS

DIAGNOSIS

(1) These occur at home, in schools and laboratories, and in industrial accidents.
(2) Most agents are strong acids or alkalis, although occasionally phosphorus and phenol are responsible.
(3) Alkali burns are generally more serious than acid as they penetrate deeper.

MANAGEMENT

(1) In the first instance, treat by copious irrigation with running water. Wear gloves to remove any contaminated clothing. Continue irrigating for at least 20 min.
(2) Do not attempt to neutralise the chemical as most resultant reactions produce heat and will exacerbate the injury, except in the case of hydrofluoric acid.
(3) Hydrofluoric acid burns should be neutralised as follows:
    (i)   Conversion of hydrofluoric acid to the calcium salt is achieved by covering the area with dressings soaked in 10% calcium gluconate solution, or by rubbing in 2.5% calcium gluconate gel (Hydrofluoric Acid Burn Jelly).
    (ii)   If the pain and burning persist, subcutaneous 10% calcium gluconate injection is advocated.
    (iii) Hypocalcaemia, hypomagnesaemia and hyperkalaemia leading to cardiac arrest may follow absorption of the fluoride ion by the skin, from as little as a 2% body surface area burn with concentrated 70% hydrofluoric acid.
(4) Refer all patients to the surgical team unless the area burnt is minimal and pain free.
(5) Remember advice is always available from the Poisons Information Centres (see p. 73).

BITUMEN BURNS

DIAGNOSIS AND MANAGEMENT

(1) Road-laying and roofing accidents are usually responsible.
(2) Irrigate the area immediately with cold water.
(3) Leave the black bitumen alone and cover it with paraffin-impregnated gauze.
(4) Await blister formation or re-epithelialisation, which will allow the bitumen to drop off.
(5) Assess subsequently for the depth of the burn, which is usually partial-thickness.

THE ACUTE ABDOMEN

The aim is to resuscitate critically ill patients and to distinguish between patients requiring surgical, gynaecological, or medical referral and patients who could be allowed home.

IMMEDIATE MANAGEMENT OF THE SERIOUSLY ILL PATIENT

(1) Clear the airway, give oxygen, and attach a cardiac monitor and pulse oximeter to the patient.
(2) Check the temperature, pulse, blood pressure and respiratory rate.
(3) Obtain a brief history of the onset, duration, nature and character of the pain, prior episodes of pain, relevant previous operations and illnesses, present medication and known drug allergies.
(4) Examine the chest and heart, then lay the patient flat to examine the abdomen, including the femoral pulses.
(5) Consider ruptured aortic aneurysm, pancreatitis, mesenteric infarction or inferior myocardial infarction in shocked patients with acute abdominal pain.

(6) Perform a rectal examination and catheterise the bladder. Test the urine for sugar, blood, protein, bile and urobilinogen, and send for microscopy and culture.

(7) Commence an i.v. infusion with normal saline. Arrange insertion of a CVP line by an experienced doctor in older patients with pre-existing cardiac disease, to avoid precipitating heart failure from fluid overload.

(8) Send blood for FBC, U&E, LFTs, blood sugar, amylase or lipase, and pregnancy test in females, and cross-match if haemorrhage is suspected. Send blood cultures if pyrexial. Check arterial blood gases.

(9) Record an ECG and request an erect CXR or lateral decubitus abdominal film if the patient is unable to sit upright, to look for free gas.

(10) Insert a nasogastric tube if there is evidence of intestinal obstruction, ileus or peritonitis.

(11) Commence broad-spectrum antibiotics such as ampicillin 1 g i.v., gentamicin 5 mg/kg i.v. and metronidazole 500 mg i.v. for generalised peritonitis.

(12) Refer the patient immediately to the surgical team.

MANAGEMENT OF THE STABLE PATIENT WITH AN ACUTE ABDOMEN

(1) *History*

   (i)   Onset and nature of pain:

      (a) Explosive and excruciating pain: consider myocardial infarction, ruptured aortic aneurysm, perforated viscus, biliary or renal colic.

      (b) Rapid, severe and constant pain: consider pancreatitis, strangulated bowel, mesenteric infarction and ectopic pregnancy.

      (c) Gradual, steady pain: consider cholecystitis, appendicitis, diverticulitis, hepatitis and salpingitis.

      (d) Intermittent pain with crescendos: consider mechanical obstruction.

   (ii) Location and radiation of pain:

      (a) Central abdominal pain radiating to the back suggests an aortic aneurysm or pancreatitis.

(b) Flank pain radiating to the genitalia suggests ureteric colic, or rarely ruptured aortic aneurysm.

(c) Otherwise pain tends to localise over the organ affected, provided there is peritoneal involvement, with radiation to a shoulder tip if the diaphragm is irritated, e.g. by cholecystitis or a ruptured spleen.

(iii) Associated nausea and vomiting:

(a) Pain tends to precede the nausea and vomiting in the surgical acute abdomen.

(b) If the nausea and vomiting precede the pain, a medical condition such as gastroenteritis or gastritis is more likely.

(iv) Fever and rigors:

(a) A low-grade pyrexia is usual in appendicitis or diverticulitis.

(b) A high fever and rigors suggest cholecystitis or cholangitis, diffuse peritonitis, pyelonephritis or acute salpingitis.

(2) *Examination*

(i) Check the temperature, pulse, blood pressure and respiratory rate.

(ii) Inspect for visible peristalsis and distension, palpate for local tenderness, guarding and masses, percuss for free gas, and listen for increased or absent bowel sounds.

(iii) Examine the hernial orifices, particularly in cases of intestinal obstruction.

(iv) Perform a rectal examination, external genitalia examination in the male, and consider a vaginal examination in the female patient.

(3) *Investigations*

(i) Send a baseline FBC, U&E, LFTs, blood sugar and amylase or lipase, although their discriminatory value in differentiating between the various conditions is limited.

(ii) Test the urine for sugar, blood, protein, bile and urobilinogen, and send for microscopy and culture in suspected UTI.

(iii)   Perform a pregnancy test in females with abdominal pain.

(iv)   Radiology. Request as indicated:

    (a)   An erect CXR. This may show evidence of pulmonary disease, a secondary pleural reaction from intra-abdominal disease and free gas under the diaphragm indicating a perforation.

    (b)   Erect and supine abdomen films. These may confirm a diagnosis, but rarely show completely unsuspected findings. Look specifically at the gas pattern, splenic shadow, renal outlines and psoas shadows, and for calcification and opacities.

    (c)   Upper or lower abdominal ultrasound. This is used increasingly to confirm or differentiate causes, particularly in females.

    (d)   CT scan. Depending on availability, this is useful for ureteric pain, other retroperitoneal pathology, e.g. aortic aneurysm, and for the difficult diagnosis.

(4) *Pain relief*

(i)   Give all patients i.v. analgesia as required, such as morphine 2.5–5 mg i.v. with metoclopramide 10 mg i.v.

(ii)   This does not interfere with the surgical diagnosis, which may even be facilitated.

(5) *Surgical referral*. Refer all cases to the surgical team if an acute surgical condition is suspected or cannot be excluded.

CAUSES OF ACUTE ABDOMINAL PAIN

These are considered under the following headings:

(1) Intestinal disorders:

    (i)   acute appendicitis

    (ii)   intestinal obstruction

    (iii)   intussusception

    (iv)   perforation of a viscus

    (v)   diverticulitis

    (vi)   gastroenteritis

    (vii) inflammatory bowel disease.

(2) Biliary and hepatic disorders:
    (i)   biliary colic
    (ii)   acute cholecystitis
    (iii)   hepatitis.
(3) Vascular disorders:
    (i)   ruptured aortic aneurysm
    (ii)   ischaemic colitis
    (iii)   mesenteric infarction
    (iv)   ruptured spleen.
(4) Pancreatic disorder: acute pancreatitis.
(5) Urinary disorders:
    (i)   renal and ureteric colic
    (ii)   pyelonephritis
    (iii)   acute urinary retention
    (iv)   acute epididymo-orchitis
    (v)   acute testicular torsion.
(6) Peritoneal and retroperitoneal disorders:
    (i)   primary peritonitis
    (ii)   retroperitoneal haemorrhage.
(7) Gynaecological disorders:
    (i)   ruptured ectopic pregnancy
    (ii)   acute salpingitis
    (iii)   ruptured ovarian cyst
    (iv)   torsion of an ovarian tumour
    (v)   endometriosis.
(8) Medical disorders presenting as acute abdominal pain:
    (i)   thoracic
    (ii)   abdominal
    (iii)   endocrine and metabolic
    (iv)   neurogenic
    (v)   skeletal
    (vi)   psychiatric.

ACUTE APPENDICITIS

DIAGNOSIS

(1) Acute appendicitis causes poorly localised central abdominal pain, worse on coughing or moving, which classically shifts to the right iliac fossa. There is associated anorexia, nausea, vomiting, and diarrhoea or constipation.

(2) A low-grade pyrexia, localised abdominal tenderness, rebound and guarding are found.

(3) A rectal examination will help diagnose a retrocaecal or pelvic appendix.

(4) Urinalysis is important to look for glycosuria, white cells and beta HCG. None of these, even if positive, rules out appendicitis.

(5) Diagnosis is most difficult in the young, elderly or pregnant patient.

MANAGEMENT

(1) Admit all patients under the surgical team if the diagnosis is definite. Give a metronidazole suppository 1 g p.r. if rupture is suspected.

(2) Refer other suspected or atypical cases to the surgical team, e.g. the confused elderly patient, the infant with diarrhoea, or the older child off their food, all of whom could have appendicitis.

    (i) WCC is frequently performed, but rarely influences decision making alone.

    (ii) Ultrasound, particularly in females, or even CT scan should be reserved for doubtful cases.

INTESTINAL OBSTRUCTION

DIAGNOSIS

(1) Intermittent colicky abdominal pain occurs with abdominal distension and vomiting in high obstruction, and constipation with failure to pass flatus in low obstruction.

(2) The causes are many, including an obstructed hernia, adhesions, diverticulitis, volvulus, intussusception, carcinoma, mesenteric infarction and Crohn's disease.

(3) Visible peristalsis may be seen, associated with tinkling bowel sounds and signs of dehydration.

(4) Always examine the hernial orifices and perform a rectal examination.

(5) Request erect and supine abdominal X-rays.

    (i) Small bowel obstruction:

(a) X-rays show an empty colon and central dilated small bowel, recognised by regular transverse bands (valvulae conniventes) extending across the entire diameter of the bowel.

(b) Fluid levels should be seen (but also occur in severe gastroenteritis). Over five are considered significant.

(ii) Large bowel obstruction: X-rays show peripheral dilated large bowel, with irregular haustral folds.

(6) If strangulation occurs (most common with a femoral hernia), the pain becomes more continuous and generalised, associated with tachycardia and signs of shock.

MANAGEMENT

(1) Check FBC, U&E, and blood sugar, and commence an i.v. infusion of normal saline to correct the dehydration from vomiting and fluid loss into the bowel.

(2) Pass a nasogastric tube. Give analgesia.

(3) Refer the patient to the surgical team.

INTUSSUSCEPTION

DIAGNOSIS

(1) Intermittent abdominal pain with sudden screaming and pallor occurs in children aged 3–18 months followed by vomiting.

(2) Abdominal distension and a mass may be felt, with blood-stained mucus ('redcurrant jelly') found on rectal examination in 50%.

(3) Request erect and supine abdominal X-rays to look for signs of intestinal obstruction.

MANAGEMENT

(1) Insert an i.v. cannula and send blood for FBC, U&E and blood sugar.

(2) Commence careful i.v. rehydration.
(3) Refer the patient to the surgical team.

PERFORATION OF A VISCUS

DIAGNOSIS

(1) Perforation may occur anywhere in the gastrointestinal tract. Common sites are a peptic ulcer, the appendix or in a diverticulum.
(2) There may be an antecedent history of alcohol or non-steroidal anti-inflammatory drug ingestion, dyspepsia or lower abdominal pain, but perforation can occur de novo.
(3) It presents with severe pain and signs of generalised peritonitis with board-like rigidity. Shock soon supervenes.
(4) An erect CXR will show gas under the diaphragm in over 70% of cases.

MANAGEMENT

(1) Send blood for FBC, U&E, blood sugar and amylase or lipase, and treat shock with i.v. saline.
(2) Pass a nasogastric tube.
(3) Commence broad-spectrum antibiotics such as ampicillin 1 g i.v., gentamicin 5 mg/kg i.v. and metronidazole 500 mg i.v.
(4) Refer the patient immediately to the surgical team.

DIVERTICULITIS

DIAGNOSIS

(1) This causes lower abdominal pain radiating to the left iliac fossa, and bloody diarrhoea, sometimes with sudden profuse rectal bleeding.
(2) There is a low-grade fever, abdominal tenderness, and guarding on the left with a palpable mass.
(3) Complications of perforation, severe bleeding, fistula formation and bowel obstruction may occur.

MANAGEMENT

(1) Send blood for FBC, U&E, blood sugar and G&S, and request an ECG and an erect CXR if perforation is suspected.
(2) Commence an i.v. infusion to treat shock.
(3) Refer the patient to the surgical team for bedrest and antibiotic therapy in uncomplicated cases, or for surgery in the remainder.

GASTROENTERITIS

See also Gastrointestinal tract infections on p. 88.

DIAGNOSIS

(1) Nausea, vomiting and diarrhoea tend to precede the pain. Close contacts may be similarly affected.
(2) There is generalised abdominal discomfort, usually without localising signs of peritonism or guarding.
(3) In severe cases, an erect abdominal film will show fluid levels.

MANAGEMENT

(1) If the patient is unwell or dehydrated (particularly children), send blood for FBC, U&E, blood sugar and blood culture. Commence an i.v. infusion and refer to the medical team.
(2) Otherwise, discharge the patient with an oral glucose/electrolyte solution such as Dioralyte or Rehidrat. If symptoms persist, ask the patient to return; send stool cultures to the laboratory then.

INFLAMMATORY BOWEL DISEASE

DIAGNOSIS

(1) Ulcerative colitis associated with bouts of diarrhoea with blood-stained mucus may present as a fulminating attack with fever, tachycardia, hypotension and a dilated

colon on plain abdominal X-ray (i.e. toxic megacolon greater than 6 cm in diameter).
(2) Crohn's disease, associated with recurrent abdominal pain, diarrhoea, malaise and perianal fistulae or abscesses, may present acutely with obstruction, perforation or right iliac fossa pain. This can mimic acute appendicitis.

MANAGEMENT

(1) Send blood for FBC, U&E, blood sugar and blood culture, and commence an i.v. infusion for shock.
(2) Refer all cases to the surgical team with shock, fever, peritonitis, severe bleeding and a dilated or obstructed bowel on abdominal X-ray.

BILIARY COLIC

DIAGNOSIS

(1) Discrete episodes of colicky pain occur in the right hypochondrium, referred to the scapula.
(2) Examination reveals right upper quadrant tenderness and possibly signs of jaundice with yellow sclerae and bilirubin in the urine, if the common bile duct is obstructed.

MANAGEMENT

(1) Send blood for FBC, U&E, LFTs and amylase or lipase. Request an upper abdominal ultrasound.
(2) Refer the patient to the surgical team if the pain is severe or acute cholecystitis is suspected.
(3) Otherwise, refer the patient to the GP or surgical outpatients for follow up.

ACUTE CHOLECYSTITIS

DIAGNOSIS

(1) Acute, constant right upper quadrant pain referred to the scapula occurs, with anorexia, nausea and vomiting.

(2) Localised tenderness is usual, sometimes with a palpable gall bladder and fever.

MANAGEMENT

(1) Send blood for FBC, U&E, blood sugar, LFTs, amylase or lipase, and blood culture, and commence an i.v. infusion of saline.
(2) Give ampicillin 1 g i.v. plus gentamicin 5 mg/kg i.v. and pethidine 0.5–1 mg/kg i.v. slowly.
(3) Refer the patient to the surgical team for bedrest, analgesics, antibiotics and cholecystectomy.

HEPATITIS

DIAGNOSIS

(1) Hepatitis presents with anorexia, nausea, vomiting, malaise and joint pain.
(2) A raised temperature, jaundice, tender hepatomegaly and splenomegaly are found.
(3) Urinalysis reveals bilirubin and urobilinogen.
(4) Causes include:
    (i) viruses, e.g. enterically transmitted hepatitis A or E, or parenterally spread hepatitis B, C, D or G, and infectious mononucleosis or cytomegalovirus (CMV).
    (ii) bacteria such as leptospirosis, or amoebae;
    (iii) toxins, such as alcohol and drugs, including methyldopa, isoniazid and paracetamol (remember the possibility of acute poisoning).

MANAGEMENT

(1) Refer unwell patients to the medical team with persistent vomiting, dehydration, encephalopathy or a bleeding tendency with a prolonged prothrombin time.
(2) Otherwise, send diagnostic bloods for LFTs and viral studies for hepatitis A, B or C.

(3) Advise the patient to avoid preparing food for others and to use their own knife, fork, spoon, cup and plate (assuming the patient could have hepatitis A or E).

(4) Advise the patient to avoid alcohol.

(5) Give the patient a referral letter to medical outpatients for definitive diagnosis and follow-up.

RUPTURED AORTIC ANEURYSM

DIAGNOSIS

(1) This classically presents with sudden abdominal pain radiating to the back or groin, faintness, collapse or unexplained shock.

(2) Abdominal examination varies from a pulsatile tender mass, to a vague fullness and discomfort. Tachycardia and hypotension occur in 50% of cases.

(3) Always consider the diagnosis in males over 55 years in particular, even when only one feature of the classic triad of abdominal or back pain, shock and a pulsatile or tender abdominal mass is present. Also consider in the older patient with apparent ureteric colic.

MANAGEMENT

(1) Give the patient oxygen by face mask, and record the ECG, as ischaemic heart disease is usually associated with or exacerbated by the hypotension.

(2) Send blood for FBC, U&E, blood sugar, amylase or lipase, cross-match 10 units of blood, and commence an i.v. infusion via a large-bore cannula.

    (i) Give minimal amounts of normal saline or a colloid such as polygeline (Haemaccel). Aim for a systolic BP of no more than 90 mm Hg.

    (ii) Arrange rapid surgical control rather than massive preoperative transfusion.

(3) Catheterise the bladder.

(4) Refer the patient urgently to the surgical team for immediate laparotomy. Contact the anaesthetist, and warn theatre and ITU.

(5) If the diagnosis is in doubt, but only if the patient is stable, consider an ultrasound scan to confirm the presence of an aneurysm, or a CT scan that will also demonstrate whether it has ruptured.

(6) Otherwise, proceed directly to theatre. Apply a pneumatic antishock garment such as MAST if the patient remains severely hypotensive, particularly if inter-hospital transfer is necessary.

ISCHAEMIC COLITIS

DIAGNOSIS

This usually occurs in an elderly patient with recurrent abdominal pain, progressing to episodes of bloody diarrhoea or intestinal obstruction from stricture formation.

MANAGEMENT

(1) Send blood for FBC, U&E, blood sugar and G&S if there is shock, and commence an i.v. infusion.

(2) Record the ECG.

(3) Perform an abdominal X-ray to look for 'thumb-printing' of the colonic wall and proximal dilation.

(4) Refer the patient to the surgical team.

MESENTERIC INFARCTION

DIAGNOSIS

(1) This is due to embolism from MI or AF, arterial or venous thrombosis, or aortic dissection.

(2) There is sudden onset of severe, diffuse abdominal pain, usually in an elderly patient, associated with vomiting and bloody diarrhoea.

(3) Abdominal distension, tenderness, shock, absent bowel sounds and rectal blood supervene.

MANAGEMENT

(1) Send blood for FBC, U&E, blood sugar, cross-match 2–4 units of blood, and commence an i.v. infusion.
(2) Record the ECG.
(3) Refer the patient to the surgical team, who will determine the need for angiography to confirm the diagnosis. The prognosis is poor.

RUPTURED SPLEEN

DIAGNOSIS

(1) Left lower rib injuries following blunt trauma are associated with splenic damage in up to 20% of cases.
(2) Occasionally, trivial injury to an enlarged spleen in glandular fever, malaria or leukaemia may cause rupture.
(3) Rupture may be acute, causing tachycardia, hypotension and abdominal tenderness with referred pain to the left shoulder.
(4) Or rupture may be delayed, occurring up to 2 weeks or more after an episode of trauma. Initial localised discomfort and referred shoulder tip pain give way to signs of intra-abdominal haemorrhage.

MANAGEMENT

(1) Send blood for a FBC and cross-match 6 units of blood for an acutely ruptured spleen. Commence an i.v. infusion and refer the patient immediately to the surgical team.
(2) In the absence of shock, insert an i.v. cannula for a delayed rupture of a subcapsular haematoma and send blood for a FBC and G&S.
    (i) Arrange an urgent upper abdominal ultrasound or CT scan.
    (ii) Delayed splenic rupture is also supported on CXR showing fractured left lower ribs and a basal pleural effusion, and on abdominal X-ray showing a displaced stomach bubble to the right and an enlarged soft-tissue shadow in the splenic area.
(3) Refer the patient to the surgical team for admission.

ACUTE PANCREATITIS

DIAGNOSIS

(1) Predisposing factors include alcohol abuse, gall stones, trauma and vasculitis.

(2) Acute pancreatitis presents with sudden, severe abdominal pain radiating to the back, eased by sitting forward, associated with repeated vomiting or retching (unlike a perforated peptic ulcer).

(3) Tachycardia with hypotension, a low-grade fever and epigastric tenderness, guarding and decreased or absent bowel sounds are found.

MANAGEMENT

(1) Send blood for FBC, U&E, blood sugar, calcium, amylase or lipase, and G&S. Check the blood gases.

(2) Commence an i.v. infusion of normal saline and pass a nasogastric tube. Give morphine 5–10 mg i.v. with an antiemetic such as metoclopramide 10 mg i.v.

(3) Record the ECG, which may show diffuse T-wave inversion, in the absence of myocardial ischaemia.

(4) Refer the patient to the surgical team. A CT abdominal scan and admission to ITU are indicated for severe pancreatitis with hypoxia and shock.

RENAL AND URETERIC COLIC

DIAGNOSIS

(1) Sudden, severe colicky pain radiating from the loin to the genitalia, associated with restlessness, vomiting and sweating is characteristic.

(2) There may be urinary frequency and haematuria.

(3) Loin tenderness in the costovertebral angle may be found, and urinalysis shows macroscopic or microscopic haematuria in over 90%.

(4) Always consider a possible ruptured abdominal aortic aneurysm in males over 55 years with a first episode of renal colic, especially if haematuria is absent (see p. 198).

MANAGEMENT

(1) Check FBC, U&E and LFTs, and send the urine for microscopy and culture.

(2) Treat pain:
   (i)   Use diclofenac (Voltarol) 75 mg i.m. or 100 mg p.r. This is as effective as pethidine, is not a controlled drug, and should discourage those who are only seeking narcotics.
   (ii) Alternatively, give pethidine 0.5–1 mg/kg slowly i.v. with an antiemetic for immediate severe pain relief.

(3) A plain abdominal X-ray KUB (kidneys, ureters, bladder) view may show a calculus in the line of the renal tract.

(4) Arrange an intravenous urogram (IVU), although a non-contrasted CT scan may be preferred, especially in older patients, to rule out other retroperitoneal pathology. Ultrasound may also be used, particularly with impaired renal function or in recurrent colic.

(5) (i)   Admit all patients with resistant pain, urinary infection, or large stones > 5 mm with an obstructed kidney.
   (ii) Discharge the remainder to their GP or urology outpatients.

PYELONEPHRITIS

DIAGNOSIS

(1) This presents with frequency, dysuria, malaise, nausea, vomiting and sometimes rigors.

(2) Raised temperature, renal angle tenderness and vague low abdominal pain are found.

(3) Dipstick urinalysis shows blood and protein. Urine microscopy shows bacteria, leucocytes and red blood cells.

MANAGEMENT

(1) Send FBC, U&E, blood sugar, blood culture and a urine culture for any patient who is significantly ill.

(i) This should include patients with vomiting, dehydration, or prostration; those who are pregnant, very young or old; and those who are known to have urinary tract abnormalities, e.g. a duplex system, horseshoe kidney or renal/ureteric stones.

(ii) Commence gentamicin 5 mg/kg i.v. and refer these patients to the surgical team for admission.

(2) Otherwise, if the symptoms are mild and consistent with predominant cystitis, send a urine culture and commence an oral antibiotic such as trimethoprim 200 mg b.d. daily for 1 week.

(3) Return the patient to their GP, with a letter requesting the GP to repeat the urine culture after the antibiotics to ensure that the infection has been eradicated.

(4) Any male with a proven urinary tract infection (UTI) must subsequently be referred to urology outpatients for investigation.

ACUTE URINARY RETENTION

DIAGNOSIS

(1) Predisposing factors include prostatic hypertrophy, urethral stricture, pelvic neoplasm, constipation in the elderly, anticholinergic drugs, pregnancy and local painful conditions such as genital herpes. Occasionally, retention is due to a neurogenic cause such as multiple sclerosis.

(2) The enlarged bladder is easily palpable, dull to percussion and is usually painful, although in the semiconscious patient it may manifest as restlessness.

(3) Always perform a rectal examination and assess perineal sensation and leg reflexes in all patients.

MANAGEMENT

(1) This depends on the suspected aetiology.

(2) Send blood for FBC, U&E and blood sugar.

(3) Carefully pass a urethral catheter as a strict aseptic procedure, and send a specimen of urine for culture.

(4) Refer the patient to the surgical team or gynaecologists as appropriate.

ACUTE EPIDIDYMO-ORCHITIS

DIAGNOSIS

(1) This occurs in sexually active men with a preceding history of urethritis, or after urinary tract infection or instrumentation, including catheterisation.
(2) Pain begins gradually, usually localised to the epididymis or testis associated with a low-grade fever.
(3) Urine microscopy shows leucocytes, and there may be a raised white cell count in the blood.

MANAGEMENT

(1) Never diagnose epididymo-orchitis in a patient under 25 years old without considering testicular torsion first.
(2) If torsion has been excluded, send urine for culture and give the patient a scrotal support, analgesics such as paracetamol 500 mg and codeine phosphate 8 mg (co-codamol 8/500) two tablets q.d.s. and an antibiotic.
(3) The choice of antibiotic depends on the suspected aetiology.
    (i) *Bacterial cystitis with epididymitis.* Give trimethoprim 200 mg orally b.d. for 2 weeks and refer to a urology clinic.
    (ii) *Nonspecific urethritis with epididymitis.* Give doxycycline 100 mg orally b.d. for 7 days and follow up in a genitourinary medicine clinic.
    (iii) *Suspected gonococcal urethritis with epididymitis.* Ideally, should be treated from the outset by a genitourinary medicine clinic.

ACUTE TESTICULAR TORSION

DIAGNOSIS

(1) Suspect this diagnosis in any male under 25 years old with sudden pain in a testicle, which may radiate to the

lower abdomen. There may be associated nausea and vomiting.

(2) The testicle lies horizontally and high in the scrotum, and is very tender. There may be a small hydrocoele.

(3) Urinalysis is typically negative and a white cell count normal.

MANAGEMENT

(1) Always refer all cases urgently to the surgical team, as the testicle becomes nonviable after 6 h of torsion.

(2) Even if more than 6 h have elapsed, still refer the patient for surgery as orchidopexy is required on the other side to prevent subsequent torsion there.

PRIMARY PERITONITIS

DIAGNOSIS

(1) Primary bacterial peritonitis occurs almost exclusively in patients with ascites, particularly due to cirrhosis or the nephrotic syndrome.

(2) Fever, abdominal pain and tenderness occur.

MANAGEMENT

(1) Send blood for FBC, U&E, LFTs, blood sugar and blood cultures. Check a urinalysis.

(2) Refer the patient to the medical team for diagnostic peritoneal tap and culture, to exclude *Mycobacterium tuberculosis* and to distinguish bacterial peritonitis from familial Mediterranean fever.

RETROPERITONEAL HAEMORRHAGE

DIAGNOSIS

(1) This condition may occur following trauma to the pelvis, kidney or back, from aortic aneurysm rupture, or from trivial trauma – even spontaneously in those with a bleeding tendency or on anticoagulants.

(2) It presents with hypovolaemic shock following trauma, in the absence of an obvious external or internal thoracic or abdominal source for haemorrhage. A paralytic ileus may develop.

(3) Plain abdominal X-ray will show loss of the psoas shadow and possibly fractures of the vertebral transverse processes in traumatic cases.

MANAGEMENT

(1) Send blood for FBC, coagulation profile, U&E, blood sugar, amylase or lipase, and cross-match blood according to the degree of shock.

(2) Insert a wide-bore i.v. cannula, and begin crystalloid infusion with normal saline.

(3) Check the urine for blood. If present, request an urgent intravenous urogram (IVU) to exclude renal damage.

(4) Organise an abdominal CT scan, which localises the bleeding in most cases. Refer the patient to the surgical team.

RUPTURED ECTOPIC PREGNANCY

See p. 353.

ACUTE SALPINGITIS

See p. 354.

RUPTURED OVARIAN CYST

See p. 355.

TORSION OF AN OVARIAN TUMOUR

See p. 356.

ENDOMETRIOSIS

See p. 356.

MEDICAL DISORDERS PRESENTING AS
ACUTE ABDOMINAL PAIN

It is rare for non-surgical causes of acute abdominal pain to present without other symptoms or signs suggesting their true origin. Always remember diabetic ketoacidosis, diagnosed by finding glycosuria and ketonuria on urinalysis (see p. 38). Causes include:

(1) *Thoracic origin*
- (i)   Myocardial infarction, pericarditis
- (ii) Pulmonary embolus, pleurisy, pneumonia
- (iii) Aortic dissection

(2) *Abdominal origin*
- (i)   Hepatic congestion from hepatitis or right heart failure
- (ii) Infection, including gastroenteritis, pyelonephritis and primary peritonitis
- (iii) Intestinal ischaemia from atheroma or sickle cell disease, vasculitis and Henoch–Schönlein purpura
- (iv) Irritable bowel syndrome
- (v)   Constipation, particularly in the elderly

(3) *Endocrine and metabolic origin*
- (i)   Diabetic ketoacidosis
- (ii) Addison's disease
- (iii) Hypercalcaemia – 'stones, bones and abdominal groans'
- (iv) Porphyria (acute intermittent)
- (v)   Lead poisoning, paracetamol or iron poisoning

(4) *Neurogenic origin*
- (i)   Herpes zoster
- (ii) Tabes dorsalis
- (iii) Radiculitis from spinal cord degeneration or malignancy

(5) *Skeletal origin.* Collapsed vertebra due to osteoporosis, neoplasm or infection, e.g. tuberculosis

(6) *Psychiatric.* Munchausen's syndrome or 'hospital hopper':
- (i)   Be suspicious of patients with multiple abdominal scars acquired at other hospitals, probably not living locally and with no GP, who present with acute abdominal pain or renal colic.

(ii)   Their aim is to gain hospital admission or narcotic analgesia by feigning illness.

(iii)   Ask for a previous hospital number or admission details, so you can 'go and verify their story'. If this does not prompt them to leave of their own accord, seek advice from a senior A&E doctor.

MANAGEMENT

This list is long and exhaustive. A careful history and examination, and request for FBC, U&E, LFTs, blood sugar, amylase or lipase, urinalysis, ECG, CXR and abdominal X-ray will avoid missing the more serious diagnoses.

REFERENCES

1   Nesathurai S. Steroids and spinal cord injury: revisiting the NASCIS 2 and NASCIS 3 trials. *J Trauma* 1998;45:1088–93.

2   Champion H, Danne P, Finelli F. Emergency thoracotomy. *Arch Emerg Med* 1986;3:95–9.

3   Boulanger BR, McLellan BA, Brenneman FD, *et al*. Prospective evidence of the superiority of a sonography-based algorithm in the assessment of blunt abdominal trauma. *J Trauma* 1999;47: 632–7.

4   Frankel H, Rozycki G, Ochsner G, *et al*. Indications for obtaining surveillance thoracic and lumbar spine radiographs. *J Trauma* 1994;37:673–6.

5   Newcombe R, Merry G. The management of acute neurotrauma in rural and remote locations. *J Clin Neurosci* 1999;6: 85–93.

6   Gentleman D, Dearden M, Midgley S, Maclean D. Guidelines for resuscitation and transfer of patients with serious head injury. *BMJ* 1993;307:547–52.

7   Braitberg G, Vanderpyl MMJ. Treatment of cyanide poisoning in Australasia. *Emerg Med* 2000;12:232–40.

ORTHOPAEDIC EMERGENCIES

INJURIES TO THE SHOULDER AND UPPER ARM

FRACTURES OF THE CLAVICLE

DIAGNOSIS

(1) These fractures are usually due to direct violence or to transmitted force from a fall on to the outstretched hand. In children, a greenstick fracture is common. In adults, a fracture between the middle and outer thirds is common.

(2) There is tenderness and local deformity. An anteroposterior (AP) X-ray of the shoulder usually shows the fracture clearly.

MANAGEMENT

(1) Support the weight of the arm in a triangular sling, and give an analgesic such as paracetamol 500 mg and codeine phosphate 8 mg (co-codamol 8/500) two tablets q.d.s.

(2) Refer the patient to the next fracture clinic.

(3) Rarely, comminuted fractures or fractures causing compression of underlying nerves or vessels may be treated operatively, and should be referred immediately to the orthopaedic team.

(4) The traditional figure-of-eight bandage has generally been abandoned as it is uncomfortable and difficult to keep tight.

ACROMIOCLAVICULAR DISLOCATION

DIAGNOSIS

(1) A fall on to the shoulder that tears the acromioclavicular ligament results in subluxation, but if the strong conoid and trapezoid coracoclavicular ligaments are torn as well, dislocation occurs, with the clavicle losing all connection with the scapula.

(2) Subluxation causes local tenderness, whereas full dislocation causes a prominent outer end of the clavicle and drooping of the shoulder, with pain on movement.

(3) X-ray of the acromioclavicular joint with the patient standing will show the displacement of the clavicle, which is highlighted by comparing the shoulders when the patient is holding weights in both hands.

MANAGEMENT

(1) Support subluxations in a sling. Give the patient analgesics and refer to the next fracture clinic.

(2) Discuss complete dislocations immediately with the orthopaedic team, as various operations are available (none of which is entirely satisfactory).

STERNOCLAVICULAR DISLOCATION

DIAGNOSIS

(1) This dislocation is rare, caused by a considerable blow to the front of the shoulder or a fall, resulting in the inner end of the clavicle displacing forwards or backwards.

(2) Anterior displacement results in local tenderness and asymmetry of the medial ends of the clavicles.

(3) Posterior displacement may impinge on the trachea or great vessels.

(4) X-rays are not easy to interpret, although AP and oblique views should be requested. A CT scan is required, particularly in posterior displacements.

MANAGEMENT

(1) A triangular sling and analgesics are suitable for subluxations. Refer the patient to the next fracture clinic.

(2) Refer posterior dislocations causing pressure symptoms immediately to the orthopaedic team.

(3) Discuss full anterior dislocations with the orthopaedic team; as with acromioclavicular dislocations, once reduced they are difficult to hold in place.

FRACTURES OF THE SCAPULA

DIAGNOSIS

(1) These can be divided into fractures of the neck, body, spine, acromion and coracoid, and are usually due to direct trauma.

(2) Their importance is to indicate that considerable trauma has been applied to the area: check for associated rib, pulmonary, spinal column and shoulder injuries.

MANAGEMENT

(1) Treat the associated injuries as a priority.

(2) Otherwise use a sling, give the patient analgesics and refer to the next fracture clinic.

ANTERIOR DISLOCATION OF THE SHOULDER

DIAGNOSIS

(1) This dislocation is caused by forced abduction and external rotation of the shoulder relative to the trunk. It is commonest in young adults from sports or traffic accidents, or in the elderly from a fall.

(2) It tends to become recurrent, when dislocation may occur with a trivial injury, movement or even spontaneously in bed.

(3) The arm appears slightly abducted and the shoulder looks 'squared off' with a prominent acromion.

(4) Always X-ray the shoulder, even if you are sure of the diagnosis, to avoid missing an associated humeral head fracture. Look for the following features:

  (i)   The humeral head is displaced medially and anteriorly with loss of contact with the glenoid fossa on the anteroposterior view.

  (ii) In doubtful cases, look at the lateral view (especially if posterior dislocation has occurred – see p. 214).

  (iii) Humeral head fracture:

    (a) A fracture of the greater tuberosity will not influence the initial reduction.

(b) A fracture through the humeral head, neck or upper humerus should be referred directly to the orthopaedic team, without any attempt at reduction.

(5) The following complications occur, and must be looked for and recorded before any attempts at manipulation:

(i)   *Axillary (circumflex) nerve damage.* Assess for sensory loss over the upper lateral aspect of the upper arm (testing for shoulder movement by the deltoid is too painful to be meaningful).

(ii) *Posterior cord of the brachial plexus.* Test wrist extension by the radial nerve. Rarely other parts of the brachial plexus are damaged.

(iii) *Axillary artery damage.* Palpate the brachial pulse.

(iv) *Fracture of the upper humerus.* Look specifically for this on the X-ray.

MANAGEMENT

(1) Give the patient morphine 2.5–5 mg i.v. with an antiemetic such as metoclopramide 10 mg i.v. if there is severe pain (unusual in recurrent dislocations). Reduce the dose of morphine in the elderly patient.

(2) Perform the reduction using i.v. midazolam 2.5–5 mg, provided that monitoring and resuscitation equipment are available, and dentures, rings, etc. have been removed. There are two methods of reduction:

(i)   *Kocher's manoeuvre*

(a) Gently apply mild traction to the arm flexed at the elbow, then slowly exert external rotation.

(b) The shoulder may 'clunk' back during external rotation. If it does not, when 90 degrees is reached adduct the arm across the chest and internally rotate it.

(c) The shoulder is felt to slip back; if not, repeat the whole procedure again.

(ii) *Hippocratic method.* Apply traction to the straight arm gently adducted over counter-traction from the physician's stockinged foot placed in the axilla.

(3) After reduction, place the arm in a sling strapped to the body, or enclosed under the patient's clothes, to prevent external rotation and a recurrent dislocation. Repeat the shoulder X-ray to confirm the reduction.

(4) Test again for neurovascular damage.

(5) Give the patient an analgesic, with instructions to keep the arm adducted and internally rotated, and refer to the next fracture clinic.

POSTERIOR DISLOCATION OF THE SHOULDER

DIAGNOSIS

(1) This condition is uncommon, occurring classically during electrocution or seizures or from a direct blow (e.g. in boxing), and is easily missed.

(2) The arm is held adducted and internally rotated, and the greater tuberosity of the humerus feels prominent. External rotation is severely limited and painful.

(3) X-rays of the shoulder must include two views, as the AP view may appear normal.

    (i)   On the AP view, look for the 'light bulb' sign due to the internally rotated humerus displaying a globular head, and for an irregular, reduced glenohumeral joint space.

    (ii)   On the axillary lateral view, look for the humeral head lying behind the glenoid. Or ask for a lateral scapular or 'Y' view, which is less painful as it does not require abduction of the shoulder. Again look for the humeral head displaced posterior to the glenoid.

MANAGEMENT

(1) Give the patient morphine 2.5–5 mg i.v. with an antiemetic such as metoclopramide 10 mg i.v.

(2) Perform the reduction using midazolam 2.5–5 mg i.v. provided that monitoring and resuscitation equipment are available.

(i)   Apply traction to the arm abducted to 90 degrees.

(ii)   Gently externally rotate the arm.

(3) Place the arm in a sling and repeat the shoulder X-ray to confirm reduction. Occasionally, the reduction may be unstable and immediate orthopaedic referral will be required.

(4) Give the patient an analgesic and refer to the next fracture clinic.

ROTATOR CUFF TEAR: SUPRASPINATUS RUPTURE

DIAGNOSIS

(1) Sudden traction on the arm may tear the rotator cuff, particularly supraspinatus. Other muscles forming the rotator cuff may also tear but are difficult to diagnose in the acute stage.

(2) There is localised tenderness under the acromion with supraspinatus rupture and inability to initiate shoulder abduction.

MANAGEMENT

(1) Refer the young patient immediately to the orthopaedic team for consideration of operative repair.

(2) Give the elderly patient a sling and analgesics, and refer to the physiotherapy department or to the orthopaedic clinic.

FRACTURES OF THE UPPER HUMERUS

DIAGNOSIS

(1) These fractures usually occur in elderly patients and may involve the greater tuberosity, lesser tuberosity, anatomical neck or the surgical neck of the humerus.

(2) There is localised pain and loss of movement, often with dramatic bruising gravitating down the arm.

(3) Complications include:

(i)   shoulder dislocation

    (ii)   complete distraction of the humeral head off the shaft

    (iii)   axillary (circumflex) nerve damage causing anaesthesia over the upper, lateral aspect of the upper arm and loss of deltoid movement

    (iv)   axillary vessel damage.

MANAGEMENT

(1) Refer patients immediately to the orthopaedic team with:

    (i)   a grossly angulated or totally distracted humeral head

    (ii)   fractures associated with a dislocation

    (iii) markedly displaced greater tuberosity fractures

    (iv) vascular damage.

(2) Otherwise, use a collar and cuff to allow gravity to exert gentle traction. Give the patient an analgesic such as paracetamol 500 mg and codeine phosphate 8 mg (co-codamol 8/500) two tablets q.d.s.

(3) Remember that the elderly patient may now need social services support in the form of 'meals on wheels', a home help and possibly a community nurse. Inform the GP by telephone and letter so he or she may visit the patient.

(4) Refer the patient to the fracture clinic for follow-up.

FRACTURES OF THE SHAFT OF THE HUMERUS

DIAGNOSIS

(1) These fractures are caused by direct trauma or a fall on to the outstretched hand.

(2) Upper third fractures tend to result in the proximal fragment being adducted by the pectoralis major, whereas in middle third fractures the proximal fragment is abducted by the deltoid.

(3) Always include views of the shoulder and elbow, remembering the old adage to X-ray the joint above and the joint below any fracture.

(4) Complications are usually seen in the middle third fractures, including:
   (i)   compound injury
   (ii) radial nerve damage in the spiral groove, causing weak wrist extension and sensory loss over the dorsum of the thumb.

MANAGEMENT

(1) Immediately refer to the orthopaedic team patients who have grossly angulated or compound fractures, and fractures involving a radial nerve palsy, where the nerve may have been severed completely (e.g. by a severely comminuted, angulated or compound injury).
(2) Otherwise support the arm for comfort in a U-slab plaster. This should not require analgesia to apply.
   (i)   Apply a 15 cm wide plaster slab medially under the axilla, around the elbow and up over the lateral aspect of the upper arm on to the shoulder, having padded the arm well with cotton wool.
   (ii) Hold the slab in place with a cotton bandage, and support the arm in a sling.
(3) Give the patient analgesics and review in the next fracture clinic. Social services support is needed for the elderly, who may require admission if they are unable to cope.

INJURIES TO THE ELBOW AND FOREARM

SUPRACONDYLAR FRACTURE OF THE HUMERUS

DIAGNOSIS

(1) This fracture occurs most commonly in children from a fall onto the outstretched hand, although it is seen in adults.
(2) There is tenderness and swelling over the distal humerus, but the olecranon and two epicondyles remain in their usual 'equilateral triangle' relationship (this is lost in dislocation of the elbow).

(3) There is a risk of the distal fragment displacing posteriorly, causing damage to the brachial artery on the lower end of the proximal fragment. Local tissue swelling will quickly worsen any ischaemia.

(4) Median nerve damage may also occur causing sensory loss over the radial three-and-a-half fingers and weakness of abductor pollicis.

(5) X-ray will show the displacement, although one-third of fractures are undisplaced, some merely greenstick. Comparison views of the other normal elbow are useful if there is difficulty in interpreting the radiographs.

MANAGEMENT

(1) Test for median nerve damage and look for any signs of arterial occlusion. These include pain, pallor, paralysis, paraesthesiae, pulselessness and cold. If arterial occlusion is suspected, refer the patient immediately to the orthopaedic team for manipulation under general anaesthesia.

(2) Even if there is no arterial damage, still refer the rest of these fractures, including the comminuted type in adults, to the orthopaedic team for admission overnight.

CONDYLAR AND EPICONDYLAR FRACTURES OF THE HUMERUS

DIAGNOSIS

(1) The lateral condyle tends to be fractured in children, and the medial epicondyle at any age, due to direct violence or forced contraction of the forearm flexors that attach to it.

(2) There is pain, swelling (which may be minimal) and loss of full elbow extension if the medial epicondyle is trapped in the joint, usually following dislocation of the elbow.

(3) The ulnar nerve may be damaged, causing sensory loss over the medial one-and-a-half digits and weakness of the finger adductors and abductors.

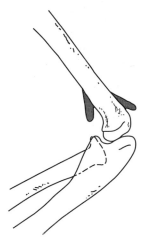

Fig. 7. Line drawing of a lateral elbow radiograph showing an anterior and posterior fat-pad sign (shaded areas) indicating a joint effusion.

(4) X-rays are often very difficult to interpret in children, as many of the structures are still cartilaginous. Helpful clues to look for are:

   (i)   The posterior fat-pad sign (see Fig. 7): this indicates a joint effusion, and is indirect evidence of significant trauma. It is also typically seen with radial head fractures.

   (ii) Comparison with the normal elbow placed in a similar anatomical position. Look for any differences between the two sides.

   (iii) Suspect displacement from injury if an epiphysis that should be visible by age is missing. The capitellum epiphysis is visible by age 1 year, the medial epicondyle epiphysis by age 6 years, and the lateral epicondyle epiphysis by age 11 years.

MANAGEMENT

Refer all these fractures to the orthopaedic team. Because the structures are mainly cartilaginous, the fractures are always more extensive than they appear on the X-ray.

DISLOCATION OF THE ELBOW

DIAGNOSIS

(1) This is caused by a fall on the outstretched hand, driving the olecranon posteriorly (rarely anterior, medial or lateral displacement occurs).

(2) The normal 'equilateral triangle' between the olecranon and two epicondyles is lost (unlike in the supracondylar fracture).

(3) The main complications are:
   (i)   ulnar nerve damage, causing sensory loss over the medial one-and-a-half fingers and weakness of the finger adductors, with the fingers held straight;
   (ii) median nerve damage, causing sensory loss over the radial three-and-a-half fingers and weakness of abductor pollicis;
   (iii) brachial artery damage, causing loss of the radial pulse with pain, pallor, paralysis, paraesthesiae and other signs of arterial occlusion.

(4) X-ray usually shows the dislocation clearly, but look for associated fractures of the coronoid process of the ulna or radial head in adults, and of the humeral epicondyles or lateral condyle in children.

MANAGEMENT

(1) Give the patient a sling and morphine 2.5–5 mg i.v. with an antiemetic such as metoclopramide 10 mg i.v., and X-ray the elbow.

(2) Call a senior A&E doctor to help perform the reduction under midazolam 2.5–5 mg i.v., provided that monitoring and resuscitation equipment are available.
   Apply axial traction to the elbow in 30 degrees of extension, and push the olecranon with the thumbs.

(3) Refer all cases to the orthopaedic team for observation or reduction under general anaesthesia if still displaced or unstable.

PULLED ELBOW

DIAGNOSIS

(1) This is typical in children aged 2–6 years following traction on the arm, such as grabbing the child's arm as it runs off or falls.

(2) The radial head is subluxed out of the annular ligament, causing local pain and loss of use of the arm, particularly supination. The arm is held with the elbow semi-flexed and pronated.

MANAGEMENT

(1) If there is pain localised over the radial head with limitation of supination, and the history is typical, perform the reduction without prior X-ray.
    (i) Gently flex the forearm upwards, alternately firmly supinating then pronating, with pressure applied over the radial head.
    (ii) The radial head is felt to click back; usually the child declines the offer of a sling.

(2) Otherwise X-ray the elbow in equivocal cases to avoid missing a supracondylar fracture.

FRACTURES OF THE OLECRANON

DIAGNOSIS

(1) These fractures follow a fall on to the point of the elbow or forced triceps contraction, which may then distract the olecranon leaving a palpable subcutaneous gap.

(2) There is therefore loss of active elbow extension.

(3) X-ray will show whether the fracture is displaced or merely hairline. Anterior dislocation of the elbow may accompany a displaced olecranon fracture.

MANAGEMENT

(1) Give the patient analgesics and a sling, and refer immediately to the orthopaedic team for operative reduction

if there is displacement of the olecranon or an associated anterior dislocation of the elbow.

(2) Otherwise, if there is an undisplaced hairline fracture only, put the patient in a long-arm plaster (with the elbow flexed) and refer to the next fracture clinic.

FRACTURES OF THE RADIAL HEAD

DIAGNOSIS

(1) These fractures are caused by direct violence or by an indirect force transmitted up the radius, which is driven against the capitellum.

(2) There is localised pain and tenderness over the radial head, and discomfort on attempted full extension and supination of the forearm.

(3) Unfortunately, this injury is commonly missed, usually because it is not thought of or because it is not seen on X-ray.

(4) It may be difficult or impossible to see a fracture on X-ray of the elbow, but look for corroborating evidence of a posterior fat-pad sign (see Fig. 7).

(5) If there is doubt, ask specifically for additional radial head views.

MANAGEMENT

(1) Place non-displaced or crack fractures in a collar and cuff, and refer the patient to the next fracture clinic.

(2) If there is severe localised pain, a plaster elbow backslab may be used for comfort and protection.

(3) Refer the patient directly to the orthopaedic team if the radial head is comminuted or grossly displaced.

FRACTURES OF THE RADIAL AND ULNAR SHAFTS

These two bones tend to act as a unit, attached proximally at the radial head by the annular ligament, throughout their length by the interosseous membrane and distally by the radio-ulnar ligaments. It is rare to fracture one bone in isolation and, as in humeral shaft fractures, it is vital to X-ray the joints above and below (here, the elbow and wrist).

DIAGNOSIS

(1) Injury is caused by direct trauma or by falling onto an outstretched hand, usually with an element of rotation fracturing both bones.
(2) There is localised tenderness, deformity and sometimes compound injury.
(3) X-ray will show the fractures. If one bone is angulated but the other is apparently unfractured, look for a second dislocation injury:
   (i) *Monteggia fracture:* fracture of the upper ulna with dislocation of the radial head.
   (ii) *Galeazzi fracture:* fracture of the lower radius with dislocation of the inferior radio-ulnar joint at the wrist.

MANAGEMENT

(1) Refer all these difficult fractures to the orthopaedic team.
(2) In the rare instance of an isolated, undisplaced, single forearm bone fracture, place the arm in a full-arm plaster cast from the metacarpal heads to the upper arm, with the elbow flexed at a right angle and the wrist in the mid-position. Refer the patient to the next fracture clinic.

INJURIES TO THE WRIST AND HAND

COLLES' FRACTURE

DIAGNOSIS

(1) This is a fracture of the distal 2.5 cm of the radius from a fall on the outstretched hand, most common in elderly females with osteoporosis.

(2) The classical 'dinner fork' deformity is due to dorsal angulation and dorsal displacement of the distal radial fragment, which may also be impacted, radially displaced and radially tilted.

(3) X-ray demonstrates the fracture, often associated with an ulnar styloid avulsion fracture from attachment to the triangular fibrocartilage.

MANAGEMENT

(1) Undisplaced or minimally displaced fractures, particularly in the elderly, may be treated directly with a Colles' backslab.

(2) Otherwise, reduce the fracture under a Bier's block, axillary block, general anaesthetic or haematoma block, according to departmental policy.

(3) *Intravenous regional anaesthesia or Bier's block technique*

    (i) Two doctors are required, allowing one to perform the manipulation and the other, with anaesthetic experience and prior training in the procedure, to perform the block.

        (a) At least one nurse attends to the patient, checks the blood pressure and assists the doctors.

        (b) Explain the technique to the patient, who should sign a written consent form.

    (ii) The technique is contraindicated in peripheral vascular disease, including Raynaud's disease, sickle cell disease, cellulitis, uncooperative patients including children, known local anaesthetic sensitivity, and hypertension with systolic blood pressure over 200 mm Hg.

    (iii) ECG and BP monitoring must be available in an area with full resuscitation facilities and a tipping trolley. The patient should ideally be starved for 4 h before the procedure.

    (iv) Use a specifically designed and properly maintained single 15-cm adult cuff, checking first for leaks or malfunction. Apply the cuff to the upper arm over cotton-wool padding.

(v)   Insert a small i.v. cannula into the dorsum of the hand on the affected side and a second cannula into the other hand or wrist.

(vi)   Elevate the affected arm for 2–3 min to empty the veins, rather than using an Esmarch bandage, which is generally too painful.

(vii)   Keeping the arm elevated, inflate the cuff to 100 mm Hg above systolic BP, but no more than 300 mm Hg. The radial pulse should no longer be palpable and the veins should remain empty.

(viii) Lower the arm and slowly inject 0.5% prilocaine 3 mg/kg (10 ml of 0.5% prilocaine contains 50 mg). Make a note of the time of injection.

(ix)   Continuously monitor the cuff pressure for leakage. Keep the cuff inflated for a minimum of 20 min to ensure the prilocaine is fully tissue bound, but with a maximum of 1 h.

(x)   Wait at least 5 min before performing the manipulation after confirming the adequacy of block. Request a check X-ray and repeat the manipulation immediately if reduction is unsatisfactory.

(xi)   If satisfactory, deflate the cuff then re-inflate for 2 min observing for signs of local anaesthetic toxicity, although the maximum safe dosage of prilocaine is 6 mg/kg (double the amount used in the block). Signs of local anaesthetic toxicity are:

  (a)   restlessness, perioral tingling, dizziness, slurred speech;

  (b)   loss of consciousness, fits, bradycardia and hypotension, which are virtually unknown with prilocaine.

(xii)   The patient then rests for at least 2 h while regular observations are made. Allow home with an accompanying adult if the plaster is comfortable and the patient feels well.

(4) *Colles' reduction and immobilisation*

  (i)   Prepare a 15-cm plaster slab measured from the metacarpal heads to the angle of the elbow.

Cut a slot for the thumb and remove a triangle to accommodate the final ulnar deviation (see Fig. 8 (a) and (b)).

(ii) Disimpact the fracture by firm traction on the thumb and fingers, while an assistant provides countertraction to the upper arm, keeping the elbow bent at a right angle. Also by hyperextending the wrist in the direction of deformity.

(iii) Next, extend the elbow and then use your thenar eminence to reduce the dorsal displacement and to rotate back the dorsal angulation, with the heel of your other hand acting as a fulcrum.

(iv) Alter grip to push the distal fragment ulnarwards to correct radial displacement.

(v) Finally, hold the hand pronated in full ulnar deviation with the wrist slightly flexed. Apply the backslab to the radial side of the forearm, which is well padded with cotton wool (see Fig. 8 (c)).

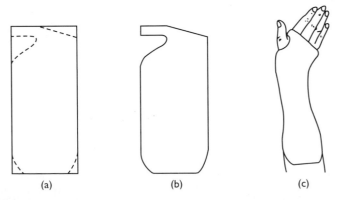

(a)   (b)   (c)

Fig. 8. The Colles' backslab plaster. (a) and (b) The backslab is prepared by trimming to permit thumb movements, full elbow flexion and to allow for the final ulnar deviation of the wrist. (c) The backslab in position.

(vi)   Hold the backslab in place with a cotton bandage, and take a check X-ray to assess the adequacy of the reduction before terminating the anaesthetic.

    (a) In a young person, reduction should be perfect.

    (b) In an elderly person, up to 10 degrees of residual dorsal angulation can be accepted, i.e. neutral position.

(5) Give the patient a sling, with instructions to keep the shoulder and fingers moving, and review in the next fracture clinic.

(6) Remember to check that the elderly patient will be able to manage at home, particularly if they already rely on a walking frame. Social services help may be needed. Inform the GP by letter and telephone.

SMITH'S FRACTURE

DIAGNOSIS

(1) This fracture is caused by a fall onto the back of the hand, resulting in a distal radial fracture with anterior displacement, i.e. a reversed Colles' fracture.

(2) Exclude median nerve damage (see p. 218).

MANAGEMENT

(1) Reduce the fracture under a Bier's block, axillary block or general anaesthetic, according to departmental policy.

(2) *Smith's reduction and immobilisation*

  (i)   Disimpact the fracture by firm traction to the forearm in supination with an assistant providing countertraction to the upper arm.

  (ii) Apply pressure with the heel of the hand to reduce the distal fragment dorsally.

  (iii) Plaster the arm in full supination and dorsiflexion, i.e. with the wrist extended.

  (iv) As the reduction is difficult to hold, a long-arm plaster is needed with the elbow at a right angle.

    (a) Mould an anterior slab around the radius with a slot cut for the thumb.

     (b)   Extend the plaster above the elbow.
   (v)   Take a check X-ray to assess the adequacy of reduction before terminating the anaesthetic. If reduction fails, internal fixation may be necessary.

(3) Give the patient a sling and analgesics, and review in the next fracture clinic.

BARTON'S FRACTURE-DISLOCATION

DIAGNOSIS

This is an intra-articular fracture-dislocation of the distal radius, with the fracture line entering the wrist joint (not parallel to it as in a Smith's fracture) and the hand displaced anteriorly.

MANAGEMENT

Refer the patient immediately to the orthopaedic team as this injury is unstable and open reduction with internal fixation is required.

DISTAL RADIAL FRACTURES IN CHILDREN

DIAGNOSIS

(1) There is marked local tenderness, sometimes with deformity.
(2) X-ray will reveal a greenstick fracture that may or may not be angulated, or a slipped radial epiphysis with dorsal displacement like a Colles' fracture, most commonly in adolescents.

MANAGEMENT

(1) Refer all angulated greenstick fractures and displaced radial epiphyses to the orthopaedic team for reduction under general anaesthesia.
(2) Otherwise, for a minimally buckled cortex that may be difficult to even see on an X-ray, place the arm in a

Colles'-type plaster backslab and refer the patient to the next fracture clinic.

FRACTURES OF THE SCAPHOID

DIAGNOSIS

(1) This common fracture is caused by a fall onto the outstretched hand, and must be considered in any patient presenting with a 'sprained wrist', particularly after a sporting injury.
(2) There is pain on dorsiflexion or ulnar deviation of the wrist and applying compression pressure along the thumb metacarpal. Localised tenderness in the anatomical 'snuff box' between extensor pollicis longus and abductor pollicis longus and weakness of pinch grip occur.
(3) The X-ray request should ask specifically for scaphoid views as well as for anteroposterior and lateral wrist views.

MANAGEMENT

(1) If the X-rays are normal and pain or tenderness are minor, place the wrist in a removable splint or a double elasticated stockinette (Tubigrip) bandage and a high-arm sling.
   (i) All X-rays must then be viewed by a senior A&E doctor within 3 days to avoid missing an unrecognised injury.
   (ii) Review the patient within 10 days and repeat the X-ray if the pain persists.
(2) Otherwise, if a fracture is confirmed on X-ray, or there is marked pain and tenderness particularly on moving the thumb or wrist, place the forearm in a scaphoid plaster.
(3) *Scaphoid plaster* (see Fig. 9):
   (i) This extends from the angle of the elbow to the metacarpal heads, including the base of the thumb to below the interphalangeal joint.

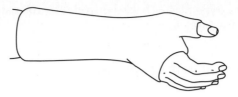

Fig. 9. The scaphoid plaster. This extends from the angle of the elbow to the metacarpal heads, and around the base of the thumb to below the interphalangeal joint.

     (ii)   The wrist should be fully pronated, radially deviated and partially dorsiflexed, and the thumb held in mid-abduction.

  (4) Give the patient a high-arm sling and refer to the next fracture clinic.

     (i)   The plaster will be reviewed and replaced if it was applied badly by the A&E department doctor.

     (ii)   It also allows the orthopaedic team to exclude other missed injuries, such as a Bennett's fracture of the base of the thumb metacarpal, a radial styloid fracture, or scapholunate dissociation.

DISLOCATIONS OF THE CARPUS

DIAGNOSIS

  (1) Dislocations of the carpus are uncommon, and are caused by a fall on the outstretched hand. Two important types are seen:

     (i)   *Dislocation of the lunate.* The distal carpal bones and hand maintain their normal alignment with the radius, but the lunate is squeezed out anteriorly, like a pip.

     (ii)   *Perilunate dislocation of the carpus.* The lunate maintains its alignment with the radius, but the distal carpal bones and the hand are driven dorsally. A displaced fracture through the scaphoid is often present.

(2) The median nerve may be compressed in dislocation of the lunate, causing loss of sensation in the radial three-and-a-half digits and weakness of abductor pollicis.

(3) X-rays are easily misinterpreted as normal in lunate dislocation, but:
- (i) on the anteroposterior view, the normal curved joint space between the distal radius and the scaphoid and lunate is disrupted and the lunate looks triangular instead of quadrilateral;
- (ii) on the lateral view, the dislocated lunate lies anteriorly in the shape of the letter 'C'.

MANAGEMENT

Refer all cases immediately to the orthopaedic team, particularly if median nerve compression is found.

FRACTURES OF THE OTHER CARPAL BONES

DIAGNOSIS

(1) These fractures are rare, and include fracture of the capitate, flake fracture of the triquetrum, hook of hamate fracture and pisiform fracture.

(2) There is localised tenderness from direct trauma, sometimes with an associated ulnar nerve palsy affecting the deep branch that supplies most of the intrinsic hand muscles.

(3) A common problem on X-ray is remembering the names of the eight carpal bones! Use the mnemonic 'Hamlet Came To Town Shouting Loudly To Polonius', corresponding to: hamate, capitate, trapezoid, trapezium, scaphoid, lunate, triquetral, pisiform (see Fig. 10).

MANAGEMENT

Place all these fractures in a scaphoid plaster and refer to the next fracture clinic.

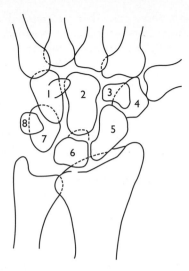

Fig. 10. The eight carpal bones. I hamate; 2 capitate; 3 trapezoid;
4 trapezium; 5 scaphoid; 6 lunate; 7 triquetral; 8 pisiform.

FRACTURES OF THE THUMB METACARPAL

DIAGNOSIS

(1) Injury usually results from forced thumb abduction, causing localised pain and tenderness.

(2) X-ray is always required and will distinguish stable from unstable injuries.

    (i)   Stable injuries include transverse shaft and greenstick fractures.

    (ii)   Unstable injuries include oblique shaft and comminuted fractures, and the fracture-dislocation of the base of the thumb (Bennett's fracture).

    (iii)   *Bennett's fracture*

        (a)   This is an oblique fracture through the base of the thumb metacarpal involving the joint with the trapezium, with subluxation of the rest of the thumb radially.

(b) Look for swelling of the thenar eminence, sometimes with local palmar bruising.

(c) Make sure X-rays include the base of the thumb to avoid missing this injury.

MANAGEMENT

(1) Refer unstable fractures (including Bennett's) to the orthopaedic team for possible open reduction and internal fixation.

(2) Otherwise, for stable fractures place the hand in a scaphoid plaster and refer the patient to the next fracture clinic.

DISLOCATION OF THE THUMB METACARPAL

DIAGNOSIS

(1) This may occur in motorcycle, skiing and soccer accidents, from forced thumb abduction or hyperextension.

(2) X-ray is needed to exclude an associated fracture.

MANAGEMENT

(1) Reduce under a general anaesthetic, a local Bier's block or with an i.v. analgesic and sedative combination.

(i) Apply traction to the thumb with pressure over the metacarpal head. After the manipulation, repeat the X-ray to confirm the reduction.

(ii) Place the forearm in a scaphoid plaster with plenty of cotton-wool padding, and refer the patient to the next fracture clinic.

(2) If the reduction fails, refer the patient immediately to the orthopaedic team. The metacarpal head may have 'button-holed' through the joint capsule between tendons, and will require open reduction.

RUPTURE OF THE ULNAR COLLATERAL LIGAMENT

DIAGNOSIS

(1) This condition ('gamekeeper's thumb', which referred to a chronic lesion) is caused by forced thumb abduction, typically now in a skiing accident.

(2) It is often missed and must be suspected whenever pain and swelling are seen around the metacarpophalangeal (MCP) joint of the thumb after an abduction injury.

(3) Look for tenderness over the ulnar aspect of the MCP joint. Test for laxity of the ulnar collateral ligament by applying an abduction stress to the proximal phalanx, although pain may prevent this.

(4) X-ray may show an avulsion fracture of the proximal phalanx or a degree of MCP joint subluxation.

MANAGEMENT

Refer all cases immediately to the orthopaedic team, as permanent disability may follow missed or untreated ruptures.

FRACTURES OF THE OTHER METACARPALS

DIAGNOSIS

(1) These are caused by direct trauma and may be multiple. The classical, isolated, little-finger metacarpal neck fracture or boxer's fracture is due to punching a hard object.

(2) All cases should be X-rayed and examined, particularly for any residual rotational deformity. On flexing the fingers into the palm, the fingertips should point to the scaphoid. If not, a rotational deformity of that finger exists.

MANAGEMENT

(1) Refer multiple fractures, rotated fractures, compound fractures and fractures associated with marked soft-tissue

swelling from crushing immediately to the orthopaedic team.

(2) Otherwise, for undisplaced, isolated fractures, give the patient a high-arm sling, an analgesic such as paracetamol 500 mg and codeine phosphate 8 mg (co-codamol 8/500) and either a padded crepe bandage or a plaster-of-Paris volar slab with the hand in the 'position of safe splintage'.

(3) *Position of safe splintage*
   (i)   The volar slab extends over the flexor aspect of the forearm, onto the palm of the hand to the fingertips well padded with cotton wool.
   (ii) The wrist is held extended, the MCP joints flexed, the interphalangeal joints extended, and the thumb abducted by the slab, which is kept in place with a cotton bandage.
   (iii) Instruct the patient to keep the hand elevated.
   (iv) Refer all patients to the next fracture clinic.

(4) *Isolated, little-finger knuckle injury*
   (i)   Many different methods of reduction have been tried, but simple neighbour-strapping of the little finger, a padded crepe bandage, a sling and analgesia are as effective as any.
   (ii) Remember that if the knuckle struck a tooth and the skin was broken, this is potentially a serious injury that may involve underlying tendons or penetration of the joint capsule:
       (a) Explore the wound in both the neutral position and with the fist clenched. If there is any suggestion of penetration into the joint space or tendon, refer the patient immediately to the orthopaedic team for surgical exploration and debridement. Give flucloxacillin 2 g i.v.
       (b) Otherwise, take a wound swab for bacterial culture and irrigate the wound with normal saline. Give the patient amoxicillin 500 mg and clavulanic acid 125 mg (Augmentin 625 mg) one tablet t.d.s. for 5 days and tetanus prophylaxis.
       (c) Review the wound within 24 h.

FRACTURES OF THE PROXIMAL AND MIDDLE PHALANGES

DIAGNOSIS

(1) Similar mechanisms of injury and rules of management apply as described previously for metacarpal fractures.
(2) All cases must be examined for rotational deformity. Check that on flexing the fingers into the palm, the tips point to the scaphoid.
(3) All injuries should be X-rayed to look for fractures, dislocations, subluxations and radio-opaque foreign bodies.

MANAGEMENT

(1) Refer all multiple, compound, angulated or rotated fractures, and those associated with marked soft-tissue damage or involving a joint surface, to the orthopaedic team.
(2) Otherwise, neighbour-strap the finger, give the patient a high-arm sling to prevent oedema, and give an analgesic such as paracetamol 500 mg and codeine phosphate 8 mg (co-codamol 8/500). Refer to the next fracture clinic.

FRACTURES OF THE DISTAL PHALANGES

DIAGNOSIS

(1) These fractures are usually caused by a crushing injury resulting in a comminuted fracture of the bone.
(2) The main problem is the associated soft-tissue injury to the nail and pulp space.

MANAGEMENT

(1) Provide adequate protection by using a plastic mallet-finger splint, elevate the hand and give analgesics.
(2) *Nail injuries*
    (i) If the nail is avulsed, cover the exposed bed with soft paraffin gauze, and give tetanus

prophylaxis and flucloxacillin 500 mg orally q.d.s. for 5 days.

(ii) If the nail is partially avulsed from the base, remove it using a ring block to exclude an underlying nail-bed injury. Debride and clean the area, then replace the nail as a splint to the nail matrix and a dressing to the nail bed.

(iii) The nail bed may need repositioning with one or two fine sutures inserted into the sides of the tip of the finger (not into the nail bed). Dress the area, give tetanus prophylaxis and antibiotics as above, and elevate the hand in a high-arm sling.

(3) *Subungual haematoma*. Relieve this by trephining the nail with a red-hot paper clip to release the blood under tension.

DISLOCATION OF THE PHALANGES

DIAGNOSIS AND MANAGEMENT

(1) Dislocations of the phalanges result from hyperextension injuries and must be X-rayed to exclude an associated fracture. They almost always displace dorsally or to one side.

(2) Reduce under a ring block by traction applied to the finger, followed by a repeat X-ray to confirm adequate reduction.

(3) Immobilise by neighbour-strapping, and encourage active finger movements. Refer the patient to the next fracture clinic.

(4) Complications include:

(i) rupture of the middle slip of the extensor tendon following proximal interphalangeal joint dislocation (see next page);

(ii) avulsion of the volar plate or rupture of one or both collateral ligaments. Accompanying small avulsion flake fractures may be seen on X-ray;

(iii)   button-holing of the head of the phalanx through the volar plate, necessitating open reduction.

EXTENSOR TENDON INJURIES IN THE HAND

DIAGNOSIS

(1) Injury can occur from a direct laceration, or by avulsion of the middle slip of the extensor tendon that inserts onto the middle phalanx or of the distal slip that inserts onto the distal phalanx.

(2) *Extensor tendon injury*
   (i)   Avulsion of the distal insertion causes a 'mallet-finger' deformity. The patient is unable to extend the distal interphalangeal joint with the middle phalanx being held.
   (ii) Avulsion of the middle slip that inserts onto the middle phalanx may be missed.
      (a) Initially, the proximal interphalangeal joint may be extended by the two lateral bands, but as they displace volarwards they then act as flexors.
      (b) Finally, the proximal interphalangeal joint becomes flexed and the distal interphalangeal joint hyperextended, resulting in the boutonnière deformity.

(3) X-ray may show an associated flake fracture of avulsed bone.

MANAGEMENT

(1) Refer a lacerated tendon or middle slip avulsion immediately to the orthopaedic team.

(2) Manage a mallet-finger deformity in a plastic mallet-finger extension splint for 6 weeks, and refer the patient to the fracture clinic.

(3) If more than one-third of the articular surface of the distal phalanx has been avulsed, refer the patient immediately to the orthopaedic team for consideration of open reduction and internal fixation.

FLEXOR TENDON INJURIES IN THE HAND

DIAGNOSIS

(1) These injuries occur from direct laceration or blunt injury.
(2) *Flexor tendon injury tests*
- (i)   Flexor digitorum profundus causes flexion at the distal interphalangeal joint.
- (ii) Flexor digitorum superficialis causes flexion of the finger at the proximal interphalangeal joint, while the neighbouring fingers are held extended.
- (iii) A partial tendon division may be suspected by pain or reduced function against resistance.

MANAGEMENT

Give tetanus prophylaxis for any penetrating wounds. Refer all suspected flexor tendon injuries directly to the orthopaedic team.

DIGITAL NERVE INJURIES

DIAGNOSIS

(1) It is mandatory to test for digital nerve function before using any local anaesthetic blocks.
(2) Sensory loss, paraesthesiae or dryness of the skin from absent sweating, demonstrated along either side of a digit, indicate digital nerve injury.

MANAGEMENT

(1) Refer immediately to the orthopaedic team nerve injuries proximal to the proximal interphalangeal joint, to the ulnar border of the little finger, the radial border of the index finger or to the thumb.
(2) Other injuries distal to the proximal interphalangeal joint rarely justify repair unless local departmental policy differs.

FINGERTIP INJURIES

MANAGEMENT

(1) Clean and debride injuries of the distal half-centimetre that do not involve the terminal phalanx and leave to granulate under a soft paraffin gauze dressing changed after 2 days.
(2) Give tetanus prophylaxis.
(3) Refer injuries involving substantial soft-tissue loss, distal phalanx exposure or degloving directly to the orthopaedic team.

CERVICAL SPINE INJURIES

See p. 141.

THORACIC AND LUMBAR SPINE INJURIES

See p. 162.

PELVIC INJURIES

See p. 159.

INJURIES TO THE HIP AND UPPER FEMUR

DISLOCATION OF THE HIP

DIAGNOSIS

(1) Dislocation of the hip occurs in violent trauma such as a traffic accident, a fall from a height or sometimes a direct fall onto the hip.

(2) The most common direction to dislocate is posteriorly (85%), as when the knee strikes the dashboard of a car. Other associated injuries from this particular accident are a fractured femoral shaft and a fractured patella.

(3) Less common are the central dislocation, fracturing through the acetabulum, or the rare anterior dislocation.

(4) In posterior dislocation, the hip is held slightly flexed, adducted and internally rotated, whereas in an anterior dislocation the hip is abducted and externally rotated.

(5) Check for sciatic nerve damage in posterior dislocation of the hip, particularly if an acetabular rim fracture is present. Assess dorsiflexion (L5) and plantar flexion (S1) of the foot, and sensation over the medial side of the foot (L5) and the lateral border of the foot (S1).

MANAGEMENT

(1) Commence an i.v. infusion of normal saline, and send blood for FBC, U&E, blood sugar and G&S.

(2) Give morphine 2.5–5 mg i.v. and an antiemetic such as metoclopramide 10 mg i.v.

(3) X-ray the pelvis, hip and the shaft of the femur.

(4) Refer all cases to the orthopaedic team for immediate reduction under general anaesthesia.

FRACTURES OF THE NECK OF FEMUR

DIAGNOSIS

(1) These fractures are most common in elderly women following a fall, and may be divided into two groups:
   (i)   *Intracapsular:* subcapital and transcervical.
   (ii) *Extracapsular:* intertrochanteric and pertrochanteric.

(2) Typically after a fall, the patient is unable to bear weight, and the leg is shortened and externally rotated.

(3) Occasionally, if the fracture impacts, the patient may be able to limp, and examination reveals localised tenderness and pain on rotating the hip.

(4) X-rays must always include the pelvis, as well as anteroposterior and lateral views of the hip. A CXR is required
as a preoperative aid for the anaesthetist. If no femoral
neck fracture is seen, look carefully for a fractured pubic
ramus, as this also presents with hip pain and a limp.

MANAGEMENT

(1) Send blood for FBC, U&E, blood sugar and G&S, and
record an ECG.
(2) Give i.v. analgesia titrated to response, and refer the
patient to the orthopaedic team.

FRACTURES OF THE SHAFT OF FEMUR

DIAGNOSIS

(1) These fractures are due to considerable violence, as in a
traffic accident, crushing injury or fall from a height.
(2) They may be associated with a hip dislocation, pelvic
fracture or fracture of the patella, and may cause concealed haemorrhage of 1–2 l in a closed injury (more if
compound).
(3) Rarely (<3%), there is damage to the femoral vessels or
sciatic nerve.
(4) Always X-ray the pelvis, hip and knee, as well as the
shaft of femur, to avoid missing these other injuries.

MANAGEMENT

(1) Give the patient oxygen, insert a large-bore i.v. cannula,
and send blood for FBC, U&E and blood sugar. Cross-
match 4 units of blood and commence an infusion of
normal saline or polygeline (Haemaccel).
(2) *Femoral nerve block*. Perform a femoral nerve block to
relieve the pain:
    (i)   Palpate the femoral artery and insert a 21 gauge
needle with syringe perpendicular to the skin,
lateral to the artery and just below the inguinal
ligament.

(ii) If paraesthesia is elicited down the leg indicating proximity of the needle to the nerve, withdraw slightly, aspirate to exclude vessel puncture, and in adults inject 10 ml of 0.5% bupivacaine, i.e. 50 mg (maximum safe dosage is 2 mg/kg).

(iii) Alternatively, a characteristic loss of resistance may be felt as the needle passes through the fascia lata then fascia iliaca:
   (a) aspirate to exclude vessel puncture;
   (b) inject 10 ml of 0.5% bupivacaine fan-wise, moving out up to 3 cm lateral to the artery.

(3) Supplement the femoral nerve block with morphine 2.5–5 mg i.v. and an antiemetic such as metoclopramide 10 mg i.v as required.

(4) Apply traction as quickly as possible to reduce the pain and blood loss, and to facilitate movement of the patient during X-ray (X-rays should be done after the splint is in place).

(5) Use a commercially available Donway traction splint.

(6) Alternatively, use a traditional skin traction device such as the Thomas splint.
   (i) Select the size of Thomas splint by measuring the oblique circumference around the top of the thigh and adding 4 cm, and the distance from the greater trochanter to the heel adding 20 cm for the length.
   (ii) Shave the lateral and medial sides of the thigh and lower leg, and spray with tincture of benzoin.
   (iii) Maintain firm traction on the leg as the adhesive strapping of the skin traction set is applied to the whole length of the leg, ensuring the malleoli are protected by the foam.
   (iv) Secure the adhesive strapping with crepe bandages.
   (v) Slip a double layer of circular elasticated stockinette (Tubigrip) over the splint, then slide the splint over the leg, which rests on the stockinette base.
   (vi) Protect the groin area with cotton-wool padding, and pad underneath the fracture and knee as well.

(vii) Tie the skin traction to the end of the splint and tighten it by twisting four wooden spatulae inserted between the ropes as a Chinese windlass.

(viii) Finally, secure the leg on the splint with further crepe bandages, and raise the leg by placing a pillow under the foot.

(ix) Check that the pulse in the foot is still present.

(7) Refer the patient to the orthopaedic team.

INJURIES TO THE LOWER FEMUR, KNEE AND UPPER TIBIA

SUPRACONDYLAR AND CONDYLAR FRACTURES OF THE FEMUR

DIAGNOSIS

(1) These injuries are caused by direct trauma or a fall in an elderly person with osteoporotic bones.

(2) The popliteal artery is rarely damaged by supracondylar fractures, although condylar fractures often cause a tense haemarthrosis.

MANAGEMENT

Give the patient analgesics and refer immediately to the orthopaedic team for aspiration of any tense haemarthrosis and operative fixation in certain cases.

FRACTURES OF THE PATELLA AND INJURY TO QUADRICEPS APPARATUS

DIAGNOSIS

(1) Damage is caused by direct trauma as in a traffic accident or fall, or by indirect violence from quadriceps contraction.

(2) Remember to always examine the shaft of femur and the hip.

(3) If the quadriceps mechanism is damaged, in most cases there is inability to extend the knee associated with local pain.

(4) X-ray will demonstrate the patella fracture.

   (i)   Confusion may arise from congenital bipartite or tripartite patellae, although these are often bilateral, unlike fractures.

   (ii) The presence of a lipohaemarthrosis causing a horizontal line fluid level on the lateral X-ray view of the knee is a helpful indicator of intra-articular fracture.

MANAGEMENT

(1) Refer a distracted or comminuted fracture or any damage to the extensor mechanism of the knee directly to the orthopaedic team.

(2) Otherwise, if there is a stable, undisplaced fracture of the patella, place the leg in a padded plaster cylinder from the thigh to the ankle and refer the patient to the next fracture clinic.

(3) If there is a tense haemarthrosis, this should be aspirated first, before applying the plaster cylinder.

(4) *Aspiration of the knee*

   (i)   Use a strict aseptic technique. Clean the skin with povidone-iodine and inject 2% lignocaine 2–3 ml into the skin, subcutaneous tissue and synovium.

   (ii) Insert a 14 gauge cannula at the midpoint of the superior portion of the patella 1 cm lateral to the anterolateral edge.

   (iii) Aim the cannula between the posterior surface of the patella and the intercondylar femoral notch.

   (iv) Withdraw the needle and attach a 50-ml syringe with three-way tap to the remaining catheter. Aspirate to dryness. Gently squeeze the suprapatellar region to 'milk' any residual fluid.

   (v)   Up to 70 ml blood-stained fluid may be removed. Look for evidence of fat globules floating on the surface of the blood to confirm an intra-articular fracture.

DISLOCATION OF THE PATELLA

DIAGNOSIS

(1) The patella commonly dislocates laterally in teenage girls and may become recurrent.
(2) Sometimes, spontaneous reduction occurs and the patient then presents with a tender knee, particularly along the medial border of the patella.
(3) A careful history and 'patella apprehension', as the patella is pushed laterally causing pain, suggest the true diagnosis.

MANAGEMENT

(1) Reduce by firm pressure with extension of the knee, pushing the patella medially under inhaled nitrous oxide with oxygen (Entonox) analgesia.
(2) Request a skyline patellar X-ray after the reduction to exclude an associated osteochondral fracture.
(3) Place the leg in a padded plaster cylinder and refer the patient to the next fracture clinic.
(4) If the dislocation is recurrent, use a pressure bandage instead of a plaster cylinder.

SOFT-TISSUE INJURIES OF THE KNEE

A careful history of the mechanism of injury and the subsequent events is crucial, as examination is often difficult in an acutely painful knee. Always lie the patient on an examination trolley and undress properly.

DIAGNOSIS

(1) Rapid swelling of the knee indicates a haemarthrosis, usually due to an anterior cruciate tear, peripheral meniscal tear or intra-articular fracture. A delayed swelling, occurring after several hours, suggests a serous effusion.
(2) Injuries may be suspected from the direction of force.
   (i) Sideways stresses will rupture the collateral ligaments or joint capsule.

(ii)   A twisting injury will damage one of the menisci, usually the medial.

(iii) Combinations may be seen. A severe lateral blow to the knee, e.g. from a car bumper, will rupture the medial collateral ligament, tear the medial meniscus, and rupture the anterior cruciate ligament (O'Donoghue's triad).

(3) Examination must include:

(i)   Palpating for the area of maximum pain.

(ii)   Assessing the medial and lateral collateral ligaments by stressing each side with the knee slightly flexed.

(iii) Assessing the cruciates by attempting to move the tibia backwards (posterior cruciate) or abnormally forwards (anterior cruciate), with the knee flexed. Be aware that a posterior cruciate tear allows the head of the tibia to slip backwards, which will then move forwards into a correct position on stressing (but not into an abnormally forward position as in an anterior cruciate tear).

(4) Meniscal tears may result in 'locking' of the knee with inability to extend the knee fully.

(5) All patients must be X-rayed to exclude associated fractures, such as:

(i)   a tibial condyle fracture;

(ii)   avulsion fracture of the tibial spines in cruciate ligament tears;

(iii) flake fractures of the lateral or medial femoral condyles in collateral ligament tears;

(iv)   vertical avulsion fracture off the lateral tibia from the lateral capsular ligament attachment (Segond fracture);

(v)   avulsion of the tibial tubercle (Osgood–Schlatter's disease due to traction apophysitis more common in young male teenagers).

MANAGEMENT

(1) Refer the following to the orthopaedic team:

(i)   a tense effusion, including all suspected haemarthroses;

    (ii)   a 'locked' knee (sudden loss of ability to extend the knee fully);

    (iii)   a suspected torn ligament;

    (iv)   an associated fracture;

    (v)   any penetrating wound of the knee suggested by air or foreign material in the joint on X-ray, although these may be absent.

(2) Otherwise, if there is only moderate swelling, a good range of joint movement and no ligamentous laxity:

    (i)   apply a double elasticated stockinette bandage (Tubigrip) to the knee;

    (ii)   give the patient anti-inflammatory analgesics such as diclofenac 50 mg orally t.d.s. or naproxen 500 mg orally b.d.;

    (iii)   lend the patient crutches to use until the acute symptoms settle;

    (iv)   review the patient within 5 days.

Note: in patients presenting with knee pain, always examine the hip and spine, as the pain may be referred, particularly in children – hence the need to undress the patient and examine on a trolley.

DISLOCATION OF THE KNEE

DIAGNOSIS AND MANAGEMENT

(1) This is a severe injury with up to 30% incidence of damage to the popliteal vessels and lateral popliteal nerve.

(2) Give the patient analgesics, check the distal pulses, X-ray and refer immediately to the orthopaedic team.

FRACTURES OF THE TIBIAL CONDYLES

DIAGNOSIS

(1) These fractures are caused by falls from a height, or severe lateral or medial stresses, which in addition may rupture the knee ligaments.

(2) A tense haemarthrosis is usual and precludes further detailed examination of the knee due to pain.

(3) Always check for vascular damage by palpating the foot pulses. Check for a lateral popliteal nerve palsy by testing for active foot dorsiflexion and eversion, and sensation over the lateral aspect of the calf.

(4) X-ray will show the tibial condyle fracture either laterally or (rarely) on the medial side although sometimes they are subtle and difficult to see. Look for a horizontal line fluid level in the suprapatellar pouch on the lateral view due to a lipohaemarthrosis, indicating an intra-articular fracture.

MANAGEMENT

Give the patient analgesics and refer immediately to the orthopaedic team.

INJURIES TO THE LOWER TIBIA, ANKLE AND FOOT

FRACTURES OF THE SHAFT OF THE TIBIA

DIAGNOSIS

(1) Direct trauma causes most of these injuries, which are often compound. Greenstick fractures in children and stress fractures in athletes are also seen.

(2) X-rays should always include the knee and ankle, as well as the shaft of the tibia.

MANAGEMENT

(1) *Compound injuries*
   (i) Send blood for FBC, U&E and blood sugar. Cross-match 2 units of blood and commence an i.v. infusion of normal saline.
   (ii) Give the patient morphine 2.5–5 mg i.v. with an antiemetic such as metoclopramide 10 mg i.v., restore anatomical alignment, and cover the exposed area with a sterile dressing.

  (iii)   Give flucloxacillin 2 g or cefuroxime 750 mg i.v.
          and tetanus prophylaxis.
  (iv)   Use a temporary plastic adjustable splint or a
          long-leg plaster backslab for support, especially if
          there are other injuries to the chest or abdomen
          requiring more urgent care.
  (v)   Refer the patient immediately to the orthopaedic
          team.
(2) Refer all other tibial shaft fractures to the orthopaedic
    team, after giving the patient analgesia and providing a
    suitable splint.

ISOLATED FRACTURE OF THE FIBULA

DIAGNOSIS AND MANAGEMENT

(1) This is caused by a direct blow, typically when playing
    soccer.
(2) Provided there is definitely no injury to the ankle, and
    no tibial fracture at another level, apply:
    (i)   a firm crepe bandage with cotton-wool padding, or
    (ii)   a below-knee walking plaster, which affords more
           protection.
(3) Refer the patient to the next fracture clinic.

PRETIBIAL LACERATIONS

DIAGNOSIS

These are most common in elderly patients, often from trivial
trauma tearing a flap of skin.

MANAGEMENT

(1) Clean the wound, remove blood clots, and trim obvi-
    ously necrotic tissue.
(2) If there is actual skin loss or marked skin retraction pre-
    venting alignment of the skin edges, refer the patient
    immediately to the surgical team for early skin grafting.
(3) Otherwise, lay the flap back over the wound and hold it
    in place with adhesive skin-closure strips (Steristrips).

Cover the wound with a single layer of paraffin-impregnated gauze and a cotton-wool and gauze combine pad.

(4) Then apply a firm crepe bandage and instruct the patient to keep the leg elevated whenever possible.

(5) Review the patient after 5 days, removing the dressing but leaving the Steristrips in place.

  (i) If the skin is now obviously nonviable, refer the patient to the surgical team for skin grafting.

  (ii) Otherwise, if healing is taking place, review the patient weekly or discharge to the care of the GP and community nurse.

INVERSION ANKLE INJURIES

DIAGNOSIS

(1) These injuries are common following sports injuries or tripping on a staircase or uneven ground.

(2) The aim is to distinguish ligament tears from bony injury, and to assess the stability of the ankle.

  (i) Immediate swelling and inability to bear weight suggest a fracture or serious ligament tear.

  (ii) Examine for the sites of maximum pain:

    (a) over the distal fibula and lateral malleolus itself;

    (b) over the anterior talofibular portion of the lateral ligament of the ankle, over the posterior talofibular portion, or the middle calcaneofibular portion;

    (c) around the medial malleolus or over the medial deltoid ligament;

    (d) over the anterior tibiofibular ligament;

    (e) over the base of the fifth metatarsal;

    (f) over the navicular;

    (g) around the calcaneus.

(3) An anteroposterior and lateral X-ray of the ankle should be requested if there is pain in the malleolar area and any of the following[1]:

  (i) bone tenderness over the posterior edge or tip of the distal 6 cm of the lateral malleolus;

    (ii)   bone tenderness over the posterior edge or tip of the distal 6 cm of the medial malleolus;

    (iii)   inability to bear weight (e.g. unable to take four steps without assistance, regardless of limping) both within the first hour of injury and in the emergency department.

(4) Additional foot X-rays should be requested only if there is pain in the mid-foot and any of the following[1]:

    (i)   bone tenderness over the base of the fifth metatarsal;

    (ii)   bone tenderness over the navicular;

    (iii)   inability to bear weight both immediately and in the emergency department.

MANAGEMENT

(1) Refer immediately to the orthopaedic team a displaced lateral malleolar fracture, an associated medial malleolar fracture, widening or diastasis of the ankle mortice, and severe pain or swelling.

(2) Otherwise, immobilise an avulsion flake fracture of the malleolus or talus and an undisplaced lateral malleolar fracture in a below-knee plaster.

    (i)   This is applied from the metatarsal heads to below the tibial tubercle, with the ankle at a right angle (not in equinus).

    (ii)   Repeat the ankle X-ray after application of the plaster.

    (iii)   Refer the patient to the next fracture clinic, with instructions to keep the leg elevated overnight.

(3) If the patient is able to bear weight and no fracture is seen, with minimal swelling:

    (i)   Apply a double elasticated stockinette (Tubigrip) bandage, give the patient crutches or a walking frame, and give an anti-inflammatory analgesic such as diclofenac 50 mg orally t.d.s. or naproxen 500 mg orally b.d.

    (ii)   Recommend initial elevation, no weight-bearing and a cold compress (e.g. a bag of frozen peas) at home, followed by gradual mobilisation.

(iii)   Warn patients that they will not be fully fit for active sports for at least 3 weeks, however much they protest.

(iv)   Review the patient after 5–10 days and refer to physiotherapy if there is persisting disability.

OTHER ANKLE INJURIES

DIAGNOSIS

(1)   Eversion injuries damaging the medial malleolus and medial deltoid ligament, hyperflexion injuries or rotational injuries tend to cause more complicated damage.

(2)   Examine the ankle as before to localise the maximum area of tenderness. In addition, palpate the upper fibula for a high (Maisonneuve) fracture associated with tibiofibular diastasis and a widened ankle mortice.

(3)   X-ray all patients meeting the criteria on p. 251, and include the upper tibia and fibula if there is proximal tenderness.

MANAGEMENT

(1)   Refer all fractures, widened ankle mortices or patients totally unable to bear weight to the orthopaedic team.

(2)   Otherwise treat as in point (3) above.

DISLOCATION OF THE ANKLE

DIAGNOSIS AND MANAGEMENT

(1)   This dislocation is most commonly posterior and is clinically obvious. It must be reduced immediately to prevent ischaemic pressure necrosis of skin stretched across the malleolus.

(2)   Give the patient morphine 5 mg i.v. and metoclopramide 10 mg i.v.

(i)   Then give midazolam 2.5–5 mg i.v. in a monitored area with resuscitation equipment available.

(ii)   Reduce the ankle dislocation by steady traction on the heel, gently dorsiflexing the foot.

(iii)   After the reduction, place the lower leg in a plastic splint or padded backslab before sending the patient for post-reduction X-ray.

(3) Refer the patient immediately to the orthopaedic team.

FRACTURES AND DISLOCATION OF THE TALUS

DIAGNOSIS

(1) The talus articulates in three joints: the ankle joint with the tibia and fibula, the subtalar joint with the calcaneus, and the midtarsal joint with the navicular (along with the calcaneus and cuboid).

(2) It is injured by falls from a height or sudden violence to the foot, as from the pedal of a car being forced upwards in a traffic accident.

(3) There is pain and swelling, and X-ray is needed to define the injuries.

(4) Complications of talar injuries include avascular necrosis and persistent pain and disability from osteoarthrosis, particularly if the injury is missed.

MANAGEMENT

(1) Refer all fractures including the osteochondral dome fracture immediately to the orthopaedic team.

(2) The only exception is an avulsion flake fracture of the neck of the talus from a ligamentous or capsular insertion. Treat this in a below-knee plaster and refer to the next fracture clinic.

(3) Occasionally, the talus can dislocate completely and lie laterally in front of the ankle joint. This requires urgent manipulation to avoid overlying skin necrosis, similar to the dislocated ankle.

FRACTURES OF THE CALCANEUS

DIAGNOSIS

(1) These are usually due to a fall from a height, and are bilateral in 20% of cases.

(2) Falls from a height are associated with a characteristic pattern of injuries, which includes fractures to the:
   (i)   calcaneus
   (ii)   ankle
   (iii)   tibial plateau
   (iv)   femoral head or hip
   (v)   thoracolumbar vertebra
   (vi)   atlas and base of the skull.
   Each of these must be looked for specifically in turn and any tender areas must be X-rayed.
(3) The heel tends to flatten following a calcaneal fracture, and is locally tender with bruising spreading onto the sole and up the calf.
(4) Request an anteroposterior and lateral ankle X-ray with an additional tangential (axial) calcaneal view to avoid missing the fracture.
(5) A CT scan may be necessary to demonstrate involvement of the subtalar joint.

MANAGEMENT

Elevate the foot and give analgesia. Refer all fractures to the orthopaedic team.

RUPTURE OF THE TENDO ACHILLIS

DIAGNOSIS

(1) This injury is most common in middle-aged men following abrupt muscular activity. There is pain and weakness of plantar flexion, although some is still possible by the long toe flexors; however, the patient is unable to walk on tiptoe.
(2) A palpable gap in the tendon may be felt, although this rapidly fills with blood.
(3) The 'calf squeeze' test shows reduced or absent foot plantar flexion compared with the uninjured side, as the relaxed calf is gently squeezed with the patient kneeling on a chair with the feet hanging free.

MANAGEMENT

Give the patient analgesics and refer to the orthopaedic team for operative repair or conservative treatment.

MIDTARSAL DISLOCATIONS

DIAGNOSIS

(1) These follow a twisting injury to the forefoot, causing pain and swelling around the talonavicular and calcaneocuboid midtarsal joint.

(2) X-ray shows disruption of the midtarsal joint, often associated with fractures of the navicular, cuboid, talus or calcaneus. These may merely be avulsion flake fractures.

MANAGEMENT

Give the patient analgesics, elevate the foot, and refer to the orthopaedic team.

METATARSAL INJURIES AND TARSOMETATARSAL DISLOCATIONS

DIAGNOSIS

(1) These are caused by direct trauma, crushing or twisting.

(2) A transverse avulsion fracture of the base of the fifth metatarsal is seen following ankle inversion, at the site of insertion of peroneus brevis.

(3) A stress fracture may occur, usually in the neck of the second metatarsal known as the 'march fracture'.

(4) Tarsometatarsal dislocation is uncommon and may be multiple, resulting in widening of the gap between the base of the hallux and second metatarsal with lateral shift of the remaining metatarsals.

　(i)　It is often missed, as the significance of the foot swelling is not appreciated and interpretation of the X-ray is difficult.

　(ii)　Circulatory impairment in the forefoot must be excluded.

MANAGEMENT

(1) Refer immediately to the orthopaedic team all compound, displaced or multiple fractures, tarsometatarsal dislocations, fractures of the first metatarsal and injuries associated with considerable crushing or oedema.

(2) Treat an avulsion fracture of the base of the fifth metatarsal as for an ankle sprain, and a 'march fracture' in a support bandage, or rarely a below-knee plaster if the pain is severe.

FRACTURES OF THE PHALANGES OF THE FOOT

DIAGNOSIS AND MANAGEMENT

(1) These fractures are usually caused by a direct blow.

(2) Clean all the wounds and release any subungual haematoma by trephining.

(3) Otherwise, give an analgesic and a support bandage after neighbour-strapping the damaged toe.

(4) If the pain is severe, particularly with injury to the great toe, apply a below-knee plaster with a toe platform extension.

(5) Refer all patients to the next fracture clinic.

SOFT-TISSUE INJURIES

The so-called 'minor injury' is of major importance to the patient and may lead to serious problems if managed incorrectly. Therefore, adopt a consistent, careful approach to every patient presenting with a soft-tissue injury.

GENERAL MANAGEMENT OF A SOFT-TISSUE INJURY

(1) *Assessment*
    (i)   Obtain a history of:
        (a) the nature of the injury, and when and where it was sustained;
        (b) current medical conditions and drug therapy;

      (c)   antibiotic allergy and tetanus immune status;

      (d)   the possibility of a foreign body, wound contamination, and damage to deeper structures;

      (e)   any crushing injury.

  (ii)   Examine nerves and tendons for evidence of damage, before infiltrating with local anaesthetic.

  (iii)   If a radio-opaque foreign body (metal or glass) is suspected, send the patient for X-rays before exploring the wound. Inform the radiographer of the nature of the foreign body.

(2) *Cleaning*

  (i)   After scrubbing up and wearing sterile gloves, remove all the dirt and debris from around the edges of the wound using normal saline or a disinfectant, e.g. chlorhexidine or cetrimide, by swabbing and gentle rubbing.

  (ii)   Trim adjacent hair for 3–5 mm, but never shave the eyebrows or eyelashes.

(3) *Local anaesthetic infiltration*

  (i)   The patient should always be lying down.

  (ii)   Use 1% lignocaine infiltrated along the edge of the wound with a 25 gauge orange needle.

  (iii)   *Ring block*. Use a ring block with plain 2% lignocaine without adrenaline for wounds around the nail, fingertip and distal finger, or similarly in the toes.

      (a)   A ring block is contraindicated in patients with peripheral vascular disease, Raynaud's phenomenon and local sepsis at the base of the finger.

      (b)   Do not use a tourniquet due to the risk of creating locally high pressures and occluding the digital vessels. First, clean the base of the finger with antiseptic.

      (c)   Insert a 25 gauge orange needle into the side of the base of the finger, and angle at 45 degrees from the vertical injecting up to 1 ml of 2% lignocaine (without adrenaline) into the lateral palmar aspect of the finger.

      (d)   Remove the needle until subcutaneous, and rotate until it is pointing to the extensor surface of the finger; inject 0.5 ml into the lateral extensor aspect of the finger.

(e) Perform the same procedure on the other side of the finger.

(f) Allow at least 5–10 min for the block to take effect.

(iv) The maximum safe dosage of lignocaine is 3 mg/kg. A 1% solution contains 10 mg/ml. Therefore, the maximum safe amounts allowed in a 67-kg patient are:

(a) 20 ml of 1% solution containing 200 mg lignocaine, or

(b) 10 ml of 2% solution containing 200 mg lignocaine.

(v) *Signs of lignocaine (or other local anaesthetic) toxicity*

(a) perioral tingling, a metallic taste, restlessness, dizziness and slurred speech;

(b) confusion, convulsions and coma;

(c) bradycardia, hypotension and circulatory collapse.

Treat convulsions with i.v. lorazepam or diazepam, and circulatory collapse by commencing cardio-pulmonary resuscitation (see p. 2).

(4) *Exploration, irrigation, debridement and haemostasis*

(i) Look carefully for evidence of foreign bodies, and severed tendons, vessels or nerves within the wound. Seek immediate senior A&E help if the latter are found.

(ii) Irrigate the wound using a 20-ml syringe filled with saline and fitted with a 23 gauge blue needle to provide a high-pressure jet. Use several syringefuls.

(iii) Excise any dead or contaminated tissue and remove local dirt on the skin by rubbing gently. It is particularly important to remove all ingrained gravel and grit to avoid permanent tattooing of the skin. A general anaesthetic may be required.

(iv) Achieve haemostasis by local pressure. Avoid the use of mosquito forceps to clamp a bleeding area, which may cause further local tissue damage.

(5) *Suture*

    (i)   The aim is to appose the edges of the wound without tension using interrupted sutures, starting in the middle of the wound and halving the remaining distance each time. Use an absorbable suture for deeper wounds such as chromic catgut or polyglactin to close the deep space first, with the knot buried at the depth of the wound.

    (ii)   The choice of material depends on local custom.

        (a)   Traditionally, silk was the most popular, although as it is braided and of animal origin, it is more likely to cause micro-abscess formation with subsequent scarring.

        (b)   Synthetic monofilament sutures such as polyamide (Ethilon) and polypropylene (Prolene) are now preferred. These are harder to tie, requiring an initial double throw and multiple knots, but elicit less of a foreign-body reaction.

    (iii)   Use the smallest practicable suture size.

        (a)   Limb laceration: use 4/0 synthetic mono-filament sutures removed at 7–10 days.

        (b)   Scalp: use 2/0 or 3/0 synthetic monofilament sutures removed at 7 days.

        (c)   Face: use 5/0 or 6/0 synthetic monofilament sutures removed at 4 days.

    (iv)   Cover the wound with a non-adherent dressing, and advise the patient to keep the area dry for at least 24 h.

    (v)   Arrange an appointment for removal of sutures in the department or with the GP.

    (vi)   Make a record in the notes of the size and nature of the wound, the deep structures involved, and the number of sutures used to close it.

(6) *Tetanus prophylaxis*

    (i)   Meticulous wound toilet is an essential part of tetanus prophylaxis, rather than simply relying on tetanus immunisation or antibiotics.

(ii) In the UK, routine tetanus immunisation was introduced in 1961, so the elderly are now the most likely to be non-immune.

(iii) Virtually any wound can become contaminated, however trivial.

(iv) Treat patients according to their immune status (see Table 5) and to the type of wound:

  (a) *Tetanus-prone wound.* Any wound that is deep, contused or penetrating, contains foreign bodies especially wood splinters, a compound fracture, a partial- or full-thickness burn, clinical evidence of pyrogenic infection and any superficial wound obviously contaminated with soil, dust or horse manure, especially if topical disinfection is delayed more than 6 h.

  (b) *Clean minor wound.* Any wound that is clean, incised or superficial, i.e. does not fulfil any criteria of a tetanus-prone wound.

(v) Local pain, redness and swelling occur with tetanus toxoid; occasionally systemic reactions, even

Table 5. Tetanus prophylaxis

Immune status category	Treatment	
	Tetanus-prone wound	Clean minor wound
Complete course of toxoid[a] or a booster[b] in last 10 years:	Nothing	Nothing
Complete course of toxoid or a booster over 10 years ago:	Toxoid booster. HTIG[c]	Toxoid booster
Never completed a course, or state of immunity unknown:	Complete course of toxoid. HTIG[c]	Complete course of toxoid

[a]A complete course of toxoid is a total of three injections of 0.5 ml adsorbed tetanus toxoid i.m. given on day 1, at 4 weeks and at 2 months.
[b]A booster is a subsequent injection of 0.5 ml adsorbed tetanus toxoid i.m.
[c]HTIG is 250 U of human tetanus immunoglobulin given i.m. at a different site to the toxoid, increased to 500 U if over 24 h have elapsed or there is heavy contamination.

anaphylaxis, occur. These reactions are much less common with tetanus immunoglobulin.

(vi) Tetanus itself is rare, with around 20 cases reported annually in the UK, but it is a frequent cause of death in parts of Asia, Africa and South America.

    (a) Incubation time from injury to first symptoms ranges from 4 to 21 days (usually about 7 days).

    (b) The commonest symptoms are jaw stiffness (trismus), dysphagia, and abdominal and back pain. Hypertonia is found on examination.

    (c) Localised or generalised painful spasms follow within 24–72 h, becoming more severe and prolonged from minimal stimuli.

    (d) Death may occur from laryngospasm, respiratory failure or autonomic dysfunction, therefore immediate admission to intensive care is mandatory.

(7) *Antibiotics.* Antibiotics should not be used indiscriminately, and are secondary to thorough surgical toilet in preventing infection. They are reserved for:

    (i) *Cellulitis*

        (a) This is usually due to a beta-haemolytic streptococcus or occasionally *Staphylococcus aureus*. Always send a swab first.

        (b) Give penicillin V 500 mg orally q.d.s. or flucloxacillin 500 mg orally q.d.s. for 1 week.

    (ii) *Dirty, contaminated wound.* Give flucloxacillin 2 g i.v., gentamicin 5 mg/kg i.v. and metronidazole 500 mg i.v.

    (iii) *Bites*

        (a) Clean with copious normal saline irrigation. Do not suture, except on the face.

        (b) Give tetanus prophylaxis.

        (c) Prescribe according to the origin of the bite:

          – Human: amoxicillin 500 mg and clavulanic acid 125 mg (Augmentin 625 mg) one tablet orally t.d.s. for 5 days. If penicillin sensitive, use doxycycline. Use erythromycin

if pregnant or breastfeeding, and in children.
- Cat: amoxicillin 500 mg orally t.d.s. for 3 days.
- Dog: treat as above for cat. Consider rabies prophylaxis if the patient was bitten abroad. Discuss this with experts at the local infectious diseases unit.

(iv) *Compound fractures*
   (a) Give flucloxacillin 2 g i.v. or cefuroxime 750 mg i.v.
   (b) Remember tetanus prophylaxis.

CRUSH INJURIES

DIAGNOSIS

(1) Crush injuries may be caused by a roller or wringer injury, a direct blow, or a vehicle wheel passing over a limb.
(2) Severe soft-tissue injury can occur with little apparent initial evidence.
(3) Test for tendon, nerve or vessel damage. Note loss of skin blanching on digital pressure, indicating shearing of capillaries, which may subsequently lead to extensive tissue necrosis.
(4) *Compartment syndrome.* Always consider the possibility of a compartment syndrome if there is marked ischaemic pain particularly on passive stretching of muscles, associated with paraesthesia and loss of motor and sensory nerve function.
   (i) Apart from crush injuries, other causes of compartment syndrome include external compression from a tight plaster, fractures, constricting burns, bleeding, vigorous exercise and prolonged local pressure in coma, e.g. following acute poisoning.
   (ii) The entire area within the closed fascial compartment feels tense.
   (iii) However, arterial pulses and even skin perfusion may initially remain deceptively normal.
(5) X-ray is required to exclude underlying fractures.

MANAGEMENT

(1) Refer all crush injuries of a limb, hand or foot to the orthopaedic team for elevation, treatment of shock, possible fasciotomy and occasionally amputation.

(2) Otherwise, in isolated finger or toe injuries, clean and debride the wound without suturing, elevate the limb, and give the patient analgesics. Review within 3 days for consideration of delayed primary suture.

PUNCTURE INJURIES

DIAGNOSIS

(1) This type of injury is caused by treading on a nail or pin, penetration of a sewing-machine needle, or through industrial accidents including those involving high-pressure guns for grease, paint, water or oil.

(2) 'Sharps injuries' within a hospital are covered on p. 113.

MANAGEMENT

(1) Refer all high-pressure gun injuries immediately to the orthopaedic team, even if no apparent damage is seen initially.

(2) Otherwise, clean the wound with antiseptic, give tetanus prophylaxis, and consider the need for antibiotics. A rusty nail injury to the foot requires amoxicillin 500 mg and clavulanic acid 125 mg (Augmentin 625 mg) one tablet orally t.d.s. for 5 days.

(3) Instruct the patient to return immediately if signs of infection or gross oedema supervene.

HAND INFECTIONS

(1) *Paronychia*
    (i)   This is pus formation adjacent to the nail, with throbbing pain.
    (ii)   Make a longitudinal incision parallel to the nail edge across the nail fold to release the pus under

a ring-block anaesthetic (see p. 258). Mop out the cavity with pledgets of cotton wool.

(iii)   Dress the finger with paraffin-impregnated gauze tucked into the cavity, and apply a plain viscose stockinette tubular bandage (Tubegauz) without tension. Use a high-arm sling for 24 h, and review the dressing after 2 days.

(2) *Pulp space infection*

(i)   This is pus formation in the distal fat pad of the finger.

(ii)   Using a ring block, make a central longitudinal incision over the middle of the abscess (take care not to cross the flexion crease of the distal interphalangeal joint). Mop out the cavity of all pus.

(iii)   Dress and review as for paronychia.

(iv)   In more extensive infections with swelling approaching the distal interphalangeal joint, the flexor tendon sheath is in danger. Refer the patient directly to the orthopaedic team, after an X-ray to exclude osteomyelitis.

(3) *Suppurative tenosynovitis of the flexor tendons*

(i)   The original wound may have been forgotten, but intense pain, swelling and tenderness develop along the line of the flexor tendon, with severe pain on passive finger flexion.

(ii)   Refer the patient directly to the orthopaedic team.

(4) *Deep palmar and web space infections*

(i)   These cause pain, swelling and loss of function with localised tenderness and the development of a 'flipper' hand, from pronounced swelling of the dorsum of the hand.

(ii)   Refer the patient directly to the orthopaedic team.

IN-GROWING TOENAILS

(1) These are common, and are associated with tight-fitting footwear or socks, poor foot hygiene and trimming off the corners of the nail. They usually afflict young people.

(2) Surgical treatment by wedge resection or total nail-bed ablation requires skill and expertise, and is only as successful as the experience of the surgeon.

(3) *Medical treatment*

    (i)   Liquid nitrogen spray cryotherapy requires special equipment that is usually not readily available.

    (ii) An alternative is to insert a pledget of cotton wool under the nail edge with a pair of forceps, and to cauterise the granulation tissue with a silver nitrate stick.

        (a)   Advise the patient to wear loose shoes and of the importance of cutting the nail straight across in future.

        (b)   Ask the patient to repeat the cotton-wool insertion and silver nitrate cautery once or twice a day at home.

        (c)   This method is effective, cheap and requires no special apparatus.[2]

BACK PAIN

This is a common problem that may be considered under four headings:

(1) direct trauma
(2) indirect trauma
(3) non-traumatic – severe or atypical pain
(4) non-traumatic – mild to moderate pain.

DIRECT TRAUMA

Back pain due to direct trauma is managed according to the principles in the appropriate chapter on multiple injuries (see p. 162).

INDIRECT TRAUMA

DIAGNOSIS

(1) Acute, severe back pain may be precipitated by bending, lifting, straining, coughing or sneezing.

(2) There is intense muscle spasm, or even complete immobility. The normal lumbar lordosis is lost, with development of a scoliosis.

(3) Examine for signs of nerve-root irritation and compression from an acute prolapsed disc.

   (i)   Diminished straight-leg raising (SLR). Remember that the ability to sit up in bed with the legs straight is equivalent to an SLR of 90° both sides.

   (ii) Motor loss occurring in the following myotomes:
      (a) L1, L2: hip flexion (iliopsoas)
      (b) S1: hip extension (gluteus maximus)
      (c) L5: knee flexion (hamstrings)
      (d) L3, L4: knee extension (quadriceps)
      (e) L5: ankle dorsiflexion (extensor hallucis longus)
      (f) S1: ankle plantar flexion (calf muscles).

   (iii) Reflex loss:
      (a) L3, L4: knee jerk
      (b) L5, S1: ankle jerk.

   (iv) Sensory loss occurring in the following dermatomes:
      (a) L3: medial lower thigh and knee
      (b) L4: medial side of calf
      (c) L5: lateral side of calf
      (d) S1: lateral border of the foot and sole.

(4) Examine in particular for signs of a central disc prolapse causing cauda equina compression:
   (i)   difficulty emptying the bladder or bowels;
   (ii) lax anal sphincter tone;
   (iii) saddle area anaesthesia over dermatomes S2, S3, S4 and S5;
   (iv) weakness in both legs.

MANAGEMENT

(1) Refer immediately to the orthopaedic team any patient with a central disc prolapse causing cauda equina compression.

(2) Also, if the patient is completely unable to move or has signs of nerve-root compression, refer to the orthopaedic team for admission.

(3) Patients with moderate pain and without nerve-root signs may be discharged.

  (i)   Give the patient a nonsteroidal anti-inflammatory analgesic such as diclofenac (Voltarol) 50 mg orally t.d.s.

  (ii) Encourage early return to ordinary activities within the limits of the pain. Bedrest should be kept to a minimum.[3]

  (iii) Request review and follow-up by the GP for back care education, including posture, exercise and lifting.

NON-TRAUMATIC – SEVERE OR ATYPICAL PAIN

DIAGNOSIS

(1) The causes vary according to the patient's age.

  (i)   *Under 30 years*
      (a) ankylosing spondylitis
      (b) rheumatoid arthritis
      (c) osteomyelitis
      (d) discitis
      (e) extradural abscess.

  (ii) *Over 30 years*
      (a) bony metastases
      (b) myeloma
      (c) lymphoma
      (d) renal or pancreatic disease
      (e) aortic aneurysm.

  (iii) *Over 60 years*
      (a) as (ii) above
      (b) osteoporosis
      (c) Paget's disease
      (d) osteoarthritis
      (e) spinal stenosis.

(2) Enquire about previous back trouble, joint trouble, unremitting symptoms, fever, weight loss, abdominal symptoms and urinary tract symptoms.

(3) Perform a full examination, including abdominal, rectal, neurological and breast examinations, and a urinalysis.

(4) X-ray the chest and thoracic and lumbosacral spine.

MANAGEMENT

Refer the patient to the appropriate specialist team according to the suspected aetiology.

NON-TRAUMATIC – MILD TO MODERATE PAIN

DIAGNOSIS AND MANAGEMENT

(1) This nebulous group with no abnormal physical signs, apyrexial with a normal urinalysis may be allowed home.

(2) Prescribe a nonsteroidal anti-inflammatory analgesic such as diclofenac (Voltarol) 50 mg orally t.d.s.

(3) Give patients a letter for their GP to follow them up and to arrange physiotherapy, an exercise regime and behaviour modification as appropriate.

REFERENCES

1 Stiell IG, McKnight RD, Greenberg GH, *et al*. Implementation of the Ottawa ankle rules. *JAMA* 1994;271:827–32.

2 Senapati A. Conservative outpatient management of ingrowing toenails. *J R Soc Med* 1986;79:339–40.

3 Malmivaara A, Häkkinen U, Aro T, *et al*. The treatment of acute low back pain – bed rest, exercises, or ordinary activity? *N Engl J Med* 1995;332:351–5.

PAEDIATRIC EMERGENCIES

Children account for one-quarter to one-third of all patients seen in the A&E department. The total number of attendances is approximately double the number attending paediatric outpatients.

NORMAL VALUES

It is impossible to know what is abnormal and to identify sick patients until the doctor recognises the normal child.

(1) *Weight and height*
- (i)   If the age is known, a simple formula for weight between age 1 and 10 years is: weight in kilograms = 2 (age in years + 4).
- (ii) Figure 11 enables an approximate weight to be derived from the age or length in centimetres (see p. 273).
- (iii) Table 6 gives some normal values for weight and height.

(2) *Drug dosages*
- (i)   Drugs should ideally be given on a per-kilogram basis after weighing the child and consulting a drug formulary.
- (ii) Figure 11 is a paediatric resuscitation chart giving all commonly used emergency drugs in millilitres according to the age, weight or body length (see p. 273).

(3) *Heart rate and blood pressure*
- (i)   A formula for the normal blood pressure is: systolic BP in mm Hg =80 + 2 (age in years). Diastolic BP =2/3 systolic BP.
- (ii) Table 7 gives some normal values for the heart rate in the awake, active child and the blood pressure using a paediatric-sized cuff (over 80% the length of the upper arm).

(4) *Circulatory blood volume*
- (i)   A formula for the normal circulatory blood volume is: 80–85 ml/kg body weight.

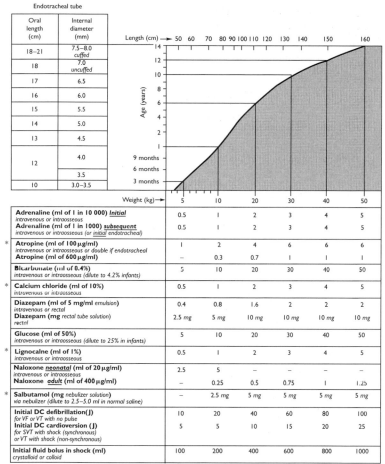

Endotracheal tube

Oral length (cm)	Internal diameter (mm)
18–21	7.5–8.0 cuffed
18	7.0 uncuffed
17	6.5
16	6.0
15	5.5
14	5.0
13	4.5
12	4.0
	3.5
10	3.0–3.5

Length (cm) → 50 60 70 80 90 100 110 120 130 140 150 160

Age (years): 14 12 10 8 6 4 2 1
9 months
6 months
3 months

Weight (kg) → 5 10 20 30 40 50

	5	10	20	30	40	50
Adrenaline (ml of 1 in 10 000) *Initial* intravenous or intraosseous	0.5	1	2	3	4	5
Adrenaline (ml of 1 in 1000) *subsequent* intravenous or intraosseous (or *initial* endotracheal)	0.5	1	2	3	4	5
* **Atropine (ml of 100 μg/ml)** intravenous or intraosseous or double if endotracheal	1	2	4	6	6	6
Atropine (ml of 600 μg/ml)	–	0.3	0.7	1	1	1
Bicarbonate (ml of 0.4%) intravenous or intraosseous (dilute to 4.2% infants)	5	10	20	30	40	50
* **Calcium chloride (ml of 10%)** intravenous or intraosseous	0.5	1	2	3	4	5
Diazepam (ml of 5 mg/ml emulsion) intravenous or rectal	0.4	0.8	1.6	2	2	2
Diazepam (mg rectal tube solution) rectal	2.5 mg	5 mg	10 mg	10 mg	10 mg	10 mg
Glucose (ml of 50%) intravenous or intraosseous (dilute to 25% in infants)	5	10	20	30	40	50
* **Lignocaine (ml of 1%)** intravenous or intraosseous	0.5	1	2	3	4	5
Naloxone *neonatal* **(ml of 20 μg/ml)** intravenous or intraosseous	2.5	5	–	–	–	–
Naloxone *adult* **(ml of 400 μg/ml)**	–	0.25	0.5	0.75	1	1.25
* **Salbutamol (mg nebulizer solution)** via nebulizer (dilute to 2.5–5.0 ml in normal saline)	–	2.5 mg	5 mg	5 mg	5 mg	5 mg
Initial DC defibrillation(J) for VF or VT with no pulse	10	20	40	60	80	100
Initial DC cardioversion (J) for SVT with shock (synchronous) or VT with shock (non-synchronous)	5	5	10	15	20	25
Initial fluid bolus in shock (ml) crystalloid or colloid	100	200	400	600	800	1000

* **CAUTION!** *Non-standard drug concentrations may be available:*
Use **atropine** *100 μg/ml or prepare by diluting 1 mg to 10 ml or 600 μg to 6 ml in normal saline.*
Note that 1 ml of calcium chloride 10% is equivalent to 3 ml of calcium gluconate 10%
Use **lignocaine** *(without adrenaline) 1% or give twice the volume of 0.5%. Give half the volume of 2% or dilute appropriately.*
Salbutamol may also be given by slow intravenous injection (5 μg/kg). but beware of the different concentrations available (e.g.50 and 500 μg/ml).

Fig. 11. Paediatric Resuscitation Chart. Drug doses, endotracheal tube sizes and defibrillator settings are read off the chart according to the age, weight or body length, whichever is known. (Reproduced by kind permission of the *British Medical Journal*.)

Table 6. Normal values for weight and height

Age (years)	Male		Female	
	Weight (kg)	*Height (cm)*	*Weight (kg)*	*Height (cm)*
Birth–1	3.5–10.3	50–75	3.4–9.6	50–74
2–5	12.5–19	85–107	12–18.5	84–106
5–12	19–38	107–147	18.5–40	106–149
14–16	49–60	160–172	51–56	160–162

Table 7. Normal values for heart rate and systolic blood pressure

Age (years)	Heart rate (beats/min)	Systolic BP (mm Hg)
<1	110–160	70–90
2–5	95–140	80–100
5–12	80–120	90–110
>12	60–100	100–120

Table 8. Normal values for circulatory blood volume

Age (years)	Circulatory blood volume (ml)
Birth–1	300–800
2–5	990–1390
5–12	1390–2700
14–16	3500–4000

- (ii) Table 8 gives some normal values for the circulatory blood volume.
- (iii) Shock therapy requires infusion of 20 ml/kg crystalloid or colloid.
- (iv) Aim for urine output of 2 ml/kg/h in infants and 1 ml/kg/h in children during therapy.
- (5) *Maintenance fluid requirements*
  - (i) Give 4% dextrose 1/5 normal saline, or 3.75% dextrose 1/4 normal saline.
  - (ii) Table 9 gives normal maintenance fluid requirements per kilogram.

Table 9. Normal maintenance fluid requirements

Weight (kg)	Requirement	
	Per hour	*Per day*
3–10	4 ml/kg	100 ml/kg
11–20	40 ml + (2 ml/kg > 10 kg)	1000 ml + (50 ml/kg > 10 kg)
>20	60 ml + (1 ml/kg > 20 kg)	1500 ml + (25 ml/kg > 20 kg)

Table 10. Normal values for respiratory rate

Age (years)	Respiratory rate (breaths/min)
<1	30–40
2–5	25–30
5–12	20–25
>12	15–20

(6) *Respiratory rate*
    (i)   Table 10 gives the normal respiratory rate/min.
    (ii)   Tidal volume is 5–7 ml/kg.
(7) *Developmental milestones*
    (i)   *6 months*
        (a)   sits erect with support
        (b)   localises sound 45 cm away
        (c)   alert and interested, friendly with strangers.
    (ii)   *1 year*
        (a)   crawls on all-fours
        (b)   understands simple commands, and babbles incessantly
        (c)   cooperates with dressing.
    (iii) *2 years*
        (a)   runs and manages stairs
        (b)   joins words in simple phrases
        (c)   dry by day.
    (iv) *3 years*
        (a)   can stand on one foot momentarily
        (b)   speaks in sentences
        (c)   dry by night.

(v)   *5 years*
      (a)   skips, hops and stands on one foot with ease
      (b)   fluent speech
      (c)   dresses and washes unaided.

GENERAL ASSESSMENT

(1) The examination commences from the first moment the child is seen, while the parent or child is giving the history or the child alone is talking.

(2) Even infants and children unable to talk will give non-verbal cues about pain, such as facial expressions and posture.

(3) Most emergencies generate fear in children, causing additional distress to the child and adding to parental anxiety.
     (i)   Always explain things as clearly as possible, in such a way that the child can understand.
     (ii)   Allow parents to stay with the child at all times.

(4) A complete examination of every child should include:
     (i)   height, weight and head circumference measurements plotted on a percentile chart;
     (ii)   an oral or rectal temperature (<2 years);
     (iii) examination of the eardrums, mouth, throat (not if epiglottitis suspected) and the skin;
     (iv)   examination of a urine sample for sugar, protein and organisms, in all cases of fever, abdominal pain, vomiting and drowsiness.

(5) Always refer the following potentially serious problems to the paediatric team, even if you yourself are unable to reach a definite diagnosis (see also under the management of a child with fever, p. 296):
     (i)   the quiet, pale child
     (ii)   the drowsy or floppy child
     (iii) the thin, malnourished child
     (iv)   the persistently crying child
     (v)   the child with difficulty breathing
     (vi)   the child with stridor
     (vii) the child under 3 years with temperature above 39°C

(viii) the baby that has stopped feeding
(ix)   the baby with repeated vomiting, especially if it is bile-stained
(x)   the baby with frank blood mixed with the stools.

CARDIOPULMONARY RESUSCITATION

DIAGNOSIS

(1) Cardiac arrest in children is usually the end result of hypoxia, hypovolaemia and acidosis. Bradycardia progressing to asystole is almost invariable.

(2) The causes include:
   (i)   hypoxia from respiratory failure due to severe asthma, bronchiolitis, poisoning, near-drowning, or upper airway obstruction from epiglottitis, inhaled foreign body, etc.;
   (ii) hypovolaemia due to haemorrhage, gastroenteritis, burns, etc.;
   (iii) septicaemia, anaphylaxis;
   (iv) sudden infant death syndrome.

(3) Ventricular fibrillation is uncommon but may occur in the following situations:
   (i)   congenital heart disease
   (ii) poisoning, especially tricyclic antidepressant ingestion
   (iii) hypothermia
   (iv) myocarditis, cardiomyopathy and hereditary prolongation of the QT interval.

MANAGEMENT

Similar principles and practice apply as for adult resuscitation (see p. 2). See Table 11 for advanced paediatric life support.[1] Significant points of detail to note include:

(1) *Assisted ventilation*
   (i)   In the event of a blocked airway from an inhaled foreign body, hold an infant or small child prone and deliver up to five blows over the back,

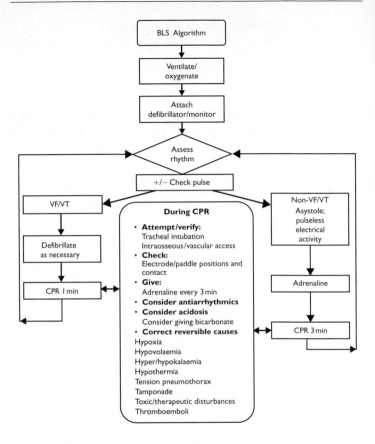

Table 11. Algorithm for paediatric cardiorespiratory arrest. (Reproduced by kind permission of *Resuscitation*).[1]

between the scapulae, followed by up to five chest thrusts. In an older child, perform the Heimlich manoeuvre (see p. 34).

(ii) Bag-and-mask ventilation is preferable to inexperienced attempts at intubation, which should be left to an airway skilled doctor.

    (a) Insert an oropharyngeal (Guedel) airway measured from the centre of the mouth to the angle of the jaw when laid on the child's face. If it is too long, it will damage the naso-pharynx, and if it is too short it will push the tongue back. An airway is unnecessary in small babies.

(b) Position the head in a neutral position in infants under 1 year, as overextension of the head may actually occlude their airway.

(c) Use a face mask that fits closely over the nose and mouth. Soft circular plastic masks are ideal.

(d) Attach a hand-ventilating device. The Laerdal Infant ventilating bag has a volume of 240 ml suitable for children up to 2 years attached to an oxygen flow rate of at least 4 l/min. The Laerdal Child ventilating bag has a volume of 500 ml suitable for children up to 10 years.

(e) Inflate the chest at a faster rate than adults, up to 20 breaths/min.

(iii) An endotracheal tube and both straight and curved-blade laryngoscopes should be made ready for the airway doctor, and the tube cut to size (see Table 12).

(a) A rough guide to internal diameter tube size is: endotracheal tube size in millimetres = (age in years/4) + 4.

Table 12. Correct size of orotracheal tube

Age	Internal diameter (mm)	Length (cm)
Birth	3.0	9
4 months	3.5	10
1 year	4.0	12
3 years	5.0	13
7 years	6.0	16
10 years	6.5	17
12 years	7.0 (+ cuff)	18
14 years	7.5 (+ cuff)	21
16 years	8.0 (+ cuff)	22
Adult	9.0 (+ cuff)	23

      (b) A rough guide to oral tube length is: oral endotracheal tube length in centimetres = (age in years/2) + 12.

      (c) A rough guide to nasal tube length is: nasal endotracheal tube length in centimetres = (age in years/2) + 15.

(2) *External cardiac massage*

    (i) In infants, use two fingers over the lower third of the sternum, depressing at a rate of at least 100/min.

    (ii) In a child, use one hand at a rate of 100/min.

(3) *Venous access*

    (i) A 20 or 22 gauge cannula is adequate, inserted into the most familiar site, such as the antecubital fossa.

    (ii) Connect this to an infusion of normal saline via a paediatric giving set slowed to a minimal rate, unless hypovolaemia is suspected, in which case an initial fluid bolus of 20 ml/kg is given rapidly.

    (iii) Other sites for venous access include the back of the hand, the external jugular, and the internal jugular vein if the doctor is suitably skilled.

    (iv) If venous access is not gained within 90 s or three attempts, perform intraosseous (bone marrow) vascular access:

      (a) This may be used up to the age of 6 years.

      (b) Use a specially designed intraosseous needle inserted into the anteromedial surface of the proximal tibia, 1–2 cm distal to the tuberosity.

      (c) Advance the needle with a gentle twisting or boring motion until it gives on entering the marrow cavity, and remove the stylet.

      (d) Aspirate blood and marrow contents to confirm correct placement, then connect an i.v. infusion giving set.

(4) *Drug administration*

    (i) If venous or intraosseous access are difficult, remember that adrenaline, atropine and lignocaine may be given via the endotracheal tube diluted in 1–2 ml (infants) or 2–5 ml (small child) normal saline:

(a) Adrenaline endotracheal dose is 10 times the initial i.v. dose, i.e. 100 µg/kg.

(b) Atropine or lignocaine dose is twice the i.v. dose, i.e. 40 µg/kg and 2 mg/kg, respectively.

(ii) Recommended drug doses are:

Drug	Intravenous or intraosseous dosage
Atropine (0.6 mg/ml)	20 µg or 0.03 ml/kg
Adrenaline (1 in 10 000)	10 µg or 0.1 ml/kg
	100 µg or 1 ml/kg (second and subsequent doses)
Bicarbonate (8.4%)	1 mmol or 1.0 ml/kg
Calcium chloride (10%)	0.2 ml/kg
Lignocaine 2% (100 mg/5 ml)	1 mg or 0.05 ml/kg
Fluid (in hypovolaemia)	20 ml/kg
Dextrose 10% (hypoglycaemia)	5 ml/kg
Dextrose 25% (hypoglycaemia)	2 ml/kg

(iii) Figure 11 is a paediatric resuscitation chart with all the drug doses calculated (see p. 273).

(5) *Defibrillation.* Ventricular fibrillation is rare but has a better prognosis than asystole.

(i) Use paediatric paddles for children under 10 kg:

(a) these are 4.5 cm in diameter;

(b) if unavailable, use adult paddles placed on the infant's back and over the left lower front of chest.

(ii) Start at 2 J/kg for the first two shocks.

(iii) Give 4 J/kg for third and subsequent shocks.

(6) *Heat loss.* Remember that in infants and small children, considerable heat loss may occur. Organise overhead heating, an incubator, warming blankets and plastic sheets to cover exposed parts of the body.

(7) *When to stop.* The senior A&E or paediatric doctor will decide at which point further attempts are futile. They will also be responsible for the distressing duty of telling the parents, who may have been present and watching.

COT DEATH (SUDDEN INFANT DEATH SYNDROME)

The cause of this syndrome is unknown, although the incidence is falling. It is more common in winter, with a peak age of 3 months. Higher rates are seen with bottle-fed males, parental smoking, and prone sleeping position.

MANAGEMENT

(1) If the child is brought in by ambulance with resuscitation in progress, always continue in the resuscitation room. Call the senior A&E doctor and paediatric team urgently (see cardiopulmonary resuscitation, p. 277).

(2) Examine the child carefully for any signs of trauma or infection, including evidence of asphyxia or petechiae. Check the temperature.

(3) Discuss the necessity for post-mortem blood tests for infection or a drug screen with the senior doctor. In addition, keep all clothes in a labelled hospital bag.

(4) Check that the parents are allowed full access to the resuscitation area, providing a senior A&E staff member is able to be with them at all times.

(5) The senior doctor should then speak in private to the parents, and encourage them to talk about the circumstances of the death and any recent illnesses in the child.

(6) Encourage the parents to see and hold their child in privacy afterwards. They may derive benefit from the presence of the hospital chaplain and social worker, and may like a photograph or a lock of the child's hair.

(7) The parents must also be told that because the death is sudden, the coroner (procurator fiscal in Scotland) will be informed, and a post mortem may be required.

(8) The coroner's officer or the police will then visit the parents later that day, and will take further details, possibly even removing the bedding for examination.

(9) Write down and give the parents the details and phone number of the Foundation for the Study of Infant Deaths. They may receive an information leaflet or arrange further

counselling and support if they wish: telephone (020) 7235 1721 (24-h helpline).

(10) The doctor should also inform by telephone:
  (i) the GP, to arrange for a home visit and to make certain all future clinic attendances for the deceased child are cancelled;
  (ii) the health visitor;
  (iii) the social work department;
  (iv) the paediatric team, if they were not present at the resuscitation;
  (v) the Community Child Health Service, to cancel immunisation appointments, etc.

CHILD ABUSE (NON-ACCIDENTAL INJURY)

Various forms are now recognised, including physical, sexual and emotional abuse, neglect and organised abuse.

DIAGNOSIS

Maintain a high index of suspicion in the following circumstances, especially in children under 4 years old:

(1) *History*
  (i) Delay between the alleged injury and the presentation to the A&E department.
  (ii) Inconsistency between the story and the actual injuries.
  (iii) Abnormal parental behaviour, poor interaction with the child, and apparent lack of parental concern.
  (iv) Frequent attendance in the A&E department by the child or a sibling, often for little apparent reason.
  (v) Previous injuries on different dates.
  (vi) Failure to thrive, or signs of neglect.

(2) *Examination*. The child must be undressed fully in stages to be examined completely, and all findings must be documented carefully. Measure bruises, scratches, burns and other skin marks with a ruler. Arrange clinical

photographs detailed in the medical notes to provide contemporaneous evidence. Look specifically for:

(i)   Torn upper-lip frenulum, or palatal haemorrhage from a feeding bottle or even a fist thrust into the mouth to prevent the baby crying, or from a direct blow.

(ii)   Human bite marks, and bruising from a fist or slapping, which may rupture the tympanic membrane.

(iii)   Deep cigarette burns, or scalds limited to the buttocks and genitalia or both feet, suggesting immersion in hot water.

(iv)   A fractured skull or long bone, particularly in a child not yet able to walk. A spiral fracture of a long bone is most suspicious, as are other healing fractures of differing ages on skeletal survey.

(v)   Subconjunctival, vitreous or retinal haemorrhage, suggesting violent shaking, or from a direct blow.

(vi)   Signs of sexual abuse to the genitalia or anus.

MANAGEMENT

(1) If you have any suspicion of child abuse, inform the senior A&E doctor and paediatric team immediately and arrange for admission of the child. Check whether the child is on the Child Protection Register already. Involve the A&E social worker.

(2) Do not confront the parents at this stage, but explain that you want a further opinion from a senior paediatric doctor.

(3) If the parent refuses admission, contact the social work department. If necessary, they can apply to a magistrate for an 8-day Emergency Protection Order, with the right of challenge for parents after 72 h.

(4) In an emergency, the police can act without requiring a magistrate's order to take a child into protection for up to 72 h (Police Protection Order).

Note: remember that osteogenesis imperfecta presents as multiple fractures, and idiopathic thrombocytopoenic purpura and leukaemia cause multiple bruising and bleeding.

However, these are rare compared with the genuine cases of child abuse.

THE BREATHLESS CHILD

The causes and management of stridor are dealt with in the next chapter. Important causes of a breathless child are:
(1) bronchiolitis
(2) bronchitis
(3) pneumonia
(4) asthma
(5) inhaled foreign body
(6) allergic and metabolic conditions.

BRONCHIOLITIS

DIAGNOSIS

(1) This condition occurs in seasonal epidemics, affecting babies under 1 year old, commonly due to the respiratory syncytial virus.
(2) It starts with fever and snuffles, but progresses rapidly to cough, irritability, fluid refusal, wheeze and marked tachypnoea.
(3) Expiratory rhonchi and fine crepitations are heard in the chest, which may appear hyperinflated. In severe cases, cyanosis develops with a raised respiratory rate and intercostal recession, or recurrent apnoeic episodes occur.

MANAGEMENT

(1) Give the child oxygen, attach a pulse oximeter, and admit under the paediatric team, particularly if there has been poor feeding, respiratory recession, cyanosis or apnoea.
(2) Request a portable CXR or X-ray on the way to the ward, with a nurse or doctor in attendance. Hyperinflation with small areas of atelectasis may be the only abnormalities seen.

BRONCHITIS

DIAGNOSIS AND MANAGEMENT

(1) This is either viral or bacterial, including atypical organisms such as mycoplasma, and may be the early feature of measles.
(2) It causes fever, cough and malaise.
(3) Refer the child to the paediatric team following a CXR.

PNEUMONIA

DIAGNOSIS AND MANAGEMENT

(1) Bronchopneumonia occurs in young children, or older children with chronic illness, e.g. cerebral palsy, and may be bacterial or viral. There is cough, fever and dyspnoea.
(2) Lobar pneumonia presents with sudden illness, fever, breathlessness and pleuritic chest pain.
(3) Staphylococcal pneumonia occurs in infants and in older children with cystic fibrosis, and presents with septicaemia, pneumothorax, empyema, etc.
(4) Remember that nonspecific presenting features of pneumonia include fever, lethargy, anorexia, abdominal pain and meningism.
(5) X-ray all the above cases and refer to the paediatric team for oxygen, fluids, antibiotics and nursing care.

ASTHMA

DIAGNOSIS

(1) Reversible airways obstruction in children is associated with infection (usually viral), allergy, atopy, exercise and emotion.
(2) It is one of the most common reasons for admission to hospital in childhood.
(3) Asthma presents with prolonged expiratory dyspnoea, wheezing and cough. A similar assessment as for adults is made, including a pulse, respiratory rate and peak flow before treatment (see p. 29).

(4) A severe attack is indicated by any one of the following:
- (i) too breathless to talk
- (ii) too breathless to feed
- (iii) respiratory rate of 50 or more breaths/min
- (iv) tachycardia 140 or more beats/min
- (v) peak expiratory flow rate 50% or less of predicted or best.

MANAGEMENT

(1) Sit the child up and give oxygen, ideally with the parent in attendance to reassure the child. Attach a pulse oximeter, aiming for an oxygen saturation above 92%.
(2) Give nebulised salbutamol 2.5–5 mg diluted to 5 ml with saline, or use multiple activations of a metered-dose inhaler with spacer device.
(3) Add ipratropium (Atrovent) 125–250 µg to the next nebuliser if the salbutamol is ineffective, and continue the nebulised salbutamol up to three doses at 20-min intervals or continuously initially, then hourly in severe cases.
(4) Refer all severe cases to the paediatric team.
- (i) Give prednisolone 1–2 mg/kg orally to a maximum of 40 mg.
- (ii) Perform CXR if the diagnosis is in doubt, infection is suspected, or there is sudden deterioration, to exclude a pneumothorax.

INHALED FOREIGN BODY

DIAGNOSIS AND MANAGEMENT

(1) This may present as upper airway obstruction with stridor or with sudden coughing and wheeze.
(2) If the object passes into the lower airways, all symptoms may disappear. Later, wheeze, infection or obstructive emphysema supervene, causing localised rhonchi, crepitations and breathlessness.
(3) Request a postero-anterior and lateral CXR. Although organic foreign bodies such as peanuts will not show, the secondary effects of compensatory hyperinflation on an

expiratory film, collapse and consolidation will gradually appear.
(4) Refer the child to the paediatric or ENT team.

ALLERGIC AND METABOLIC CONDITIONS

DIAGNOSIS AND MANAGEMENT

(1) Acute allergy to antibiotics or nuts, etc. may present as breathlessness and wheeze as part of angioneurotic oedema or an anaphylactic reaction.
   (i) Management is similar to that for adults (see p. 102).
   (ii) Give 1:1000 adrenaline 0.01 mg/kg (0.01 ml/kg) i.m. in severe cases.
(2) Diabetic ketoacidosis presents with deep, sighing respirations. Peritonitis presents with rapid, shallow breathing. The child will be severely ill and other features will alert the doctor to the underlying diagnosis.
(3) Finally, remember poisoning with salicylates, methanol, ethylene glycol, etc. may cause breathlessness.
(4) Refer all these patients immediately to the paediatric team.

STRIDOR

This is noise predominantly on inspiration originating from airway obstruction above the level of the larynx. There are three important causes:
(1) acute laryngotracheobronchitis or 'croup'
(2) epiglottitis
(3) inhaled foreign body.

ACUTE LARYNGOTRACHEOBRONCHITIS (CROUP)

DIAGNOSIS AND MANAGEMENT

(1) Croup usually occurs between the ages of 1 and 3 years due to a virus such as parainfluenza.

(2) Hoarseness, a barking cough and harsh inspiratory stridor develop, typically in the middle of the night, preceded by an upper respiratory tract infection.
(3) The child is irritable and tired, but lacks the drooling, dysphagia and toxic appearance of epiglottitis.
(4) Give nebulised 1:1000 adrenaline 0.5 ml/kg to a maximum of 5 ml (5 mg) with oxygen in severe cases, and call the senior A&E doctor and paediatric team[2].
(5) Commence steroids with prednisolone 1 mg/kg orally, dexamethasone 0.3–0.6 mg/kg orally or i.m., or nebulised budesonide 2 mg according to local policy.
(6) Admit all moderate or severe cases for observation, humidification and occasionally endotracheal intubation.

EPIGLOTTITIS

DIAGNOSIS

(1) This is a life-threatening illness with sudden onset of sore throat, dysphagia and difficulty in breathing usually due to *Haemophilus influenzae*, in unimmunised or HiB vaccine-failure children.
(2) The child looks severely ill and pale, and sits up leaning forwards and drooling. The voice is muffled and the stridor is softer than with croup.

MANAGEMENT

(1) Do not examine the child further. Do not request or perform a rectal temperature, BP or X-ray, and do not attempt to visualise the throat.
(2) Leave the child with the parent, sitting upright with an oxygen mask held near its face.
(3) Summon urgent senior A&E, paediatric, anaesthetic and ENT help, and warn ITU.
(4) Stay with the child until help arrives. If sudden respiratory arrest occurs, be prepared to attempt intubation with a small endotracheal tube and an introducer. If this fails, insert a large-bore i.v. cannula through the cricothyroid membrane as an emergency airway (see p. 34).

INHALED FOREIGN BODY

DIAGNOSIS

(1) There is sudden onset of cough, spluttering and choking noises, appropriate to the degree of airway obstruction. Hoarseness or aphonia may occur.

(2) The child may progress to complete airway obstruction or remain unchanged, or all the symptoms may disappear as the foreign body passes into the lower airways.

MANAGEMENT

(1) *Complete airway obstruction*
   (i)   Hold infants or small children head down and deliver up to five blows to the back between the shoulder blades, followed by up to five chest thrusts. In an older child, perform the Heimlich manoeuvre (see p. 34).
   (ii) If the above two fail, attempt removal of the impacted object using a laryngoscope and a pair of long-handled forceps, or proceed directly to emergency cricothyroid puncture (see p. 34).

(2) *Stable airway obstruction*
   (i)   Summon urgent anaesthetic and ENT help.
   (ii) Await their arrival before considering a lateral soft-tissue X-ray of the neck or a CXR.

(3) *Disappearance of the symptoms of obstruction*
   (i)   Consider the possibility that the foreign body has passed further into the lower airways.
   (ii)   Request a postero-anterior and lateral CXR if the object is radio-opaque.
   (iii) Otherwise, if the object is radiolucent, request an inspiratory and expiratory CXR. Look for compensatory hyperinflation on the expiratory film, or the development of collapse and consolidation.
   (iv)   Refer the child to the paediatric team if the history is convincing, even when the CXR appears normal.

ABDOMINAL PAIN, DIARRHOEA AND VOMITING

Abdominal pain may present acutely, or may become chronic and recurrent. Diarrhoea and vomiting are common problems that may both lead to dehydration.

ACUTE ABDOMINAL PAIN

DIAGNOSIS

(1) *History*
- (i)   Ask about the onset of the pain, the site, duration and previous similar episodes.
- (ii)   Enquire about associated vomiting or diarrhoea, and the time of the last bowel motion or the passage of flatus.
- (iii) Record any medication given or known allergy.
- (iv)   Children aged over 2 years should be able to indicate the site of their pain. In infants, pain may be inferred from spasms of crying, restlessness, drawing up of the knees and refusal to feed.

(2) *Examination*
- (i)   The whole child should be examined fully undressed to look for signs of a raised temperature, rash, upper respiratory tract infection, and localising signs in the abdomen, including inspection of the genitalia.
- (ii)   The urine must always be tested for sugar and, if urinary tract infection is suspected, should be sent for microscopy and culture. White cells may also be seen in the urine in pelvic peritonitis and appendicitis.
- (iii) Erect and supine abdominal films are requested for suspected intestinal obstruction.

(3) *Causes of acute abdominal pain.* These are best considered in two groups:

    (i)   Surgical:
        (a)   appendicitis
        (b)   Meckel's diverticulitis
        (c)   peritonitis
        (d)   intestinal obstruction, including intussusception and sigmoid volvulus
        (e)   strangulated inguinal hernia
        (f)   testicular torsion
        (g)   trauma, including child abuse.
    (ii)   Medical:
        (a)   mesenteric adenitis
        (b)   gastroenteritis
        (c)   urinary tract infection
        (d)   hepatitis
        (e)   Henoch–Schönlein purpura
        (f)   diabetic ketoacidosis
        (g)   pneumonia
        (h)   tonsillitis
        (i)   meningitis
        (j)   poisoning, such as lead.

MANAGEMENT

(1) Ideally, refer all cases to the senior A&E doctor or paediatric team.
(2) Significant features include pain for over 3 h, associated pyrexia and vomiting.
(3) If the child is allowed home, inform the GP by telephone and letter, and arrange for review of the child the next morning.

RECURRENT ABDOMINAL PAIN

DIAGNOSIS

(1) The vast majority of cases (over 90%) do not appear to have an organic cause, but remember the possibility of:
    (i)   urinary tract infection and hydronephrosis
    (ii)   inflammatory bowel disease
    (iii) recurrent volvulus

(iv)   peptic ulcer
(v)   constipation, including Hirschsprung's.
(2) Recurrent abdominal pain of childhood or 'periodic syn-drome' is the usual cause. A child with this condition may, however, present with a new acute organic illness at any time.

MANAGEMENT

(1) Examine the child fully as for an acute attack of abdom-inal pain. Discuss investigations with the senior A&E doctor.
(2) Refer the child back to the GP if nothing is found, or to the paediatric outpatient department.
(3) Instruct the parents to return with the child at the start of the next attack of abdominal pain.

DIARRHOEA, VOMITING AND DEHYDRATION

DIAGNOSIS

(1) Diarrhoea and vomiting are common problems that require investigation and treatment. Dehydration is a serious end result.
(2) *Causes of diarrhoea*
   (i)   Gastroenteritis: this is usually viral due to a rota-virus, but it can be due to *Escherichia coli*, *Salmonella* or campylobacter, etc.
   (ii)   Surgical conditions, such as appendicitis, peritonitis, or occasionally intussusception.
   (iii)   Drugs, e.g. ampicillin.
   (iv)   Other infections such as tonsillitis or otitis media.
   (v)   Malabsorption, ulcerative colitis, Crohn's disease.
   (vi)   Dietary indiscretion, including too much or too little food.
   (vii)   'Toddler diarrhoea'.
(3) *Causes of vomiting*
   (i)   Causes in the newborn:
      (a)   infection, including meningitis and urinary tract infection (UTI);

          (b)   intestinal obstruction from duodenal atresia, Hirschsprung's disease or a meconium plug;

          (c)   cerebral haemorrhage or oedema;

          (d)   metabolic, such as galactosaemia or congenital adrenal hyperplasia.

  (ii)   Causes in infants (up to 1 year):

          (a)   pyloric stenosis, typically in males aged 3–8 weeks;

          (b)   infections, including gastroenteritis, tonsillitis, otitis media, meningitis and UTI;

          (c)   intestinal obstruction from intussusception, or an obstructed hernia, etc.;

          (d)   gastro-oesophageal reflux and hiatus hernia;

          (e)   feeding problems due to overfeeding or excessive wind;

          (f)   poisoning.

  (iii)   Causes after infancy:

          (a)   infections – see point ii (b) above;

          (b)   intestinal obstruction or appendicitis;

          (c)   metabolic, such as ketoacidosis or uraemia;

          (d)   raised intracranial pressure;

          (e)   migraine or periodic syndrome;

          (f)   poisoning.

MANAGEMENT

(1) Take a careful history and examine for possible causes listed above. Refer any patient with suggestive features to the paediatric team for investigation.

(2) *Assessment of dehydration.* Regardless of the suspected cause, assess and treat dehydration in its own right.

    (i)   Mild dehydration (<5% body weight lost): the child is in good general condition, with dry mouth, thirst and mild oliguria.

    (ii)   Moderate dehydration (5–10% body weight lost): the child looks ill, is floppy and apathetic with sunken eyes and fontanelle, has a dry mouth, decreased skin tissue turgor, tachycardia, marked thirst and oliguria.

(iii)   Severe dehydration (10% or more body weight lost): the child is drowsy, cool, cyanosed, tachypnoeic, tachycardic, hypotense and may become comatose. There is a risk of sudden death.

Note: beware missing the diagnosis of dehydration in an overweight baby presenting with tachycardia alone.

(3) *Treatment of mild dehydration*

(i)   Stop all milk and solid food for 24 h but continue breastfeeding, supplemented by extra water or glucose-electrolyte solution between feeds.

(ii)   Use an oral glucose-electrolyte solution, e.g. Dioralyte or Rehidrat.

   (a)   Make up the sachet with water according to the instructions. In infants, give 1–1.5 times the volume of their usual feed.

   (b)   In older children, give 200 ml of solution after each loose motion, or enough to quench the thirst, given in frequent small amounts.

   (c)   Aim to replace the normal maintenance fluid requirement, plus an extra 20–50% fluid to cover continuing losses.

   (d)   Normal maintenance fluid requirement per hour according to the usual body weight is:

Up to 10 kg	4 ml/kg
10–20 kg	40 ml + (2 ml/kg for each kg over 10 kg)
Over 20 kg	60 ml + (1 ml/kg for each kg over 20 kg).

(iii)   After 24–48 h, begin graduated feeds with half-strength milk for a day in infants, and a bland diet gradually reintroducing solids in the older child.

(iv)   Give the parents a letter for the GP, and instruct them to return if the child's condition deteriorates.

(4) *Treatment of moderate or severe dehydration*

(i)   Send blood for U&E, blood sugar and FBC, and start an infusion of half-normal 0.45% saline in 2.5% dextrose. Give 20–25 ml/kg over 1–2 h while waiting for the electrolyte results. If the child is shocked, give 20 ml/kg of a plasma expander such as polygeline (Haemaccel) rapidly over 10–20 min, repeated as necessary to restore the circulation.

(ii) Further fluid management will depend on the blood results and degree of dehydration. In hyper-natraemic dehydration, give fluid and electrolyte replacement slowly over 2–3 days aiming to reduce serum sodium by no more than 5 mmol/day, to avoid precipitating cerebral oedema.

(iii) Refer the child to the paediatric team for immediate admission.

FEVER

The normal oral temperature is 37°C, and the normal rectal temperature is 37.5°C. A fever is defined as a rectal temperature above 38°C.

DIAGNOSIS

(1) Look for the following common causes of fever in a child:
  (i) upper and lower respiratory tract infection
  (ii) otitis media
  (iii) tonsillitis
  (iv) gastroenteritis
  (v) viral exanthema, even before the rash appears (see Table 13)
  (vi) urinary tract infection (UTI)
  (vii) appendicitis
  (viii) meningitis and septicaemia
  (ix) malaria, particularly if the child has been abroad to an endemic area in the previous 2 years.

(2) Serious bacterial infections including meningitis, septi-caemia, bone and joint infections, UTI, pneumonia and enteritis may all present with fever and no localising signs.

MANAGEMENT

(1) Refer the following febrile patients to the paediatric team:

Table 13. Common childhood exanthematous diseases

Disease	Incubation period (days)	Prodrome	Rash	Other features and infectivity
Chickenpox	10–20	None	Macules, papules, vesicles and pustules of differing ages	Infective until all vesicles are crusted over (usually 6 days after last crop)
Glandular fever	5–14	Fever, sore throat, malaise	Transient maculopapular (rare); itchy drug rash with ampicillin (common)	Palatal petechiae, cervical lymphadenopathy; hepatosplenomegaly; tonsillar exudate; infective for many months by close physical contact
Measles	9–14	3 days of cough, cold and conjunctivitis	Red, confluent, maculopapular lasts 7–11 days	Koplik's spots; cough predominates; may be quite ill; infective for 5 days after rash appears
Rubella	14–21	None	Pink, maculopapular discrete; lasts 3–5 days	Occipital and preauricular lymphadenopathy; infective until rash disappears
Scarlet fever	2–5	1–2 days sore throat, fever, vomiting	Minute, red, punctate papules lasts 7 days	Unwell; circumoral pallor; 'strawberry tongue'; infective until negative throat swabs following penicillin

(i)   Children aged under 6 months, particularly if they are drowsy or pale, have difficulty breathing or have taken less than half their normal feeds over 24 h or produced less than four wet nappies in 24 h.

(ii)   Children under 3 years who appear toxic, e.g. are lethargic, poorly perfused and hypoventilating or hyperventilating.

(iii)   Any signs of meningism, irritability, drowsiness or a history of seizure (see p. 300).

(iv)   An unexplained rash, particularly if petechial or purpuric.

(v)   Any signs of dehydration (see p. 294).

(vi)   Children with a temperature of 39°C or more.

(2) Discuss the role of urinalysis, WCC, CXR and empirical oral or parenteral antibiotics in children under 3 years with fever without source with the senior A&E doctor or paediatric team[3].

(3) If there is no obvious cause for the fever, and the child looks well and does not fulfil any of the above criteria, advise the parents to adopt symptomatic measures including:

(i)   regular fluid intake – 'little but often';

(ii)   minimal clothing;

(iii)   paracetamol elixir at a dose of 15 mg/kg 4-hourly. Paracetamol suspension is available in various strengths, including 120 mg paracetamol/5 ml or 250 mg paracetamol/5 ml.

(4) Always write a letter to the GP listing your findings, even if they were negative, and arrange for the child to be seen again within 24–48 h.

FITS AND FEBRILE CONVULSIONS

FITS

Fits must be distinguished from other causes of brief loss of consciousness, such as syncope, pallid breath-holding, and cyanotic breath-holding.

DIAGNOSIS

Consider the likely cause of the fit according to the age of the child.

(1) *Newborn*. Seizures tend to be mere twitching of a limb, fluttering of an eyelid or conjugate eye deviation. Causes include:
- (i) hypoglycaemia
- (ii) hypocalcaemia
- (iii) hypoxia, especially from birth injury
- (iv) cerebral haemorrhage and subdural haematoma
- (v) infection
- (vi) drug withdrawal.

(2) *Preschool child*. The commonest cause is a febrile convulsion. Other possibilities include:
- (i) idiopathic epilepsy
- (ii) sudden reduction in epilepsy medication
- (iii) meningitis or encephalitis
- (iv) head injury, including injury from child abuse
- (v) dehydration from gastroenteritis, etc.
- (vi) hypoglycaemia
- (vii) poisoning.

(3) *Older child*. Causes include:
- (i) idiopathic epilepsy
- (ii) sudden reduction in epilepsy medication
- (iii) head injury
- (iv) meningitis or encephalitis
- (v) hypoglycaemia
- (vi) poisoning, including lead, iron and tricyclic antidepressants.

MANAGEMENT

(1) Clear the airway, place the child on their side, and give oxygen via a face mask.

(2) Check for hypoglycaemia using a Glucostix. If the reading is low, give 5 ml/kg of 10% dextrose i.v. having saved 10 ml serum for subsequent laboratory investigation.

(3) Record the rectal temperature. If it is raised, tepid sponge the child and use a fan.

(4) If the child fits again or is still fitting:

(i)　　Gain i.v. access and give lorazepam 0.1 mg/kg i.v. or give diazepam (Diazemuls) 0.1–0.2 mg/kg i.v. at 1 mg/min up to a maximum of 0.5 mg/kg.

(ii)　　Follow this with phenytoin 18 mg/kg i.v. at no faster than 1 mg/kg/min for recurrent fits, providing the child is not on oral phenytoin.

　　(a)　If already on oral phenytoin, give phenobarbitone 15–20 mg/kg i.v. slowly instead.

　　(b)　Both drugs must be given with ECG monitoring.

(iii)　　If i.v. access is impossible, give rectal diazepam 0.5 mg/kg. Use the parenteral diazepam solution (Valium) given via a syringe with a short, plastic catheter.

(iv)　　An alternative if venous access is still unavailable is paraldehyde: give 0.4 ml/kg rectally diluted 1:1 with olive oil or normal saline.

(5) Refer all children with a fit to the paediatric team.

FEBRILE CONVULSIONS

These are the most common cause of fits in preschool children.

DIAGNOSIS

(1) Features that favour the diagnosis of febrile convulsion are:

(i)　　age between 6 months and 5 years;

(ii)　　the child is unwell before the fit, with a rising temperature;

(iii)　　a generalised, non-focal fit that lasts under 10 min;

(iv)　　a fit that does not recur (except a few hours after the first), and that does not leave any focal neurological signs, or residual weakness such as a Todd's palsy.

(2) If there are features different from the above, do not label the episode a febrile convulsion.

MANAGEMENT

(1) Undress the child, tepid-sponge and use a fan.

THE LIMPING CHILD

DIFFERENTIAL DIAGNOSIS

(1) Exclude trivial local causes such as a painful shoe, verruca, foreign body in the foot or groin lymphadenopathy.
(2) Hip pain is referred to the knee and vice versa, so always examine both.
(3) Typical causes according to age are:
    (i) *Age 0–5 years*
        (a) congenital dislocation of the hip
        (b) transient synovitis 'irritable hip'.
    (ii) *Age 5–10 years:* Perthes' disease.
    (iii) *Age 10–15 years:* slipped upper femoral epiphysis.
    (iv) *Any age*
        (a) trauma
        (b) osteomyelitis, septic arthritis (including TB)
        (c) Still's disease and leukaemia.

MANAGEMENT

(1) X-ray all these children and refer to the orthopaedic team if the limp is confirmed and an innocent local cause is not found.
(2) Arrange an ultrasound scan to demonstrate any hip effusion, which, if positive, may be followed by aspiration under anaesthesia to exclude a septic arthritis.

REFERENCES

1   Paediatric Life Support Working Group. European Resuscitation Council guidelines 2000 for advanced paediatric life support. *Resuscitation* 2001;48:231–4.
2   Advanced Life Support Group. *Advanced Paediatric Life Support*, 3rd edn. BMJ Books, London; 2001.
3   Baraff LJ. Management of fever without source in infants and children. *Ann Emerg Med* 2000;36:602–14.

ENT EMERGENCIES

TRAUMATIC CONDITIONS OF THE EAR

SUBPERICHONDRIAL HAEMATOMA

DIAGNOSIS

(1) Blunt trauma to the ear causes bleeding between the peri-chondrium and auricular cartilage, known as a subperi-chondrial haematoma.

(2) If untreated, this will lead to a 'cauliflower ear' deformity from proliferative fibrosis.

MANAGEMENT

(1) Aspirate small clots under local anaesthesia, and apply firm pressure by packing around the interstices of the ear with cotton wool under a turban dressing. Refer the patient to the next ENT clinic, since the bleeding may recur.

(2) Protect against perichondritis with flucloxacillin 500 mg orally q.d.s. for 5 days.

(3) Refer the patient with a large and extensive bleed directly to the ENT team for immediate drainage through multiple small incisions.

WOUNDS OF THE AURICLE

MANAGEMENT

(1) Perform minimal debridement of devitalised tissue under local anaesthesia.

(2) Refer the patient to the ENT team or plastic surgeons if there are extensive lacerations or skin loss leaving exposed cartilage.

(3) Otherwise, appose the edges of the cartilage with 5/0 chromic catgut or polyglactin (Vicryl) through the peri-chondrium.

(4) Suture the skin with 6/0 synthetic monofilament and apply a firm dressing. Remove the sutures after 7 days.

(5) Protect against perichondritis with flucloxacillin 500 mg orally q.d.s. for 5 days, and give tetanus prophylaxis.

FOREIGN BODY IN THE EXTERNAL EAR

DIAGNOSIS AND MANAGEMENT

(1) A foreign body in the external ear causes pain, deafness and discharge if left.
(2) If the foreign body is superficial, attempt gentle removal with a loop or wax hook.
(3) Do not attempt any further manoeuvres if the object is not freed instantly, or if the patient is uncooperative, as the object may be pushed further in and the eardrum damaged.
   (i)   Refer the patient to the next ENT clinic.

PERFORATED EARDRUM

DIAGNOSIS

(1) The eardrum may be perforated by direct injury from a sharp object, such as a hairpin, or indirectly by pressure from a slap, blast injury, scuba diving, or from a fracture of the base of the skull (see below).
(2) There is pain, conductive deafness and sometimes bleeding.
(3) If there is tinnitus, vertigo or complete hearing loss, suspect inner ear involvement.

MANAGEMENT

(1) Refer the patient immediately to the ENT team if inner ear damage is suspected.
(2) Otherwise, do not put anything into the ear or attempt to clean it out. Advise the patient to keep water out of the ear canal.
(3) Give an antibiotic such as amoxicillin 500 mg orally t.d.s., and refer the patient to the next ENT clinic.

BASAL SKULL FRACTURE

Most basal skull fractures (see also p. 170) involve the temporal bone. Fractures may be divided into tympanic bone fracture, longitudinal fractures and transverse fractures.

DIAGNOSIS

(1) The temporal bone forms the glenoid fossa of the temporomandibular joint, and is damaged if the mandibular condyle is driven upwards into the middle ear or external auditory canal, causing bleeding or laceration of the canal.

(2) Alternatively, a longitudinal fracture of the temporal bone will tear the eardrum and cause dislocation of the ossicular chain, with conductive deafness, haemotympanum and cerebrospinal fluid leakage. Occasionally, delayed facial nerve damage is seen.

(3) A transverse fracture of the temporal bone results in complete sensorineural deafness associated with tinnitus, nystagmus and vertigo. Facial nerve palsy is more common than with longitudinal fractures.

MANAGEMENT

(1) Do not insert an auriscope to examine obvious bleeding from the external auditory meatus, as infection may be introduced.

(2) Remember that basal skull fracture is a clinical diagnosis. X-rays may have to wait until the patient is stable on the ward and other injuries to the head, neck and chest have been assessed fully.

   (i)   Request an immediate CT scan if the patient has been stabilised.

   (ii) Intracranial air or a fluid level in the sphenoid sinus on lateral skull X-ray are suggestive of fracture when CT is unavailable.

(3) Admit the patient under the surgical team for head injury care and advice from the neurosurgical unit or ENT specialist.

NON-TRAUMATIC CONDITIONS OF THE EAR

All these conditions present with pain and/or hearing loss.

OTITIS EXTERNA

DIAGNOSIS

(1) A bacterial or fungal infection is usually responsible, often following exposure to water 'swimmer's ear'.
(2) There is pain, desquamation of skin, and a thin, offensive discharge that may become frankly purulent.

MANAGEMENT

(1) Perform aural toilet using a cotton wick to gently remove the debris.
(2) Give the patient a proprietary anti-infective and steroid preparation, e.g. 1% clioquinol with 0.02% flumethasone (Locorten-Vioform) three drops b.d. to the external auditory canal.
(3) Refer the patient to the ENT clinic for follow-up.
(4) If the otitis externa is severe with occlusion of the canal, refer the patient directly to the ENT team.

FURUNCULOSIS OF THE EXTERNAL EAR

DIAGNOSIS

(1) A furuncle may develop in the outer part of the external auditory canal causing extreme pain.
(2) Movement of the pinna and introduction of a speculum exacerbate the pain. Deafness is minimal.

MANAGEMENT

(1) Insert a wick soaked in 10% ichthammol in glycerine to encourage discharge of the pus, start flucloxacillin 500 mg orally q.d.s. and give an analgesic such as

paracetamol 500 mg and codeine phosphate 8 mg (co-codamol 8/500) two tablets orally q.d.s.
(2) Test the urine for sugar, and refer the patient to the ENT clinic for follow-up.

ACUTE OTITIS MEDIA

DIAGNOSIS

(1) This is common in children, due to viral or bacterial infection, such as pneumococcus or *Haemophilus influenzae* (in children under 6 years).
(2) There is intense earache, conductive deafness, fever and, on examining the eardrum in the early stages, there is loss of the light reflex and injected vessels are seen around the malleus.
(3) As the infection progresses, a bulging, immobile drum is seen, which may perforate, discharging pus.

MANAGEMENT

(1) In the early stages, give amoxicillin 250–500 mg orally t.d.s. for 5 days and an analgesic such as paracetamol elixir 15 mg/kg 4-hourly.
(2) Give erythromycin 500 mg orally q.d.s for 5 days if the patient is allergic to penicillin.

MASTOIDITIS

DIAGNOSIS AND MANAGEMENT

(1) There is extension of infection from acute otitis media into the mastoid air-cell system.
(2) The patient is ill and feverish, with tenderness over the mastoid, and the pinna is pushed down and forwards.
(3) Refer the patient immediately to the ENT team for X-ray, CT scan and parenteral antibiotics.
(4) Complications include cranial nerve palsy, meningitis and subperiosteal abscess.

VERTIGO

DIAGNOSIS

(1) Two main groups occur:
   (i)   *Central vertigo*. This is due to lesions in the CNS, such as a vertebrobasilar transient ischaemic attack (TIA), cerebellar or brainstem stroke, cerebral tumour, demyelination, vertebrobasilar migraine, or drug toxicity.
   (ii) *Peripheral vertigo*. This is due to lesions in the vestibular nerve and inner ear, such as vestibular neuronitis, Ménière's disease, benign paroxysmal positional vertigo, acoustic neuroma, otosclerosis, cholesteatoma or ototoxic drugs.
(2) Central vertigo is usually dominated by associated neurological signs, whereas peripheral vertigo causes nystagmus, deafness, nausea, vomiting and sweating.

MANAGEMENT

(1) Incapacitating vertigo may be controlled symptomatically by diazepam (Diazemuls) 5–10 mg i.v. or prochlorperazine (Stemetil) 12.5 mg i.m.
(2) Refer patients with central causes of vertigo to the medical team, and patients with peripheral causes of vertigo to the ENT team.

FACIAL NERVE PALSY

DIAGNOSIS

(1) *Upper motor neurone paralysis*
   (i)   There is weakness of the lower facial muscles, often associated with other neurological signs such as hemiplegia.
   (ii) The cause is usually a stroke.
(2) *Lower motor neurone paralysis*
   (i)   There is weakness of the whole side of the face, including the forehead muscles.

    (ii)   Causes include:
- (a) Bell's palsy with an abrupt onset sometimes associated with postauricular pain, hyperacusis and abnormal taste;
- (b) trauma to the temporal bone or a facial laceration in the parotid area;
- (c) tumours, such as an acoustic neuroma or parotid malignancy;
- (d) infection, such as acute otitis media, chronic otitis media with cholesteatoma or geniculate herpes zoster, the Ramsay Hunt syndrome;
- (e) miscellaneous, including Guillain–Barre syndrome, sarcoidosis, diabetes.

(3) Examination must therefore include assessment of the external auditory canal, eardrum, parotid region and a full neurological examination.

MANAGEMENT

(1) Refer all acute cases with associated signs immediately to the medical, surgical or ENT team according to the likely aetiology.

(2) Give prednisolone 50 mg orally daily to a patient with Bell's palsy if seen within 2 days of onset, hypromellose artificial tears, eye padded or taped closed at night, and refer to the next ENT clinic.

TRAUMATIC CONDITIONS OF THE NOSE

FRACTURED NOSE

DIAGNOSIS

(1) This injury is usually obvious following a direct blow, causing swelling, deformity and epistaxis.

(2) Exclude a more serious facial bone fracture, e.g. with cerebrospinal rhinorrhoea from cribiform plate damage (see p. 170).

(3) Look carefully for a septal haematoma, which will lead to necrosis of the nasal cartilage and septal collapse if it

is not drained. The nasal passage is blocked by a dull-red swelling replacing the septum, associated with marked nasal obstruction.

MANAGEMENT

(1) Refer a grossly deformed or compound fracture, and any patient with a septal haematoma, to the ENT team. Refer more serious facial bone fractures to the maxillo-facial surgery team.
(2) Otherwise, refer the patient to the ENT clinic within the next 5–10 days if operative treatment to straighten the nose for cosmetic reasons is requested.
(3) Do not take an X-ray as this will not alter the clinical management.

FOREIGN BODY IN THE NOSE

DIAGNOSIS AND MANAGEMENT

(1) This may be quite asymptomatic, or it may lead to a serosanguinous, offensive, unilateral nasal discharge.
(2) If the object is easily accessible in the anterior part of the nose, attempt removal with a bent hook or pair of forceps after the patient has vigorously blown the nose.
(3) However (as with the foreign body in the ear), if removal is difficult, or a child is uncooperative, refer immediately to the ENT team. Sudden posterior dislodgement with inhalation of the foreign body is a real danger.

NON-TRAUMATIC CONDITIONS OF THE NOSE

EPISTAXIS

DIAGNOSIS

(1) This is usually spontaneous in children, occurring from vessels in Little's area on the anterior part of the septum,

possibly precipitated by rhinitis or minor trauma (e.g. picking).

(2) In adults, the bleeding occurs posterior to Little's area and may be associated with hypertension or a bleeding diathesis, including anticoagulant drugs.

(3) In the elderly, bleeding occurs high in the posterior part of the nose from arteriosclerotic vessels, and leads rapidly to haemorrhagic shock if profuse.

MANAGEMENT

(1) *Bleeding from Little's area*

    (i)   Pinch the anterior part of the nose for 10 min with the patient sitting forward until the bleeding stops. Forbid the patient to pick, blow or sniff through the nose to prevent recurrence of the epistaxis.

    (ii)   If a bleeding point persists, identify it with suction or by swabbing, and anaesthetise the area with a cotton-wool pledget soaked in 4% lignocaine with adrenaline or in 5% cocaine (see below for maximum recommended dosage).

    (iii) Cauterise the bleeding point with a silver nitrate stick touched onto the area for 10 s. Avoid over-zealous application or cauterising both sides of the septum, as this will lead to septal necrosis.

(2) *Persistent anterior bleeding and failed cautery*

    (i)   *Anterior nasal pack*

        (a) Cover the patient and yourself with protective drapes, and wear a face mask and goggles.

        (b) Apply local anaesthetic with cotton-wool pledgets soaked in either 4% lignocaine with adrenaline (maximum dose 12 ml or approximately 500 mg lignocaine in a 65-kg patient, i.e. 7 mg/kg) or 5% cocaine (maximum dose 2 ml or 100 mg in a 65-kg patient, i.e. 1.5 mg/kg).

        (c) Use 2 cm Vaseline gauze or a calcium alginate (Kaltostat) 2-g pack.

(d) Insert successive layers horizontally along the floor of the nose using Tilley's nasal dressing forceps.

(e) Remember in the adult that the nose extends 6.5–7.5 cm backwards to the posterior choanae (see Fig. 12).

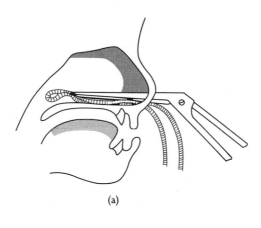

(a)

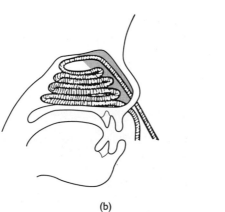

(b)

Fig. 12. (a) Anterior nasal packing, introducing the first loop along the floor of the nose and building upwards. (b) The pack in place.

(ii) *Anterior nasal tamponade.* Alternatively, use a balloon catheter or nasal tampon, both of which are much easier to insert.

(iii) Refer the patient to the ENT team for admission and removal of the pack within 48 h.

(3) *Severe posterior bleeding*

(i) Send blood for FBC, clotting study and G&S. Establish an i.v. infusion before the patient becomes hypotensive, and restore the circulation.

(ii) Attempt to stem posterior nasal bleeding by inserting a Foley urethral catheter far back along the floor of the nose, inflate the retaining balloon with air, and pull the catheter forwards to occlude the back of the nose. Tape the catheter to the cheek to prevent it slipping backwards.

(a) Insert an anterior nasal pack as described previously.

(b) Occasionally, both sides of the nose require packing to stop the bleeding.

(iii) Refer the patient immediately to the ENT team for admission.

TRAUMATIC CONDITIONS OF THE THROAT

See Neck injuries: airway injury on p. 146.

NON-TRAUMATIC CONDITIONS OF THE THROAT

TONSILLITIS

DIAGNOSIS AND MANAGEMENT

(1) This is either viral or bacterial, usually due to the beta-haemolytic streptococcus.

(2) There is sore throat, dysphagia, fever and fetor. A febrile convulsion may be precipitated in a child under 5 years old.

(3) Clinically, it is impossible to distinguish a viral from a bacterial cause, as glandular fever may present with a grey, exudative tonsillitis.

(4) Give the patient penicillin V 250–500 mg orally q.d.s. for 10 days and an antipyretic analgesic such as paracetamol. Return the patient to their GP.

PERITONSILLAR ABSCESS (QUINSY)

DIAGNOSIS AND MANAGEMENT

(1) This may follow tonsillitis and is more common in adults.

(2) There is a worsening of the illness, with high temperature, muffled voice, dysphagia, referred earache and trismus.

(3) Examination shows unilateral swelling of the soft palate, with displacement of the tonsil downwards and medially, and deviation of the uvula to the unaffected side.

(4) If difficulty in breathing supervenes, particularly in children, consider whether this could be epiglottitis and manage accordingly (see p. 289).

(5) Give benzylpenicillin 1.2 g i.v. q.d.s. and metronidazole 500 mg i.v. 12-hourly. Refer the patient immediately to the ENT team for operative drainage.

FOREIGN BODY IN THE PHARYNX

DIAGNOSIS

(1) Fish or meat bones are the most common objects to cause symptoms.

(2) Usually, a fish bone will impact in the tonsil, base of the tongue, or posterior pharyngeal wall, and may be seen by depressing the tongue to visualise the tonsil, or using a laryngeal mirror to see the back of the tongue and posterior pharynx.

(3) If no bone is seen despite symptoms, request a lateral soft-tissue X-ray of the neck. Calcification of superimposed

hyoid, thyroid, cricoid and laryngeal cartilages may cause confusion.

MANAGEMENT

(1) Attempt to remove the fish bone from the tonsil or the back of the tongue using Tilley's curved forceps.
   - (i)   If this fails in a patient with pain or salivating excessively, refer the patient immediately to the ENT team.
   - (ii) Alternatively, the pharyngeal mucosa may only have been scratched. If symptoms are minimal, prescribe an antibiotic such as amoxicillin 500 mg orally t.d.s., and ask the patient to return in 24 h for review.
(2) Refer other patients immediately to the ENT team for oesophagoscopy if oesophageal impaction with dysphagia, excessive salivation, local tenderness or retrosternal pain is suspected (see below).

SWALLOWED FOREIGN BODY

DIAGNOSIS

(1) Coins are the most common objects swallowed by pre-school children, although small children swallow almost anything, and the elderly may swallow their dentures.
(2) Oesophageal impaction, usually around the cricopharyngeus at the level of C6, is suggested by dysphagia, excessive salivation, local tenderness or retrosternal pain, but may be totally asymptomatic[1].
(3) Button batteries pose a particular risk, as they may cause local mucosal pressure necrosis or corrosive effects.
(4) Occasionally, airway obstruction occurs from upper oesophageal impaction, or the object may in fact have been inhaled rather than swallowed (see p. 290).

MANAGEMENT

(1) Request X-rays of the neck and chest to look for oesophageal impaction.

(i) Include postero-anterior (PA) and lateral views both to avoid missing a radio-opaque object super-imposed over the skeletal or cardiac shadows on the PA view, and to differentiate tracheal lodgement.

(ii) An abdominal X-ray is indicated only for button-battery ingestion, or for symptoms such as abdominal pain, distension or gastrointestinal bleeding.

(2) Refer the following patients immediately to the ENT team:

(i) airway obstruction or foreign body inhalation;

(ii) oesophageal impaction suspected clinically;

(iii) oesophageal lodgement seen on X-ray or inferred from prevertebral soft-tissue swelling, soft-tissue gas or air in the upper oesophagus;

(iv) button battery seen in the oesophagus or stomach.

(3) Otherwise, if the patient is asymptomatic, and neck and chest X-rays are normal, allow the patient home.

(i) Reassure the parents that most objects will pass spontaneously.

(ii) Request immediate review if symptoms develop.

(iii) Consider a repeat abdominal X-ray after 4 days in button-battery ingestion if it has not been passed in the stools.

(iv) Otherwise, repeat X-rays are required only if the patient develops symptoms.

STRIDOR

See p. 288 in the paediatric section.

REFERENCE

1 Mackway-Jones K. Towards evidence based emergency medicine: best BETS from the Manchester Royal Infirmary. Signs and symptoms of oesophageal coins. *J Accid Emerg Med* 2000;17:126–7.

OPHTHALMIC EMERGENCIES

Ophthalmic emergencies may be conveniently grouped into traumatic or non-traumatic, then subdivided further according to whether the eye is red, painful or has diminished visual acuity.

VISUAL ACUITY

(1) Visual acuity must always be recorded, with distance glasses if they are worn, at the start of every eye examination before any drops or dyes have been introduced.
   (i)   Acuity is measured by reading a Snellen chart at a distance of 6 m.
   (ii) Each eye is tested separately, and the lowest line that can be read accurately is recorded. Normal vision is 6/6.
(2) Ask patients with refractive errors who have left their glasses at home to look through a pinhole to optimise their visual acuity.

TOPICAL OPHTHALMIC PREPARATIONS

The following preparations are indicated when referred to in the text:
(1) Antibiotic drops: 0.5% chloramphenicol solution, 2 drops 2–3-hourly.
(2) Antibiotic ointment: 1% chloramphenicol ointment, one application to the lower lid conjunctival sac 4-hourly, or at night (if eye drops are used during the day).
(3) Local anaesthetic: 1% amethocaine solution or 0.4% oxybuprocaine solution, 1 or more drops as required.
   (i)   The patient must then wear a protective eye pad for 1–2 h until corneal sensitivity returns.
   (ii) Never give a course of drops or allow the patient to take them home.

(4) Fluorescein corneal stain: fluorescein sodium strips, or 2% fluorescein solution (do not use with soft contact lenses).

(5) Short-acting mydriatic dilating drops to examine the fundus: 1% tropicamide, 2 drops repeated after 15 min if necessary (do not use in patients with narrow anterior chambers, to avoid precipitating glaucoma).

(6) Miotic to constrict the pupil or reverse a mydriatic: 2% pilocarpine 1 or 2 drops.

Note: steroid preparations should not be used except by an experienced ophthalmologist. Any condition diagnosed that needs treatment with steroid drops also requires an ophthalmic opinion first.[1]

TRAUMATIC CONDITIONS OF THE EYE

PERIORBITAL HAEMATOMA (BLACK EYE)

DIAGNOSIS AND MANAGEMENT

(1) This is caused by a direct blow. If bilateral, suspect local trauma to the nose or a basal skull fracture (see p. 170).

(2) Always perform a thorough step-wise assessment:

   (i) Check that the patient can see, if necessary by opening the eyelids manually. Test visual acuity using distance glasses if they are worn, or a pin-hole aperture if they are unavailable.

   (ii) Check the eyeball for damage. Examine the cornea for abrasions, the anterior chamber for hyphaema, and the pupil size and reactions. Also check for the presence of a red reflex through the pupil and a normal fundus.

   (iii) Refer any abnormal findings suggestive of one of the above complications immediately to the oph-thalmology team.

   (iv) Test that the eye movements are full and the eyeball is not tethered, suggesting a 'blow-out' fracture of the orbital floor (see p. 346).

    (v)   Palpate to see whether the bony margin of the orbit is intact.

(3) If a 'blow-out' or a malar fracture is suspected, request appropriate facial X-rays and refer the patient to the maxillofacial surgery team.

(4) Otherwise, give the patient an analgesic such as paracetamol 500 mg and codeine phosphate 8 mg (co-codamol 8/500), and chloramphenicol eye ointment if the eye is shut.

(5) Review the patient within 48 h when the swelling has decreased to confirm the absence of significant ocular damage.

SUBCONJUNCTIVAL HAEMATOMA

DIAGNOSIS AND MANAGEMENT

Two types are recognised – spontaneous and traumatic.

(1) *Spontaneous*

    (i)   This may arise from coughing or from atherosclerotic vessels, particularly in the elderly, and is occasionally associated with hypertension or a bleeding diathesis.

    (ii)   Measure the BP and reassure the patient that the blood will disperse within 2 weeks. No treatment is needed.

(2) *Traumatic*

    (i)   This may be due to a surface conjunctival foreign body, a penetrating foreign body, or a scleral perforation. Gentle digital assessment may reveal reduced eyeball tone in penetration of the globe.

    (ii)   Refer all patients immediately to the ophthalmology team with one of the suspected serious causes listed above.

    (iii)   If the posterior margin cannot be seen, this suggests a basal skull fracture. Refer this patient to the surgical team (see p. 170).

    (iv)   Otherwise most cases are minor and require reassurance only.

EYELID LACERATION

DIAGNOSIS AND MANAGEMENT

(1) If the laceration involves the tarsal plate, upper eyelid, lid margin or the medial canthus and the lacrimal apparatus, refer the patient directly to the ophthalmology or plastic surgery team.

(2) Otherwise, suture the eyelid under local anaesthesia using fine 6/0 synthetic monofilament sutures, removed after 4 days.

EYELID BURN

DIAGNOSIS AND MANAGEMENT

(1) The eye must be examined carefully for evidence of corneal or scleral damage before oedema makes the examination impossible, although the blink reflex usually protects the globe.

(2) Give the patient antibiotic drops, analgesia and tetanus prophylaxis, and refer immediately to the ophthalmology team.

CHEMICAL BURNS TO THE EYE

DIAGNOSIS AND MANAGEMENT

(1) Alkalis are far more dangerous than acids, and include common agents such as cement, plaster powder, and oven and drain cleaners.

(2) The mainstay of treatment is immediate, copious, prolonged irrigation with normal saline from an i.v. giving set. Local anaesthetic drops will be needed to initially open the eye.

(3) Take care to irrigate all corners of the eye and to evert the upper eyelids to remove any particulate matter and to irrigate the superior fornix of the conjunctiva.

(4) Refer the patient immediately to the ophthalmology team, unless fluorescein staining reveals no corneal damage and the surrounding conjunctiva appears normal and is pain free.

(5) Provide adequate analgesia if necessary with morphine 5 mg i.v. plus an antiemetic such as metoclopramide 10 mg i.v.

CONJUNCTIVAL FOREIGN BODY

DIAGNOSIS AND MANAGEMENT

(1) Usually a piece of grit blows into the eye, causing pain, redness and watering.

(2) The object is seen easily by direct vision, and is removed with a moistened cotton-wool bud after instilling local anaesthetic. An eye pad is then worn for 1–2 h until the return of normal sensation.

(3) If the object impacts on the upper subtarsal conjunctiva, nothing will be seen immediately but the eye will be red and painful to blink. Fluorescein staining will reveal multiple linear corneal abrasions.

(4) Evert the upper eyelid.
    (i)   Stand behind the patient to evert the upper lid, supporting the head against your body.
    (ii)   Instruct the patient to look downwards, pull the upper lid eyelashes down and then up and over the tarsal plate, which is held depressed by a glass rod or orange stick (see Fig. 13).
    (iii) Remove the foreign body with a moistened cotton-wool bud.

(5) Always stain the cornea with fluorescein for evidence of corneal abrasion. If this is present, give the patient antibiotic drops for 2 days.

(6) Remember the possibility of intraocular penetration, e.g. by a metal fragment (see p. 329).

CORNEAL FOREIGN BODY

DIAGNOSIS AND MANAGEMENT

(1) The foreign body may be obvious, or may be revealed by fluorescein staining.

(2) Instil local anaesthetic drops and attempt removal of the foreign body with a moistened cotton-wool bud or the edge of a hypodermic needle, introduced from the side.

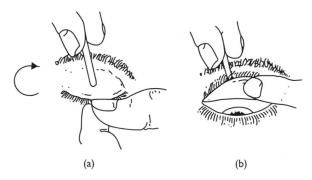

Fig. 13. (a) Eversion of the upper eyelid; (b) demonstrating the subtarsal conjunctiva.

(3) However, deep or recalcitrant foreign bodies, and those with extensive rust rings, should be left alone. Refer the patient to the ophthalmology team to avoid causing further damage during attempted removal.

(4) If local anaesthetic was used, pad the eye for 1–2 h until the return of normal sensation. Treat any residual corneal epithelial defect demonstrated with fluorescein as for a corneal abrasion (see below).

(5) Review the patient within 2 days to exclude infection. If there is evidence of an infected corneal ulcer, refer the patient immediately to the ophthalmology team.

CORNEAL ABRASION

DIAGNOSIS AND MANAGEMENT

(1) Corneal abrasion is due to a foreign body or to direct injury from a finger, stick or a piece of paper.

(2) There is intense pain, watering and blepharospasm. Local anaesthetic drops may be needed before the eye can be opened properly.

(3) Fluorescein staining will reveal the damage. Give the patient 0.5% chloramphenicol eye drops and mydriatic drops, and review within 2 days. An eye pad is no longer recommended, other than for 1–2 h following local anaesthetic use.[2]

(4) The cornea should be fully healed by then, but if there is delayed healing or a recurrence, refer the patient to the ophthalmology team.

FLASH BURN (ARC EYE)

DIAGNOSIS AND MANAGEMENT

(1) A superficial keratitis that occurs after exposure to ultraviolet light, from welding without using protective goggles, or from a sun lamp.
(2) There is pain, watering and blepharospasm occurring after a few hours. Fluorescein staining reveals a pitted corneal surface.
(3) Instil local anaesthetic drops and mydriatic drops, and double-pad the eyes until the return of normal sensation and the blepharospasm settles. Give an analgesic such as paracetamol 500 mg and codeine phosphate 8 mg (co-codamol 8/500).
(4) Recovery occurs within 12–24 h.

BLUNT TRAUMA TO THE EYE

DIAGNOSIS AND MANAGEMENT

(1) Injury to the eye should always be considered in any trauma to the face. It must not be forgotten when other injuries appear more dramatic, or periorbital oedema obscures the eye.
(2) Blunt trauma may cause a sequence of injuries from the front to the back of the eye:
    (i) periorbital haematoma or subconjunctival haemorrhage;
    (ii) corneal abrasion or laceration;
    (iii) bleeding into the anterior chamber, called hyphaema. This may be microscopic or macroscopic with formation of a fluid level;
    (iv) a fixed pupil or torn iris, known as traumatic mydriasis and iridodialysis, respectively;
    (v) a dislocated lens or subsequent traumatic cataract;

(vi)   vitreous haemorrhage, causing a dull or absent red reflex and obscuring the fundus;

(vii) a retinal tear, with retinal detachment seen as a dark, wrinkled, ballooned area diametrically opposite any resultant visual field defect;

(viii) retinal oedema (commotio retinae) seen as whitish areas of oedema, usually associated with haemorrhage;

(ix)   optic nerve damage, causing blindness with no direct pupillary response to light;

(x)   ruptured globe, with marked visual loss, a soft eye and shallow anterior chamber;

(xi)   retrobulbar haematoma, with pain, proptosis and a fixed, dilated pupil.

(xii) orbital fracture, usually a 'blow-out' fracture of the orbital floor (see p. 346).

(3) All these conditions require immediate examination by the ophthalmology team. The patient must not be allowed home in the meantime, but should lie quietly semi-upright pending expert assessment.

(i)   Ideally, pad both eyes and give appropriate analgesia.

(ii) Protect a suspected ruptured globe with an eye shield, not a pad.

PENETRATING TRAUMA TO THE EYE

DIAGNOSIS AND MANAGEMENT

(1) Penetrating trauma is usually obvious, although on occasions it may be difficult to recognise initially.

(2) The following injuries are possible:

(i)   Corneal laceration, often with prolapse of the iris into the defect.

(ii) Scleral perforation with chemosis or local haemorrhage. This must be differentiated from a trivial subconjunctival bleed.

(iii) Collapse of the anterior chamber, hyphaema or vitreous haemorrhage, pupil irregularity and lens dislocation.

(3) *Intraocular foreign body*

    (i)   This is usually a metal fragment from using a hammer and chisel, metal drill or grinding wheel.

    (ii)   Sudden sharp pain is followed by localised redness, or the outside of the eye may appear normal and the incident forgotten.

    (iii) Examine carefully for a puncture wound, and use an ophthalmoscope to inspect the inner eye, although a traumatic cataract may preclude this.

    (iv) Always X-ray the orbit in all suspected cases if there is the remotest possibility of penetration. Two soft-tissue films, with the eye looking up and down, should identify a radiodense intraocular foreign body.

(4) Instil antibiotic eye drops (not ointment), protect the eye from further damage with an eye shield, and give tetanus prophylaxis.

    (i)   Provide analgesia if required, e.g. morphine 5 mg i.v. with an antiemetic such as metoclopramide 10 mg i.v.

    (ii)   Give gentamicin 5 mg/kg i.v. plus cefotaxime 1 g i.v.

(5) Refer all cases of documented penetrating injury to the eye and actual or suspected intraocular foreign bodies immediately to the ophthalmology team.

CONDITIONS AFFECTING THE EYELIDS

BLEPHARITIS

DIAGNOSIS AND MANAGEMENT

(1) Blepharitis is an infection of the eyelid margin, causing red, itchy, crusted lids, which may become chronic with an allergic element. Styes and chalazions are commonly associated.

(2) Prescribe antibiotic ointment, but refer the patient to the ophthalmology clinic for follow-up if this condition becomes persistent or recurrent.

EXTERNAL STYE (HORDEOLUM)

DIAGNOSIS AND MANAGEMENT

(1) This is due to an infection of a lash follicle pointing on the lid margin.
(2) Give the patient antibiotic ointment and remove any protruding eyelash. Warm bathing may help.

INTERNAL STYE

DIAGNOSIS AND MANAGEMENT

(1) This is an infected Meibomian gland within the tarsal plate. It does not discharge as easily as an external stye, and it may leave a residual Meibomian cyst.
(2) Alternatively, it may point and discharge inwards through the tarsal plate, causing conjunctivitis and discharge.
(3) Commence flucloxacillin 500 mg orally q.d.s. and refer the patient to the ophthalmology clinic. Warm bathing is unhelpful.

MEIBOMIAN CYST (CHALAZION)

DIAGNOSIS AND MANAGEMENT

(1) This feels like a hard pip within the tarsal plate.
(2) Refer the patient to the ophthalmology clinic for incision and curettage.

DACRYOCYSTITIS

DIAGNOSIS AND MANAGEMENT

(1) Dacryocystitis is inflammation of the lacrimal sac in the inner canthus of the lower eyelid (dacryoadenitis is inflammation of the lacrimal gland in the outer upper eyelid).
(2) There is a localised, tender, red swelling and watering of the eye due to the blocked lacrimal duct.
(3) Start a systemic antibiotic such as flucloxacillin 500 mg orally q.d.s. after sending a swab of any exuding pus.
(4) Refer the patient to the next ophthalmology clinic.

ORBITAL CELLULITIS

DIAGNOSIS AND MANAGEMENT

(1) This condition follows sinusitis or a periorbital injury, with intense pain, swelling, reduced eye movements and exophthalmos.

(2) There is generalised malaise, a raised temperature, and a discharging, congested eye. Adjacent sinuses are tender when associated with the infection.

(3) Take blood cultures and give flucloxacillin 2 g i.v. and cefotaxime 1 g i.v.

(4) Refer the patient immediately to the ophthalmology team, and obtain a CT scan and ENT opinion if the paranasal sinuses are involved.

(5) Complications, particularly in children, can occur within hours, including meningitis, central retinal vein occlusion, optic nerve compression and cavernous sinus thrombosis.

BASAL CELL CARCINOMA (RODENT ULCER)

DIAGNOSIS AND MANAGEMENT

(1) Basal cell carcinoma is the commonest malignancy of the eyelid, more frequent on the lower lid and following prolonged exposure to sunlight.

(2) An early, opalescent pink papule with surface telangiectasia progresses slowly to an ulcerated nodule with a pearly, rounded edge that is locally invasive.

(3) Refer the patient to the next ophthalmology clinic for treatment by excision, curettage, cryotherapy or radiotherapy in the elderly.

HERPES ZOSTER OPHTHALMICUS (OPHTHALMIC SHINGLES)

DIAGNOSIS AND MANAGEMENT

(1) This presents as a vesicular rash over the distribution of the ophthalmic division of the trigeminal (fifth) cranial nerve. Pain and tingling often precede the rash.

(2) The patient is usually unwell and in pain. The eye may be affected, resulting in blepharitis, conjunctivitis, keratitis, uveitis, secondary glaucoma, ophthalmoplegia or optic neuritis.

(3) Treatment of the varied ocular problems is awkward, as eyelid swelling makes topical therapy difficult and pain may be incapacitating.

(4) Therefore refer the patient to the ophthalmology team for inpatient care.

(5) Start aciclovir 800 mg orally five times daily with 3% aciclovir ophthalmic ointment or famciclovir 250 mg orally t.d.s. to decrease pain, corneal damage and uveitis.

THE PAINFUL, RED EYE

There are five important causes to consider:
(1) acute conjunctivitis
(2) acute episcleritis and scleritis
(3) acute keratitis
(4) acute iritis
(5) acute glaucoma.

ACUTE CONJUNCTIVITIS

DIAGNOSIS

(1) The causes are:
    (i)   allergic
    (ii) bacterial, such as staphylococci, pneumococci, gonococci or *Haemophilus*
    (iii) viral, particularly adenovirus or enterovirus
    (iv) chlamydial.

(2) There is generalised conjunctival injection, with gritty discomfort, mild photophobia and variable discharge. Vision should be normal.

MANAGEMENT

(1) Clean away the discharge with moist cotton-wool balls, and avoid irritating cosmetics and eye lotions.

(2) Allergic conjunctivitis responds to steroid drops, but these must only be prescribed by an ophthalmologist. Initially, prevent secondary bacterial infection with antibiotic drops and refer the patient to the ophthalmology clinic.

(3) Bacterial conjunctivitis requires frequent antibiotic drops, as often as hourly in severe cases, and ointment at night. Refer the patient to the ophthalmology clinic if the infection does not settle.

(4) Viral conjunctivitis, due to the adenovirus or enterovirus, is highly contagious and person-to-person spread is rapid unless scrupulous care is taken with hand washing.

  (i) Give antibiotic drops and ointment to prevent secondary bacterial infection.

  (ii) Refer the patient to the next ophthalmology clinic for a definitive diagnosis and to monitor for the development of keratitis.

(5) Chlamydial conjunctivitis usually occurs in young adults, causing chronic bilateral conjunctivitis with mucopurulent discharge. The cornea may be involved (keratitis).

  (i) The diagnosis is difficult but should be suspected when conventional antibiotic therapy fails.

  (ii) Associated urethritis or salpingitis may suggest the aetiology.

  (iii) Take special swabs for antigen detection, polymerase chain reaction (PCR) or culture, and treat with azithromycin 1 g orally. Discuss with the Special Clinic (genitourinary medicine clinic).

ACUTE EPISCLERITIS AND SCLERITIS

DIAGNOSIS

(1) Episcleritis is localised inflammation beneath the conjunctiva adjacent to the sclera. Scleritis is a more painful inflammation of the sclera itself. Rheumatoid arthritis may be associated.

(2) The eye is locally red and sore with reflex watering but no discharge. Progression to eyeball perforation occurs in scleritis.

MANAGEMENT

(1) Send blood for FBC, ESR and rheumatoid factor, and commence a nonsteroidal anti-inflammatory agent such as diclofenac (Voltarol) 50 mg orally t.d.s.
(2) Refer the patient to the ophthalmology team for definitive treatment, including steroid eye drops.

ACUTE KERATITIS

DIAGNOSIS

(1) This is inflammation of the cornea due to many possible causes, including viruses such as herpes simplex and the adenovirus, bacterial infection of a corneal ulcer, abrasion, exposure or wearing contact lenses.
(2) The main distinguishing feature from conjunctivitis is the prominent pain, with diminution of vision if there is a central ulcer or a hypopyon (pus in the anterior chamber).
(3) Fluorescein staining will demonstrate a marginal or central ulcer. Where herpes simplex is implicated, the ulcer is typically branching or dendritic.

MANAGEMENT

(1) Steroid eye drops are absolutely forbidden.
(2) Commence antibiotic drops or 3% aciclovir ointment five times daily for herpes simplex ulceration. Refer the patient immediately to the ophthalmology team.

ACUTE IRITIS

DIAGNOSIS

(1) This is occasionally due to exogenous infection from a perforating wound or corneal ulcer.
(2) Otherwise ill-understood endogenous mechanisms some linked with HLA-B27 and sero-negative arthropathy are involved, as in ankylosing spondylitis, Reiter's syndrome, ulcerative colitis, Crohn's disease and Still's

disease. Other causes include sarcoidosis, toxoplasmosis, TB, syphilis and herpes zoster ophthalmicus.

(3) There is circumcorneal ciliary injection, constant pain, photophobia and impaired vision. The pupil contracts, and tiny aggregates of cells, known as keratic precipitates, may be seen on the inner surface of the cornea.

(4) In severe cases, pus forms in the anterior chamber causing a hypopyon, and the iris may adhere to the anterior lens surface causing posterior synechiae.

MANAGEMENT

(1) Refer the patient immediately to the ophthalmology team for treatment with steroid drops and cycloplegics.

(2) Attacks may become recurrent and progress to secondary glaucoma.

ACUTE GLAUCOMA

DIAGNOSIS

(1) Glaucoma is associated with a narrowed anterior chamber with obstruction to the outflow of aqueous humour.

(2) It is more common in middle-aged or elderly hypermetropes (long-sighted people), and it is precipitated by pupillary dilation.

(3) There is severe throbbing, boring pain accompanied by headache, nausea, vomiting and prostration. Vision is reduced with haloes around lights, and the cornea becomes hazy with a fixed, semi-dilated oval pupil. On gentle palpation the eye feels hard.

MANAGEMENT

This is an ocular emergency requiring urgent referral to the ophthalmology team. On their advice commence:

(1) miotic drops such as pilocarpine every 5 min for up to 1 h;

(2) acetazolamide 500 mg slowly i.v., then 250 mg i.v. or orally t.d.s. – but contraindicated in sulphonamide allergy;

(3) an antiemetic such as metoclopramide 10 mg i.v., and analgesia such as morphine up to 2.5 mg i.v. for severe pain.

SUDDEN LOSS OF VISION IN THE UNINFLAMED EYE

Conditions to be considered include:
(1) central retinal artery occlusion
(2) central retinal vein occlusion
(3) vitreous haemorrhage
(4) retinal detachment
(5) optic neuritis.

CENTRAL RETINAL ARTERY OCCLUSION

DIAGNOSIS

(1) This condition is most common in the elderly arteriosclerotic patient, but it may occur due to emboli or in association with temporal arteritis.
(2) There is sudden blindness associated with a relative afferent pupillary defect (Marcus Gunn pupil):
    (i)   A swinging light directed into one eye then briskly into the other produces apparent dilation of the pupil in the affected eye, as the relaxing consensual reflex in the good eye is dominant.
    (ii)   It is an excellent sign of a unilateral or asymmetrical optic nerve or retinal lesion.
(3) The fundus is milky white, the optic disc is pale and swollen, and a cherry-red spot develops at the macula in 1–2 days.

MANAGEMENT

(1) Commence acetazolamide 500 mg slowly i.v. to reduce intraocular pressure.
(2) Give gentle pulsed ocular massage and advise rebreathing into a paper bag to dilate the retinal vessels by CO_2 retention.

(3) Refer the patient urgently to the ophthalmology team, as treatment within 1–2 h including anterior chamber paracentesis may restore the retinal circulation.

(4) If there is a prodromal history of headache, scalp tenderness and malaise, consider temporal arteritis. Measure an ESR; if raised, give the patient prednisolone 60 mg orally to prevent the other eye becoming involved (see p. 66).

CENTRAL RETINAL VEIN OCCLUSION

DIAGNOSIS

(1) This condition is most common in elderly patients with atherosclerosis, hypertension and simple glaucoma. Diabetes and hyperviscosity also predispose.

(2) Visual loss is less abrupt but may be noticed suddenly. A relative afferent pupillary defect may be seen in extensive cases.

(3) The fundus shows congested veins with scattered flame haemorrhages and optic disc swelling.

MANAGEMENT

(1) There is no specific treatment, although predisposing conditions must be looked for.

(2) Refer the patient to the ophthalmology clinic to monitor for the development of secondary acute glaucoma (some weeks later) from neovascularisation.

VITREOUS HAEMORRHAGE

DIAGNOSIS

(1) This may be traumatic or spontaneous, associated with diabetes, various blood disorders and retinal detachment.

(2) There is a reduced or absent red reflex and diminution in vision, preceded by floaters.

MANAGEMENT

(1) Refer the patient to the ophthalmology team to exclude retinal detachment and to look for other predisposing conditions.

(2) Vitrectomy may be necessary if the haemorrhage fails to clear.

RETINAL DETACHMENT

DIAGNOSIS

(1) This may be traumatic, or spontaneous in myopes (short-sighted people), or may follow a vitreous haemorrhage.
(2) There is peripheral visual loss, like a curtain, which may be profound if the macula is affected. A preceding history of floaters or sudden flashes of light is common.
(3) The retina is dark, wrinkled and ballooned, and the choroid may be seen as a red tear. A relative afferent pupil defect is seen if the detachment is large.

MANAGEMENT

Refer the patient immediately to the ophthalmology team for possible surgical repair.

OPTIC NEURITIS

DIAGNOSIS

(1) This may be idiopathic, post-viral or associated with demyelination from multiple sclerosis.
(2) There is more gradual loss of central, particularly colour vision, with pain on moving the eye, and a relative afferent pupillary defect (see p. 337).
(3) If the optic disc is involved, there is papillitis, which must be distinguished from papilloedema. Papilloedema tends to be bilateral, pain-free with normal pupil responses. There is no visual loss, but an enlarged blind-spot is found on field testing.

MANAGEMENT

(1) Examine the patient for other signs of demyelination, but never inform him or her of your suspicions at this early stage.
(2) Refer the patient to the ophthalmology clinic.

REFERENCES

1   Lavin MJ, Rose GE. Use of steroid eye drops in general practice. *BMJ* 1986;292:1448–50.
2   Campanile TM, St Clair DA, Benaim M. The evaluation of eye patching in the treatment of traumatic corneal epithelial defects. *J Emerg Med* 1997;15:769–74.

SECTION VIII

MAXILLOFACIAL AND DENTAL EMERGENCIES

TRAUMATIC CONDITIONS OF THE FACE AND MOUTH

LACERATIONS

MANAGEMENT

(1) *Face*. Meticulously debride facial cuts under local anaesthesia, and suture using fine 5/0 synthetic monofilament nylon (Ethilon) sutures, removed by 4 days.

(2) *Lips*
  (i)   Use 3/0 or 4/0 absorbable sutures such as polyglactin (Vicryl) for intra-oral lesions, and 5/0 synthetic monofilament nylon sutures for external lacerations.
  (ii) If the full thickness of the lip is lacerated vertically, breaching the vermilion border, refer the patient to the oral surgery team to avoid cosmetic deformity from inexperienced repair.

(3) *Tongue*
  (i)   Most lacerations may be left unless large and through the edge, or bleeding profusely, when an absorbable suture such as 3/0 catgut or polyglactin (Vicryl) is used.
  (ii) Advise regular mouthwash of warm saline.

TOOTH INJURIES

MANAGEMENT

(1) *Chipped tooth*
  (i)   Enamel or dentine damage: the tooth will be sensitive but viable. Advise the patient to avoid hot or cold drinks and refer to the patient's own dentist.
  (ii) Pulp space exposed: the tooth may be bleeding from the pulp, and sensitive to light touch. Refer the patient immediately to the oral surgery team, as there is a risk of pulp infection or necrosis.[1]

(2) *Displaced tooth*

(i)   Do not manipulate unless the tooth is about to fall out, in which case it should be firmly replaced in its socket.

(ii)   Refer the patient to a dental surgeon as soon as possible for immobilisation of the tooth.

(3) *Avulsed permanent incisor tooth*. Reposition of a dry, avulsed tooth within 30 min outside its socket or up to 2 h if stored in saliva or milk gives the best chance of successful re-implantation.

(i)   If immediate re-implantation is not performed, transport the tooth in the buccal sulcus of the patient's own cheek, or in milk if the patient is uncooperative or unconscious.

(ii)   On arrival in the A&E department, handle the tooth by the crown only, rinse it in saline, and replace back into the socket with firm pressure. No analgesia is necessary.

(iii)   Splint the tooth with aluminium foil, give the patient an antibiotic such as amoxicillin 500 mg orally t.d.s., and give tetanus prophylaxis.

(iv)   Refer the patient to a dental surgeon as soon as possible.

Note: if a tooth or denture is actually missing following trauma, perform a postero-anterior (PA) and lateral CXR to exclude inhalation into the lung or PA and lateral neck X-rays if obstruction in the upper oesophagus is suspected (see p. 318).

(4) *Bleeding tooth socket*

(i)   This can be post-traumatic or post-extraction.

(ii)   Clear out clots and arrest haemorrhage using a calcium alginate (Kaltostat) dressing or gauze roll. Ask the patient to bite on it for 15–30 min.

(iii)   If the bleeding persists, infiltrate with 1% lignocaine with 1:200 000 adrenaline, and close the mucosa over the socket using 3/0 absorbable polyglactin (Vicryl) sutures. If this fails, refer the patient to the oral surgery team.

(5) *Broken dentures*. Always save these, as they will be invaluable to the maxillofacial surgeon to aid in the fixation of jaw fractures or if a splint is needed.

FRACTURED MANDIBLE

DIAGNOSIS

(1) This injury is due to a blow on the jaw causing a unilateral or frequently bilateral fracture. Occasionally, the temporomandibular joint may be dislocated or the condylar process driven back into the temporal bone, causing bleeding and deformity of the external auditory canal.

(2) There is localised pain, particularly on attempted jaw movement and malocclusion. Inside the mouth, bruising or bleeding of the gum and discontinuity of the teeth occur if there is a displaced fracture.

(3) There will be numbness of the lower lip if the inferior dental nerve has been damaged in its course through the mandible.

(4) X-rays should include an anteroposterior view, with a panoramic orthopantomogram (OPG) or lateral views of the mandible.

MANAGEMENT

(1) Clear the airway of any clots or debris, and ensure that the tongue or a portion of the mandible does not slip back and occlude the pharynx.

(2) Refer any unstable or grossly displaced injuries immediately to the maxillofacial surgery team.

(3) Otherwise, for an undisplaced fracture give the patient tetanus prophylaxis and antibiotics, as most fractures are compound into the mouth. Use amoxicillin 500 mg and clavulanic acid 125 mg (Augmentin 625 mg) one tablet orally t.d.s for 5 days.

(4) Refer the patient to the next maxillofacial surgery clinic.

DISLOCATED MANDIBLE

DIAGNOSIS

(1) Dislocation may occur spontaneously after yawning or it may follow a blow to the jaw. It may be unilateral or more commonly bilateral and may become recurrent.

(2) The mouth is stuck open and is painful.

(3) Exclude drug-induced dystonia due to metoclopramide or phenothiazines on direct questioning, as this may mimic or even predispose to dislocation. It is treated with benzatropine (Cogentin) 1–2 mg i.v.

MANAGEMENT

(1) Request an anteroposterior and lateral X-ray of the temporomandibular joints to exclude an associated fracture, unless the dislocation was spontaneous or recurrent.

(2) In the absence of a fracture, try to reduce without sedation. If unsuccessful, use i.v. midazolam 2.5–5 mg with full resuscitation facilities available.

    (i) Stand in front of the patient and press firmly downwards by applying pressure with your thumbs inside the mouth to the angle of the jaw to distract the condyle, placing your fingers under the chin. Then push backwards to relocate the condyle in the fossa.

    (ii) In bilateral dislocations, reduce one side at a time.

    (iii) Repeat the X-ray to confirm reduction, and refer to the next maxillofacial surgery clinic. Advise the patient to avoid excessive mouth opening.

    (iv) Apply a barrel bandage to discourage wide opening if the dislocation is recurrent or required i.v. midazolam.

FRACTURE OF THE ZYGOMATIC OR MALAR COMPLEX

DIAGNOSIS

(1) This injury is due to a direct blow to the cheek, which may fracture the zygomatic arch in isolation, but more usually causes a 'tripod' fracture through three structures:

    (i) superiorly through the zygomaticofrontal suture;

    (ii) laterally through the zygomatic arch or zygomaticotemporal suture;

    (iii) medially through the zygomaticomaxillary suture or the infraorbital foramen region.

(2) There is flattening of the malar process best seen from above (which may be masked by oedema), epistaxis, sub-conjunctival haemorrhage extending posteriorly, and infraorbital nerve paraesthesia. Jaw movement may be limited if the coronoid process obstructs under the zygo-matic arch.

(3) Although these fractures are best diagnosed clinically, particularly by finding local bony tenderness, request facial X-rays including occipitomental views (OM 10° and OM 30°).

    (i)   Look carefully for the fractures comparing with the normal side.

    (ii)   Or look for secondary evidence of injury, e.g. opa-city of the maxillary antrum from bleeding into the maxillary sinus or overlying soft-tissue swelling.

MANAGEMENT

(1) Advise the patient not to blow his or her nose, as subcu-taneous emphysema may occur if the paranasal sinuses are involved.

(2) Commence amoxicillin 500 mg orally t.d.s. (or erythro-mycin 500 mg orally q.d.s. if the patient is allergic) as most fractures are compound into the maxillary sinus, and an analgesic such as paracetamol 500 mg and codeine phosphate 8 mg (co-codamol 8/500).

(3) Refer the patient to the maxillofacial surgery team within 24 h for elevation of the depressed cheekbone within 7 days.

'BLOW-OUT' FRACTURE OF THE ORBITAL FLOOR

DIAGNOSIS

(1) This uncommon fracture is due to blunt trauma to the eye from a small object the size of a squash ball, driving the eyeball backwards and rupturing the weak bony floor of the orbit. Orbital fat and occasionally the inferior rectus muscle herniate through the defect into the maxil-lary sinus.

(2) It is essential to initially exclude blunt trauma to the eye (see p. 328). The fracture itself causes enophthalmos, which may be masked by periorbital oedema, infra orbital nerve loss and diplopia with restricted upwards gaze due to trapping of the inferior rectus muscle.

(3) Facial X-ray often fails to show the fracture, but it can be inferred from an opaque maxillary sinus or a fluid level from the bleeding, and a 'tear drop' soft-tissue opacity hanging from the roof of the sinus. CT scan demonstrates the fracture more clearly.

MANAGEMENT

(1) Refer blunt eye damage immediately to the ophthalmology team.

(2) Commence amoxicillin 500 mg orally t.d.s. and 1% chloramphenicol eye ointment 4-hourly.

(3) Refer the patient to the maxillofacial surgery team within 24 h.

MIDDLE-THIRD-OF-FACE FRACTURES

DIAGNOSIS

These complicated fractures are usually bilateral and are divided into three groups:

(1) *Le Fort I*
    (i) This is due to a blow to the maxilla causing a horizontal fracture separating the alveolar bone and teeth from the maxilla.
    (ii) There is epistaxis and malocclusion, and crepitus may be elicited.

(2) *Le Fort II*
    (i) This is a pyramidal fracture extending up from a Le Fort I fracture to involve the nasal skeleton and the middle of the face. The middle of the face is thus 'stove in', elongating the face and causing malocclusion.
    (ii) The airway may be compromised and cerebrospinal fluid may leak from the nose.

(3) *Le Fort III*
   (i)   This dislocates the entire midfacial skeleton from the base of the skull (craniofacial dysjunction).
   (ii) There is massive facial swelling and bruising, and often brisk pharyngeal bleeding that may cause haemorrhagic shock. The airway is again in danger.

MANAGEMENT

(1) Attend urgently to the airway.
   (i)   Sometimes, if the face is stove in, the whole segment may be lifted forwards manually to relieve the airway.
   (ii) Otherwise, orotracheal intubation or even cricothyrotomy is required if there is difficulty maintaining an adequate airway.
(2) Remember that the direct force to the face may have caused an additional cervical spine injury or head injury.
   (i)   Lateral cervical spine X-ray and a head CT scan are therefore the priority.
   (ii) Specific facial-view X-rays must wait until all the other major injuries are stabilised and a cervical spine injury is excluded.
(3) Refer all fractures immediately to the maxillofacial surgery team.

NON-TRAUMATIC CONDITIONS OF THE MOUTH

TOOTHACHE

DIAGNOSIS AND MANAGEMENT

(1) Toothache is usually due to inflammation of the pulp space in a carious tooth.
(2) Exclude a dental abscess (see below) and give the patient an analgesic such as paracetamol 500 mg and codeine

phosphate 8 mg (co-codamol 8/500). Return the patient to his or her own dentist.

DENTAL ABSCESS

DIAGNOSIS AND MANAGEMENT

(1) An apical or periapical abscess is an extension of a pulp space infection.
    (i)   The tooth is tender to tapping, with associated soft-tissue swelling and continuous pain.
    (ii)   There may be systemic malaise and fever.
(2) If the patient is severely ill, or the abscess is pointing extra-orally, refer to the oral surgery team.
(3) Otherwise, commence an antibiotic such as amoxicillin 500 mg orally t.d.s., give an analgesic (e.g. codeine phosphate 30–60 mg orally q.d.s.), and return the patient to his or her own dentist.

LUDWIG'S ANGINA

DIAGNOSIS AND MANAGEMENT

(1) This condition is a bilateral, fulminant, brawny cellulitis of the sublingual and submandibular areas, associated with poor dental hygiene or dental instrumentation.
(2) There is trismus, dysphagia, submandibular pain and swelling, and a risk of sudden respiratory obstruction from upwards displacement of the tongue.
(3) Give benzylpenicillin 1.8 g i.v. and metronidazole 500 mg i.v., and admit the patient immediately under the ENT team for careful observation of the airway.

SUBMANDIBULAR SWELLINGS

DIAGNOSIS AND MANAGEMENT

Several causes are possible:
(1) *Submandibular stone.* This intermittently blocks the submandibular duct, causing pain and swelling aggravated

by food. The stone is palpable on bimanual examination in the floor of the mouth and is seen on X-ray. Refer the patient to the oral surgery team.

(2) *Submandibular abscess.* The pain is constant with associated malaise, swelling in the angle of the jaw, and trismus. Refer the patient to the oral surgery team.

(3) *Mumps.* This affects the parotids and is usually bilateral, but can affect the submandibular glands. Remember the association with orchitis. Give the patient paracetamol elixir, and reassure them.

(4) *Dental abscess.* This may point downwards from a molar tooth to the submandibular area.

(5) *Lymph node enlargement.* The most common causes of cervical adenopathy in this area are tonsillitis and pharyngitis.

(6) *Rare causes.* These include carcinoma, lymphoma, sarcoid, TB, osteomyelitis, and a bony cyst or fibrous dysplasia.

REFERENCE

1   Roberts G, Scully C, Shotts R. ABC of oral health: dental emergencies. *BMJ* 2000;321:559–62.

GYNAECOLOGICAL EMERGENCIES

VAGINAL EXAMINATION

(1) Most gynaecological emergencies that present with abdominal pain or vaginal bleeding will require the opinion of the gynaecology team, who should be asked to perform the vaginal examination if the A&E department doctor is inexperienced.

(2) However, in every case make a detailed history and examination, send urgent blood samples to the laboratory, perform a urine or serum beta-HCG pregnancy test, and institute resuscitative procedures as necessary. Also consider possible non-gynaecological conditions.

PRESCRIBING IN PREGNANCY

(1) Consult the prescribing information first before giving any drug to a pregnant patient. Look at the appendix at the back of the British National Formulary (BNF). Ideally, all drugs should be avoided in the first trimester unless absolutely necessary.

(2) Therefore, it is essential to enquire about the possibility of pregnancy in every female of reproductive age.

(3) This is also relevant when requesting X-rays, although most hospital radiology departments have their own guidelines to minimise the risk of irradiation in early pregnancy.

(4) The BNF also has another appendix of drugs to avoid when breastfeeding.

GYNAECOLOGICAL CAUSES OF ACUTE ABDOMINAL PAIN

The following conditions may present with acute abdominal pain:

(1) ruptured ectopic pregnancy
(2) acute salpingitis
(3) ruptured ovarian cyst

(4) torsion of an ovarian tumour

(5) endometriosis.

RUPTURED ECTOPIC PREGNANCY

DIAGNOSIS

(1) Ectopic pregnancy is more common in patients with a previous ectopic pregnancy, pelvic inflammatory disease or tubal surgery, and in patients using an intrauterine contraceptive device (IUCD).

(2) Ectopic pregnancy usually presents from 5 to 9 weeks of pregnancy. Patients presenting early may not realise they are pregnant, although there may be breast tenderness, nausea or a history of recent unprotected intercourse. It must always be considered in every female patient with menstrual irregularities, vaginal bleeding, lower abdominal pain or collapse.

(3) The unstable form presents with sudden abdominal pain, often referred to the shoulder tip, followed by scanty vaginal bleeding, proceeding to circulatory collapse and haemorrhagic shock.

(4) The stable form has a prodromal history of lower abdominal pain and slight vaginal bleeding that is typically dark brown ('prune juice'), although the bleeding can be fresh red.

(5) Examination in the unstable form reveals a pale, collapsed, hypotensive patient with a tender, rigid silent abdomen.

(6) In the stable form, there is localised lower abdominal tenderness and guarding to one side, with discomfort and swelling in that lateral fornix on vaginal examination, and a smaller uterus than expected for the duration of amenorrhoea.

MANAGEMENT

(1) *Unstable ectopic pregnancy*
   (i)   Give the patient oxygen, insert a large-bore i.v. cannula, send blood for FBC, U&E, blood sugar and beta-HCG, and cross-match 4 units of blood.

  (ii)   Commence an infusion of crystalloid such as normal
         saline or colloid such as polygeline (Haemaccel),
         and refer the patient immediately to the gynaecology
         team. Inform theatre and the duty anaesthetist.

(2) *Stable ectopic pregnancy*
  (i)   Insert an i.v. cannula and send blood for FBC,
         U&E, blood sugar and G&S. Send serum for a
         pregnancy test if a urinary test kit is unavailable
         (see below).
  (ii)   Perform a pregnancy test.
         (a) A serum radioimmunoassay pregnancy test
              for beta-HCG in blood is extremely sensitive,
              with a negative test ruling out a recent ectopic
              or abortion, although it takes time to do and
              may not be available after hours.
         (b) Alternatively, use a urinary beta-HCG mono-
              clonal antibody immunoassay. This can be
              done rapidly in the A&E department, and
              may be positive even before the first missed
              period. Again, a negative test virtually rules
              out an ectopic.
  (iii) Request a transabdominal ultrasound scan to
         demonstrate a gestation sac within the uterus, which
         effectively excludes an ectopic pregnancy. Trans-
         vaginal ultrasound scan is even more sensitive as it
         identifies signs of the extra-uterine pregnancy
         itself.
  (iv)   Refer all cases to the gynaecology team. Ultimately,
         a laparoscopy or laparotomy confirms the condi-
         tion and allows definitive management.
  (v)   Give rhesus-negative mothers anti-D immuno-
         globulin 250 units i.m. to prevent maternal forma-
         tion of antibodies from isoimmunisation.

ACUTE SALPINGITIS

DIAGNOSIS

(1) This is usually a sexually transmitted disease caused
    principally by chlamydial or gonococcal infection.

Recurrent infections are increasingly likely to cause infertility.

(2) It presents acutely with fever, malaise, bilateral lower abdominal pain, dyspareunia, menstrual irregularities and vaginal discharge.

(3) On examination there is an elevated temperature with bilateral lower abdominal tenderness and guarding.

(4) On vaginal examination adnexal tenderness and pain on moving the cervix, known as a positive cervical excitation test are found, with cervical or vaginal discharge.

(5) The white blood cell count is raised, and a serum or urine beta-HCG pregnancy test is negative.

MANAGEMENT

(1) Send blood for FBC and blood culture, and send a midstream specimen of urine (MSU). Perform a pregnancy test.

(2) Remove an IUCD if it is present and send it for culture.

(3) Send an endocervical and urethral swab for gonococcal culture in a suitable transport medium such as Stuart's, and an endocervical swab for chlamydia antigen, polymerase chain reaction (PCR) or culture.

(4) Refer all patients who are systemically unwell, unable to rest at home, pregnant (unusual) or in whom the diagnosis is uncertain to the gynaecology team.

(5) In the remainder, commence doxycycline 100 mg orally b.d. and metronidazole 400 mg orally b.d. (avoiding alcohol), both for 2 weeks, plus ciprofloxacin 500 mg orally as a single dose.

(6) Review the patient in the next gynaecology clinic, or refer her to the genitourinary medicine Special Clinic for follow-up.

(7) Advise abstinence from sexual intercourse until the partner has also been seen and treated in a Special Clinic.

RUPTURED OVARIAN CYST

DIAGNOSIS AND MANAGEMENT

(1) There is sudden, moderate, lower abdominal and pelvic pain without gastrointestinal symptoms.

(2) The patient is afebrile with localised tenderness, but no mass is felt. A pregnancy test is negative, and pelvic ultrasound confirms the diagnosis.

(3) Refer the patient to the gynaecology team.

TORSION OF AN OVARIAN TUMOUR

DIAGNOSIS AND MANAGEMENT

(1) Fibroids or cysts that twist or suddenly distend from a bleed cause sudden lower abdominal pain, often with preceding episodes of milder pain.

(2) The patient may have nausea, a low-grade fever and localised abdominal tenderness with a palpable mass.

(3) Send blood for FBC, collect a midstream specimen of urine (MSU), and exclude pregnancy with a pregnancy test.

(4) Arrange a pelvic ultrasound, and refer the patient to the gynaecology team for possible laparoscopy.

ENDOMETRIOSIS

DIAGNOSIS AND MANAGEMENT

(1) There is a preceding history of recurrent abdominal and flank pain, worse at the time of menstruation and immediately following the period, dyspareunia, painful defecation, infertility and acquired dysmenorrhoea.

(2) This is a difficult diagnosis requiring review by the gynaecology team and laparoscopy.

BLEEDING IN EARLY PREGNANCY

Two important causes are ectopic pregnancy and spontaneous abortion. Induced septic abortion is now rare. Spontaneous abortion is the expulsion of the products of conception before the 24th week of pregnancy. In practice, this presents as vaginal bleeding or abdominal pain.

Refer any bleeding or abdominal pain in a patient over 18–20 weeks pregnant directly to the labour ward (this rule may differ from hospital to hospital).

SPONTANEOUS ABORTION

DIAGNOSIS

There are five recognised stages of spontaneous abortion:

(1) *Threatened abortion*
- (i)   This is most common up to 14 weeks gestation, causing mild cramps and transient vaginal bleeding.
- (ii) The uterine size is compatible with the duration of pregnancy. A guide to the expected size of the uterus is given by:
  - (a)   bimanual examination: the uterus is the size of a hen's egg at 7 weeks, an orange at 10 weeks, and a grapefruit at 12 weeks;
  - (b)   abdominal palpation: the fundus reaches the symphysis pubis at 12 weeks and the umbilicus at 24 weeks.
- (iii) The external cervical os is closed on speculum examination.

(2) *Inevitable abortion*
- (i)   The bleeding is heavier, followed by cramps that are more persistent.
- (ii) The external cervical os is open 0.5 cm or more, and the products of conception may be found in the vagina or protruding from the cervical canal.
- (iii) The symptoms and signs of pregnancy will disappear. These include amenorrhoea, nausea, vomiting, breast enlargement, tenderness, tingling, areolar pigmentation, and frequency of micturition.

(3) *Incomplete abortion*
- (i)   Bleeding remains heavy and the cramps persist, with the passage of clots and the products of conception. These may be found on examination or may have been noted previously by the patient.

(4) *Complete abortion*
    (i)   The bleeding and cramps stop after the conceptus has been passed and the signs of pregnancy disappear.
    (ii)   The cervical os is closed.
(5) *Missed abortion*
    (i)   The products of conception are retained, although cramps and bleeding are replaced by a brownish vaginal discharge.
    (ii)   The uterus is small and irregular, and ultrasound fails to detect fetal heart motion.
    (iii) Infection and disseminated intravascular coagulation may occur.

MANAGEMENT

(1) Send blood for FBC and G&S if the bleeding is heavy, and commence an infusion of normal saline. Confirm recent pregnancy with a serum or urine beta-HCG immunoassay pregnancy test.
(2) Remove the products of conception with sponge forceps if they are blocking the cervical canal, to help relieve pain, bradycardia and hypotension. Send them for histology to exclude a hydatidiform mole.
(3) Arrange a pelvic ultrasound to rule out an ectopic pregnancy and to assess fetal viability.
(4) Refer all patients to the gynaecology team for bedrest (threatened abortion), or evacuation of retained products of conception (ERPC) for inevitable or incomplete abortion.
(5) Remember all rhesus-negative mothers must be given anti-D immunoglobulin 500 units i.m. within 72 h to prevent maternal formation of antibodies to fetal rhesus-positive cells.

INDUCED SEPTIC ABORTION

DIAGNOSIS AND MANAGEMENT

(1) This is usually the result of criminal abortion or occasionally therapeutic abortion.

(2) There is rapidly spreading pelvic infection, with salpingitis, peritonitis, septic pelvic and pulmonary thrombophlebitis, leading to septicaemic shock and death.

(3) The patient is unwell with fever, abdominal pain, foul vaginal discharge and bleeding, leading to hypotension, oliguria, confusion then coma.

(4) Give the patient oxygen, start an i.v. infusion, and send blood for FBC, coagulation profile, U&E, LFTs, blood sugar and blood culture.

(5) Commence ampicillin 2 g i.v., gentamicin 5 mg/kg i.v. and metronidazole 500 mg i.v., and refer the patient urgently to the gynaecology team for evacuation of the uterine contents or emergency hysterectomy.

CONDITIONS IN LATE PREGNANCY

Ideally, all patients over 18–20 weeks pregnant should be sent straight to the labour ward. Occasionally, they are too unstable or there is not time to get them there. Thus the following conditions may be seen, all requiring prompt obstetric help.

CONFUSING TERMINOLOGY

Two terms are easy to confuse in obstetric practice:

(1) *Gravida*. This is the number of pregnancies of any gestation, including the current pregnancy, with twins counting as one.

(2) *Parity*

    (i) This is the number of previous pregnancies of 28 weeks or more, whether live or stillborn. Distinction is made between events after and before 28 weeks.

    (ii) It is described as 'para $x + y$', where x is deliveries after 28 weeks, whether stillborn or live, with twins counting as two, and y is pregnancies ending before 28 weeks, whether by spontaneous or therapeutic abortion.

ANTEPARTUM HAEMORRHAGE

DIAGNOSIS AND MANAGEMENT

(1) Vaginal bleeding after 24 weeks pregnancy is a life-threatening emergency when due to placenta praevia or placental abruption.

(2) Never examine the patient vaginally or with a speculum, for fear of precipitating torrential vaginal haemorrhage.

(3) Give oxygen, place the patient in the left lateral position, and start an i.v. infusion if the patient is hypotensive or shocked. Send blood for FBC and coagulation profile, and cross-match 4 units.

(4) Refer the patient immediately to the obstetric team.

PRE-ECLAMPSIA AND ECLAMPSIA

DIAGNOSIS AND MANAGEMENT

(1) Pre-eclampsia is diagnosed on finding oedema, protein-uria and hypertension, with a systolic blood pressure over 140 mm Hg and a diastolic blood pressure over 90 mm Hg in the third trimester of pregnancy (or greater than a 25 mm Hg systolic rise or 15 mm Hg diastolic rise compared with early pregnancy).

(2) If pre-eclampsia becomes fulminating, there is headache, visual symptoms, nausea, vomiting and abdominal pain. Irritability and hyper-reflexia may herald generalised eclamptic convulsions. Oliguria, thromboctopoenia, abnormal liver function tests and disseminated intravascular coagulation occur.

(3) Call the senior A&E doctor and obstetric team urgently. Give oxygen, gain venous access, and send blood for FBC, coagulation profile, U&E, LFTs and uric acid.

(4) Catheterise the patient. Place a wedge under the right hip, or nurse in the left lateral position.

(5) Control fits with magnesium sulphate 4 g i.v. over 5 min, followed by an infusion at 1 g/h. This is the drug of choice for eclampsia and possibly seizure prophylaxis in pre-eclampsia.[1] An alternative regime is diazepam (Diazemuls) 5–10 mg i.v. followed by phenytoin 15 mg/kg by infusion. Take the advice of the obstetric team.

(6) Initiate BP control with hydralazine 5 mg i.v. slowly, aiming for a diastolic BP of 90–100 mm Hg.

EMERGENCY DELIVERY

MANAGEMENT

(1) Call the obstetric team and paediatric or neonatal team immediately.

(2) Allow the mother to lie or sit semi-upright, and give her 50% nitrous oxide with oxygen (Entonox) during the first half of the contractions.

(3) A mediolateral episiotomy may be needed in primiparous women.

(4) Ask the mother to pant and thus to stop pushing as the head crowns, usually with the occiput upwards, which is followed by rotation (restitution) of the head.

(5) The next contraction delivers the anterior shoulder by gentle downward traction on the head, which is followed by the posterior shoulder and trunk.

(6) The baby is then delivered by lifting the head and trunk up and over the symphysis pubis, to lie on the mother's abdomen.

(7) Cut the cord immediately if it is wound tightly around the baby's neck. Otherwise it is clamped off or tied with two 2/0 silk ties after delivery, and divided.

(8) Aspirate mucus from the baby's nose and mouth, and keep the baby warm by wrapping it in a blanket. Be prepared to intubate if there is apnoea.

(9) Leave the placenta to deliver itself. Avoid the temptation to pull on the cord for fear of causing uterine inversion. Try gentle abdominal massage to stimulate a uterine contraction, or give syntocinon 5 units and ergometrine

0.5 mg (Syntometrine) 1 ml i.m. to prevent postpartum haemorrhage and aid delivery of the placenta.

(10) The mother can commence suckling her baby immediately. This will stimulate uterine contraction to help expel the placenta and reduce the risk of haemorrhage.

CARDIOPULMONARY RESUSCITATION IN LATE PREGNANCY

DIAGNOSIS

(1) Causes of cardiac arrest in late pregnancy include utero-placental bleeding, cerebrovascular haemorrhage, pulmonary embolus, amniotic fluid embolus and cardiac disease.

(2) Impaired venous return from inferior vena caval compression by the gravid uterus, with the patient supine, renders resuscitation ineffectual unless deliberately minimised.

MANAGEMENT

(1) Tilt the patient laterally using a wedge or pillow under the right side, and displace the uterus by lifting it manually upwards and to the left off the great vessels.

(2) Perform basic and advanced life support as for adult cardiac arrest (see p. 2), but compared with the non-pregnant patient:
   (i)   intubation is more tricky due to large breasts, short neck, laryngeal oedema, etc.;
   (ii) there is increased risk of regurgitation and pulmonary aspiration;
   (iii) effective external chest compression is more difficult due to flared ribs, raised diaphragm, breast enlargement and inferior vena caval compression.

(3) Consider immediate caesarean section if the resuscitation is not rapidly successful, having called the obstetric and paediatric team on the arrival of the patient.
   (i)   Ideally, surgical intervention should be within 5 min of cardiac arrest for optimum maternal and neonatal survival.[2]

(ii)   Continue cardiopulmonary resuscitation throughout the procedure and afterwards until a stable
rhythm with a sustained cardiac output is obtained.

TRAUMA IN PREGNANCY

The best treatment for the fetus is to rapidly stabilise the
mother. Treatment priorities for trauma in a pregnant patient
are the same as for the non-pregnant patient.

MANAGEMENT

(1) Follow the immediate management guidelines as for
multiple injuries (see p. 134), but note the following
additional considerations:
   (i)   Tilt the supine patient laterally using a wedge or
pillow under the right hip, and manually displace
the gravid uterus upwards and to the left to minimise impaired venous return from inferior vena
caval compression in the third trimester.
   (ii)   Protect the airway from the increased risk of gastric
regurgitation and pulmonary aspiration.
   (iii)   Larger amounts of blood may be lost before
obvious signs of hypovolaemia such as tachycardia,
hypotension and tachypnoea occur, as both maternal blood volume and cardiac output increase in
pregnancy.
   (iv)   Fetal distress without signs of maternal shock
occurs readily, as blood is shunted preferentially
away from the uterus to maintain the maternal circulation following blood loss.
   (v)   Perform peritoneal lavage when indicated,
using a supra-umbilical approach with the mini-
laparotomy technique, after first inserting a nasogastric tube and urethral catheter.
   (vi)   Retroperitoneal bleeding with pelvic fracture after
blunt trauma may be massive from the engorged
pelvic veins.
(2) After initial resuscitation of the patient, assess the fetus
during the secondary survey, including fundal height,
uterine tenderness, contractions, fetal movement, and

fetal heart rate. Use a fetal stethoscope or Doppler ultrasound for the heart rate.

(i)   Fetal distress is indicated by:
   (a)   bradycardia less than 110 beats/min (normal 120–160 beats/min);
   (b)   loss of fetal heart acceleration to fetal movement, or late deceleration after uterine contractions.

(ii)   Important causes of fetal distress or fetal death in trauma include maternal hypovolaemia, placental abruption and uterine rupture.
   (a)   Signs of placental abruption vary, from vaginal bleeding, abdominal pain, tenderness, increasing fundal height and premature contractions, to maternal shock.
   (b)   Signs of traumatic uterine rupture, which occurs more commonly in the second half of pregnancy, range from abdominal pain to maternal shock or a separately palpable uterus and fetus.

(iii)   Arrange continuous fetal monitoring, e.g. by cardiotocography for a minimum of 6 h, even after apparently minor maternal trauma.

(iv)   Give all rhesus-negative mothers anti-D immunoglobulin 500 units i.m.

(3)   Therefore, call the obstetric team to review and admit all pregnant trauma cases. Call the paediatric team in addition if the fetus is over 24–26 weeks gestation and immediate delivery is indicated. Emergency caesarean section performed within 5 min of maternal cardiac arrest maximises the chance of fetal survival and may also improve maternal outcome.

POST-COITAL CONTRACEPTION

Occasionally, patients present for emergency contraceptive measures after unprotected intercourse. There are two possibilities:

(1)   *Post-coital pill*. This may be used up to 72 h after unprotected intercourse.

(2) *Intrauterine contraceptive device.* This may be used up to 5 days after unprotected intercourse. Refer the patient to the family planning clinic or specialist pregnancy advice service for this.

POST-COITAL PILL

MANAGEMENT

(1) Give levonorgestrel 750 μg (Levonelle-2) one tablet immediately, followed by a second tablet 12 h later.
- (i)   This has fewer side effects than the combined hormonal (Yuzpe) method taking ethinyl oestradiol 50 μg and levonorgestrel 250 μg two tablets 12 h apart (Schering PC4).
- (ii) Do not use levonorgestrel 750 μg in women with severe liver disease or active acute porphyria.
- (iii) Double the first dose to levonorgestrel 1.5 mg followed by the usual dose of 750 μg 12 h later in women on enzyme-inducing drugs such as carbamazepine, rifampicin, phenytoin and phenobarbitone.

(2) Warn the patient that her next period may be early or late, and advise the use of a barrier contraceptive device until then.

(3) Refer all patients for follow-up to their GP or a family planning clinic to check that:
- (i)   the pregnancy test is negative 3–4 weeks later;
- (ii) there is no ectopic pregnancy (slight increased risk if the method fails);
- (iii) the patient receives proper contraceptive advice for the future.

MISSED ORAL CONTRACEPTIVE PILL

Usually a frantic call on the telephone requests advice on what to do following a missed oral contraceptive pill.

(1) *If the patient is on the combined oral contraceptive*

    (i)   *Up to 12 h late.* Take the missed pill and carry on as usual.

    (ii)   *Over 12 h late*

        (a)   Continue normal pill taking, but for the next 7 days either abstain from sex or use an alternative barrier method of contraception such as the condom.

        (b)   If these 7 days run beyond the end of the packet, start the next packet immediately the present one is over, i.e. no gap between packets.

        (c)   This will mean that no period may occur until the end of two packets, but this is not dangerous.

        (d)   If everyday (ED) pills are being used, miss out the seven inactive pills.

        (e)   Remember that missing a pill at the beginning or end of a cycle is potentially more critical than missing one in the middle.

(2) *If the patient is on the progestogen-only pill.* Over 3 h late: continue normal pill taking, but abstain from sex or use an alternative barrier method of contraception for the next 7 days.

DOMESTIC VIOLENCE

DIAGNOSIS

(1) Most victims are women, although a similar management approach is applicable to both sexes, including in the elderly.

(2) Domestic violence affects women of every class, race and religion. It may commence at times of acute stress such as unemployment, first pregnancy or separation.

(3) The victim may present with injury, abdominal pain, substance abuse, attempted suicide, rape or with multiple somatic complaints.

(4) Victims may delay attending, and may be evasive and embarrassed. Their partner may answer for them or act unconcerned.

MANAGEMENT

(1) Ensure privacy by interviewing alone without the partner. Ask gently but directly about the possibility of violence, which may initially be denied.
(2) Record all injuries, measuring bruises or lacerations with a ruler, and institute any urgent treatment to save life.
(3) Enquire about any additional risk of physical or sexual abuse to other members of the household, particularly children (see p. 283).
(4) Offer admission if it is unsafe for the patient to return home or if acute psychiatric illness is present, e.g. depression.
(5) Call the duty social worker. However, if in the meantime the patient wishes to return home, give written contact numbers, including:
    (i)   GP
    (ii)   social worker
    (iii) local police
    (iv)   local domestic violence 24-h specialist helplines in the telephone book.

RAPE

Follow a standard procedure in all cases of alleged rape in which the patient requests or accepts police involvement.

MANAGEMENT

(1) Be accompanied by a senior female nurse escort at all times.
(2) Record a careful history of exactly what occurred and when, and a description of the assailant.

(3) Institute any urgent treatment to save life, e.g. cross-match and starting a transfusion for haemorrhage.

(4) Contact the police and inform the duty police surgeon, who will perform the forensic examination with the patient's consent aimed at meticulously collecting evidence regarding:

    (i)   proof of sexual contact

    (ii)   lack of consent

    (iii) identification of the assailant.

(5) Examine the patient for associated injuries, measuring bruises or lacerations with a ruler. Request informed, written consent to keep all clothing for forensic analysis.

    (i)   Then undress the patient on a sheet to collect any debris.

    (ii)   Wrap each garment in a brown paper bag fastened with tape and labelled with the patient's name, the date, the nature of the sample, and the name of the person taking the sample.

(6) Request a senior gynaecology doctor to perform the examination of the external genitalia and vagina if the duty police surgeon is unavailable.

(7) Check whether the police have been able to arrange for a designated sexual offences unit to attend (usually non-uniformed women police officers who have received special training).

(8) Call the duty social worker or give the patient written contact telephone numbers/addresses if a social worker is not available immediately.

(9) Offer admission to the patient and discuss the following issues:

    (i)   the need for the post-coital pill to prevent pregnancy;

    (ii)   the need to exclude a sexually transmitted disease or to provide prophylactic treatment and follow-up;

    (iii) specialist counselling from various external organisations, such as the local Rape Crisis Centre – telephone (020) 7837 1600 available 24 h (London);

(iv)   written aftercare instructions with details of all the tests performed, treatments provided and other arrangements made.

REFERENCES

1   Munro PT. Management of eclampsia in the accident and emergency department. *J Accid Emerg Med* 2000;17:7–11.
2   Oates S, Williams GL, Rees GAD. Cardiopulmonary resuscitation in late pregnancy. *BMJ* 1988;297:404–5.

PSYCHIATRIC EMERGENCIES

DELIBERATE SELF-HARM

DIAGNOSIS

(1) The most common method of deliberate self-harm is by acute poisoning.

    (i)   This may be admitted freely, or may be evident from finding a suicide note or an empty bottle beside the patient.

    (ii)   The possibility should also be considered in any unconscious or confused patient, or in patients with unexplained metabolic, respiratory or cardiac problems (see p. 69).

(2) Other methods of deliberate self-harm include cutting the wrists or throat, shooting, hanging, drowning, gassing, and jumping from a height.

MANAGEMENT

(1) Perform the necessary investigations and resuscitative procedures to save life, and refer the patient directly to the medical, surgical or orthopaedic team if there is serious illness or injury.

(2) A medically unimportant acute poisoning, including a patient intoxicated with alcohol, may have been a serious self-harm attempt and should still be admitted for 24 h, possibly to the department's own observation ward.

(3) A full assessment may then be made the next day to decide on the further management of the patient[1].

    (i)   *Assessment of current suicidal intent.* Enquire specifically about:

        (a)   present suicidal thoughts

        (b)   previous deliberate self-harm

        (c)   evidence of a premeditated act without the intention of being found.

    (ii)   Consider other high-risk factors, including:

        (a)   mental illness, including depression and schizophrenia

        (b)   violent self-harm attempt, such as jumping, hanging or shooting

    (c)   chronic alcohol abuse, drug dependence, unemployment, homelessness

    (d)   older, single, urban, lonely male

    (e)   puerperium.

(iii)   Refer any patients considered to have a continuing suicide risk immediately to the psychiatric team.

(iv)   Make a psychiatric outpatient appointment for less acute problems, and refer problems with a domestic or social basis to the social work team.

(4) In all cases, inform the GP by telephone and letter if the patient is allowed home (preferably accompanied by a relative or friend).

THE CONFUSED PATIENT

'Confusion' should be reserved to describe a state of clouding of consciousness or disturbed awareness, which may fluctuate.

DIAGNOSIS

(1) There is a wide spectrum of confusional states between the following two extremes:

    (i)   difficulty maintaining attention, irritability, emotional lability and illusions;

    (ii) delirium: disorientation in time and place, impaired memory, restlessness, hallucinations and poor comprehension.

(2) *Causes of confusion*

    (i)   Drugs:

        (a)   intoxication or withdrawal from alcohol, LSD, cocaine and amphetamines

        (b)   side effects (especially in the elderly) of analgesics, anticonvulsants, digoxin, psychotropics, anticholinergics and antiparkinsonian drugs such as benzhexol and levodopa.

    (ii) Hypoxia:

        (a)   after head injury or chest injury

        (b)   chest infection, pulmonary embolus, cardiac failure

      (c)   respiratory depression from drugs or muscle disorders, e.g. myasthenia gravis or muscular dystrophy.

(iii) Metabolic:
- (a) renal, liver, respiratory and cardiac failure
- (b) vitamin deficiency, e.g. thiamine or B_{12}
- (c) electrolyte imbalance, such as hyponatraemia, hypernatraemia or hypercalcaemia
- (d) acute intermittent porphyria.

(iv) Endocrine:
- (a) hypoglycaemia or hyperglycaemia
- (b) thyrotoxicosis, myxoedema, Cushing's syndrome, steroids, Addison's disease.

(v) Cerebral:
- (a) trauma
- (b) postictal state, complex partial (temporal lobe) seizures
- (c) cerebrovascular accident, subarachnoid haemorrhage
- (d) meningitis, encephalitis
- (e) space occupying lesion, e.g. tumour, abscess or haematoma
- (f) hypertensive encephalopathy
- (g) systemic lupus erythematosus.

(vi) Other infections, e.g. biliary tract, urinary tract or malaria.

(vii) Faecal impaction and urinary retention in the elderly.

MANAGEMENT

(1) A detailed history and examination will help build up a picture of which condition(s) is responsible.

(2) Always exclude hypoglycaemia, and perform some or all of the following investigations based on the suspected aetiology:
- (i) FBC, coagulation profile
- (ii) U&E, blood sugar, calcium, liver function tests, thyroid function tests, drug screen
- (iii) arterial blood gases

(iv)   blood cultures, MSU
(v)   CXR, ECG
(vi)   CT scan
(vii) lumbar puncture.

(3) Admit all patients under the appropriate specialist team. Avoid the temptation to simply sedate the confused patient, without looking carefully for the underlying cause.

THE VIOLENT PATIENT

DIAGNOSIS

(1) Much of the violence encountered by staff in the A&E department will be the result of alcohol intoxication, either by the patient or by their relatives or friends, who may be irritated and angry at having to wait if the department is busy.

(2) Other causes for violent behaviour include:
   (i)   hypoglycaemia (including as the patient recovers from a hypoglycaemic episode after i.v. dextrose administration)
   (ii)   hypoxia
   (iii) drugs, including amphetamines, LSD and cocaine
   (iv)   withdrawal syndromes from alcohol or barbiturates
   (v)   postictal state
   (vi)   mental illness, especially mania and paranoid schizophrenia, personality disorder
   (vii) other organic confusional state (see p. 373).

MANAGEMENT

(1) Explain what is happening at all times, reassure the patient, and avoid confrontation. Never turn your back on a patient or allow them between you and the cubicle door.

(2) Attempt verbal restraint by defining acceptable and unacceptable behaviour and their likely consequences.

(3) If verbal restraint fails, consider physical restraint.
  (i) Call the police or security guards, and await adequate numbers (ideally five or six people).
  (ii) Never try to restrain a patient single-handedly, particularly if they have a weapon.
  (iii) Conversely, never remove physical restraints until a full evaluation has been made and help is standing by.
(4) If chemical restraint is now indicated, give haloperidol or droperidol 5–10 mg i.m. or slowly i.v. This may be supplemented with midazolam 5–10 mg i.v. for more rapid control.
  (i) Such treatment may be given without consent under common law in an emergency if the patient is a danger to others or themselves.
  (ii) Every sedated patient must then be monitored in a resuscitation area until the risks of respiratory depression and hypotension have passed.
  (iii) Complete a full physical examination, looking for evidence of organic disease (see p. 375).
(5) Record exact details of events and the necessary action taken in the notes.
(6) Admit the patient under the medical or psychiatric team if further treatment is indicated.
(7) Debrief A&E staff, and consider immediate support for staff injury or intimidation and future strategies for violence prevention and management.

ALCOHOL-RELATED PROBLEMS

Alcohol is causally related to all types of trauma, including motor vehicle accidents, accidents in the home, deliberate self-harm, assaults, drownings, child abuse and falls in the elderly.

MEASUREMENT OF ALCOHOL LEVEL

Various methods are available, including a breath test, a urine test and a blood level test. This may not be available out of hours, therefore an approximate blood alcohol level may be derived by measuring the serum osmolality and using the following formula:

Approximate blood alcohol in mg % (divide by 1000 for g %) = 5 × (measured osmolality − calculated osmolality) where calculated osmolality = 2(Na + K) + urea + glucose.

Units: measured osmolality in mosmol/kg; Na, K, urea, glucose in mmol/l.

Note: the British legal limit for driving is a blood alcohol level below 80 mg %. Intoxication is marked above a level of 150 mg %, and coma usually occurs above a level of 300 mg %.

THE PATIENT WITH AN ALTERED CONSCIOUSNESS LEVEL AND SMELLING OF ALCOHOL

MANAGEMENT

Never assume that a confused, obtunded or unconscious patient smelling of alcohol is simply drunk until you have excluded all of the following:
(1) *Hypoglycaemia*
    (i) Check a blood sugar on all 'drunks', and give 50 ml of 50% dextrose if it is low.
    (ii) Occasionally, this may precipitate worsening of the confusion. Suspect Wernicke's encephalopathy, a condition associated with alcohol abuse and malnutrition causing ataxia, nystagmus and bilateral lateral rectus palsy. Give thiamine 100 mg i.v. immediately for this.
(2) *Head injury*
    (i) Always remember the possibility of an extradural or subdural haematoma.
    (ii) Commence neurological observations and perform a CT head scan if confusion persists or there is a deteriorating conscious level (see p. 171). A skull X-ray is useful only in the absence of a CT scan, but even if normal it does not exclude intracranial injury.
(3) *An additional medical problem*
    (i) epileptic fit

      (ii)   acute poisoning
      (iii)   cerebral haemorrhage
      (iv)   meningitis, chest infection, etc.
      (v)   hypothermia
      (vi)   rib fracture, wrist fracture, abdominal trauma.

(4) *An acute condition more prevalent in alcoholics*
      (i)   aspiration or pneumococcal pneumonia, TB
      (ii)   gastrointestinal haemorrhage
      (iii)   pancreatitis
      (iv)   liver failure
      (v)   withdrawal fits or delirium tremens
      (vi)   cardiac arrhythmia, cardiomyopathy
      (vii) hypokalaemia, hypomagnesaemia, hypocalcaemia
      (viii) renal failure
      (ix)   lactic acidosis
      (x)   Wernicke's encephalopathy.

(5) Thus, many patients will require admission to exclude the above conditions. If in doubt, always admit for observation.

ALCOHOL WITHDRAWAL

This is caused by an absolute or relative decrease in the usual intake of alcohol through lack of funds or by detention in hospital or by the police.

DIAGNOSIS AND MANAGEMENT

Two conditions are recognised: the alcohol withdrawal syndrome, and the progression to delirium tremens.

(1) *Alcohol withdrawal syndrome*
      (i)   This is common, occurring within 12 h of abstinence and lasting a few days. It is characterised by agitation, irritability, fine tremor, sweats and tachycardia.
      (ii)   Commence diazepam 10–20 mg orally 2–6-hourly until the patient is comfortable, plus thiamine 100 mg i.v. or i.m. daily.

- (iii) Control fits with lorazepam 4 mg i.v. or diazepam (Diazemuls) 5–10 mg i.v., after excluding hypoglycaemia.
- (iv) Refer the patient to the medical team.

(2) *Delirium tremens*
- (i) This is uncommon, occurring 72 h after abstinence. There is clouding of consciousness, terrifying hallucinations, gross tremor, autonomic hyperactivity with tachycardia, dilated pupils, fever, sweating, dehydration, and grand mal fits that may be prolonged (status epilepticus).
- (ii) Delirium tremens is a medical emergency. Give lorazepam 4 mg i.v. or diazepam (Diazemuls) 5–10 mg i.v. for fits, and exclude other causes of status epilepticus such as head injury and meningitis (see p. 57).
- (iii) Replace fluid and electrolyte losses, avoiding excessive normal saline in liver failure. Give thiamine 100 mg i.v. daily.
- (iv) Refer all patients immediately to the medical team or intensive care unit.

Note: never dispense chlormethiazole (Heminevrin) capsules in the A&E department to take home. They are reserved for inpatient detoxification programmes only.

PROBLEM DRINKING

MANAGEMENT

(1) Alcohol-dependent patients may request help or be brought in by concerned others to stop drinking.
- (i) If there is actual suicidal depression or total inability to cope at home, refer the patient immediately to the psychiatric team.
- (ii) Otherwise, refer the patient to the appropriate hospital or community clinic for outpatient assessment, or to the social work department.
- (iii) Meanwhile, give the patient the telephone numbers of local support organisations to contact,

such as:
- (a) Alcoholics Anonymous: telephone (020) 7352 3001 (London)
- (b) Al-Anon – provides help and advice for the family and friends of problem drinkers: telephone (020) 7403 0888.

(2) Always write to the GP to enlist their help and support.

DRUG DEPENDENCY AND DRUG ABUSE

DIAGNOSIS

(1) Patients may be seen who are dependent on or abuse the following classes of drugs:
- (i) opiates
- (ii) barbiturates
- (iii) benzodiazepines
- (iv) alcohol
- (v) stimulants, including amphetamines and cocaine
- (vi) miscellaneous substances, including cannabis, LSD and solvents.

(2) Abrupt withdrawal of many of these drugs causes acute symptoms.
- (i) Opiate withdrawal causes restlessness, excitability, muscle cramps, diarrhoea, tachycardia and sweating, known as 'cold turkey'.
- (ii) Barbiturate withdrawal causes hallucinations and epileptic fits.
- (iii) Benzodiazepine withdrawal causes a rebound increase in tension, anxiety and apprehension, with anorexia, insomnia and epileptic fits.

OPIATE ABUSE

MANAGEMENT

(1) Patients may need admission under the medical team for acute poisoning (see p. 78), cellulitis, abscesses

including pulmonary and cerebral, septicaemia, bacterial endocarditis, hepatitis B, C or D, and, increasingly, HIV infection.

(2) Otherwise, if a regular opiate user needs admission to the A&E observation ward, perhaps following an orthopaedic or minor operative procedure:

    (i)   give salicylate or paracetamol for mild or moderate pain, and methadone orally or i.m. for severe pain;

    (ii)   if signs of opiate withdrawal occur, such as agitation, cramps, pupillary dilatation, tachycardia and sweating, give the patient diazepam 5–10 mg orally, repeated as required;

    (iii)   if the patient should demand a controlled drug, explain that it is actually an offence for a doctor to administer or authorise the supply of a drug of addiction, except in the treatment of an organic disease or injury, unless licensed to do so.

(3) Look at the front of the BNF for more detailed information on drugs of dependence, prescriptions and the Misuse of Drugs Act, 1971.

(4) Refer patients wishing to stop their habit and seeking help to:

    (i)   a drug dependency clinic

    (ii)   a drug dependency 24-h emergency organisation such as Narcotics Anonymous: telephone (020) 7351 6794

    (iii)   the social work department

    (iv)   the patient's own GP.

BARBITURATE, BENZODIAZEPINE AND SOLVENT ABUSE

MANAGEMENT

Patients who abuse these groups of drugs all require referral to specialist clinics to coordinate their withdrawal regime. Help and advice is available from:

(1) psychiatric outpatient clinics

(2) a local drug dependency organisation, such as the self-help groups organised by MIND: telephone (020) 7637 0741

(3) the social work department
(4) the patient's own GP.

COMPULSORY ADMISSION

It is rarely necessary to detain a patient against his or her will in the A&E department under the Mental Health Act (MHA) 1983 Part II (England and Wales). However, if a patient is suffering from a mental disorder that is severe enough to endanger his or her own health or safety, or that of others, detention will be required.

(1) Always request the help and advice of the psychiatric team in such circumstances. It is unusual to have to act in their absence.
(2) *Section 4: Admission for assessment in cases of emergency*
   (i)   This lasts for 72 h.
   (ii)   Application may be made by the nearest relative or preferably by an approved social worker, either of whom must have seen the patient within the previous 24 h.
   (iii) One medical recommendation only is required from a doctor, ideally with prior knowledge of the patient. If this is not possible, it should be stated clearly on the medical recommendation why such a doctor is not available.
(3) *Section 136: Police admission order*
   (i)   This lasts for 72 h.
   (ii)   Application is by any police officer.
   (iii) It allows a police officer to move any person apparently suffering from a mental disorder from a public place to a designated place of safety, such as the local A&E department or a police station.
   (iv)   Assessment is then made by a doctor and an approved social worker.
(4) *Section 2: Admission for assessment*
   (i)   This is a 28-day order.

(ii) Application to the hospital may be made by the nearest relative (as defined in Section 26 of the MHA) or an approved social worker.

(iii) Two medical recommendations are required:
  (a) a doctor approved under Section 12 of the MHA;
  (b) a doctor preferably with previous knowledge of the patient, e.g. the GP.

(5) Similar arrangements provide for compulsory detention under local legislation in Scotland and Northern Ireland.

REFERENCE

1 Isacsson G, Rich CL. Management of patients who deliberately harm themselves. *BMJ* 2001;322:213–15.

ADMINISTRATIVE AND LEGAL CONSIDERATIONS

TRIAGE

(1) All patients presenting to A&E should be sorted or triaged on arrival, usually by an experienced, specially trained A&E nurse in order to direct resources to the more seriously ill first. The triage nurse allocates an acuity category from the UK National Triage Scale following assessment of current physiological disturbance and the risk of serious underlying illness or injury.

(2) The triage category answers the question 'this patient should receive medical care from a doctor or nurse practitioner ...' within an ideal time period embodied in the treatment acuity (see Table 14).

(3) Children and patients in pain may be up-triaged to a more acute category to facilitate expeditious care.

(4) Triage category underpins sentinel A&E performance indicators, such as waiting times (by triage category), admission rates, and did not wait (DNW) rates, and aids the prediction of optimal staffing levels, resources, space and budgetary requirements.

Table 14. UK National Triage Scale

UK National Triage Scale	Treatment acuity	Numeric code
Immediate resuscitation	Immediately	1
Very urgent	Within 10 min	2
Urgent	Within 60 min	3
Standard	Within 120 min	4
Non-urgent	Within 240 min	5

ACCIDENT AND EMERGENCY DEPARTMENT RECORDS

The following is a guide to recording accurate and concise information for every patient examined in the department. Details will obviously vary according to the nature and layout of each department's records. Even if computerisation of the medical record is established, the same high standards of recording must still be adhered to.

(1) Ensure all the boxes at the top of the page have been filled in (usually by the reception staff) to identify the patient fully.

(2) Start by printing your own name and designation, and the date and time you commenced seeing the patient.

(3) Write legibly throughout. Other members of staff will be reading your notes, which will be meaningless if they are illegible.

(4) Record all the positive clinical findings in the history and examination, and relevant negative findings.

(5) Avoid the use of abbreviations, except for unambiguous, approved examples, such as 'BP'. Digits should be named not numbered, and 'left' and 'right' should be written in full.

(6) Make detailed notes in assault or traffic accident cases of the patient's recall of events, or from a witness. Document the exact size of bruises or lacerations measured with a ruler.

    (i) Statements may subsequently be required by the police or a solicitor, and could be requested months or even years later, so you cannot rely on your memory.

    (ii) A photograph is an ideal record and may save a detailed description. Unfortunately, few doctors have access to a suitable camera at the necessary time.

(7) Record your diagnosis and differential diagnosis.

(8) Record any investigations performed, and put down the results, including your own interpretation of the X-ray or ECG.

(9) Record if you discussed the case with a senior A&E doctor, their name and grade, the time, and exactly what they advised.

(10) Detail your proposed treatment plan, printing drug names and quantities.

(11) Document any verbal or written instructions or advice given to the patient.

(12) Record the disposal of the patient.

  (i) If you hand the patient over to another A&E department doctor at the end of your shift, record on the notes to whom clinical responsibility has been transferred.

  (ii) If you refer to an inpatient team, record the name and seniority of the doctor concerned and the time the patient was referred.

  (iii) If the patient is referred to outpatients, record the clinic name and the consultant if possible.

  (iv) If the patient is admitted, write the ward and the consultant under whom the patient was admitted on the records.

  (v) If the patient is referred back to the GP, attach a copy of any discharge letter to this doctor onto the A&E department record. Computerisation of the medical record may now enable a printed letter to be generated for every patient.

(13) Sign your name clearly at the end of the record, and print your name and initials underneath for future identification.

Most of the above points may appear obvious, but they are essential to the quality and continuity of the medical care of the patient, and underpin good risk management practice.

RISK MANAGEMENT AND INCIDENT REPORTING

Risk management is defined as 'the activities required to minimise financial loss for hospitals and doctors who work in them. The five mainstays of effective risk management include credentialling of medical staff, incident monitoring and tracking, complaints monitoring and tracking, infection control, and documentation in the medical record.[1] Whether any or all of these activities are adopted at your hospital, you can begin to empower yourself.

(1) Know the types of A&E situations that lead to incidents and claims, or a doctor requiring medico-legal assistance:
    (i)   failure to correctly diagnose the patient's medical condition
    (ii)   dissatisfaction with treatment
    (iii)   inquiry regarding death of a patient
    (iv)   dissatisfaction with medical practitioner's conduct
    (v)   delay in diagnosis
    (vi)   requirement for a medical report regarding diagnosis and treatment
    (vii) failure to treat patient.

(2) Some of the common A&E conditions that are reported as incidents include:
    (i)   failure to diagnose all other fractures, e.g. scaphoid, phalanx, neck of femur, talus, calcaneus, etc.
    (ii)   failure to diagnose cerebral haemorrhage, particularly subarachnoid
    (iii)   failure to diagnose spinal fracture
    (iv)   medication errors
    (v)   failure to diagnose/treat appropriately tendon/nerve injury, particularly lacerations to the hand or foot
    (vi)   failure to diagnose torsion of the testis
    (vii) failure to diagnose/treat appropriately wounds/wound infections, particularly inadequate debridement and cleaning
    (viii) failure to diagnose appendicitis
    (ix)   failure to diagnose myocardial infarction
    (x)   failure to diagnose foreign body, including glass and intraocular.

(3) Therefore, adopt the following strategies to minimise your medico-legal risk:
    (i)   Always ask more senior A&E staff for advice when you are unsure.
    (ii)   Never stereotype a patient, trivialise their complaint, or jump to an easy conclusion.
    (iii)   Follow the guidelines above for good A&E record keeping.

(iv) Learn to be an excellent communicator – with the patient, your medical colleagues, nursing staff and with the GP (see Good Communications with the General Practitioner below).

(v) Become a team player and use the supports available to you.

(4) If an incident does occur that you think could turn into a complaint or claim, notify the senior A&E doctor and contact your medical defence organisation (MDO) immediately. Include the following situations:

(i) an adverse outcome

(ii) angry/disgruntled patient

(iii) communication breakdown

(iv) missed or delayed diagnosis

(v) a 'gut feeling' that something is not quite right.

(5) Your initial reaction to the incident may help ameliorate the likelihood of a claim being lodged. Do make sure you:

(i) talk the problem through with the patient in layperson's language;

(ii) express regret and empathy for the adverse outcome;

(iii) continue to liaise with the medical team to ensure proper follow-up;

(iv) document meticulously, and never backdate, alter or delete a medical record;

(v) be positive not defensive;

(vi) contact your MDO early.

GOOD COMMUNICATIONS WITH THE GENERAL PRACTITIONER

It is essential to communicate whenever possible with the GP.

(1) Ring the GP to clarify current management, including medications and allergies, when the patient is unsure, or for a recent past history in complex or atypical presentations.

(2) Ring and/or write a letter, keeping a copy in the patient's notes, if:
   (i)   the GP writes a referral letter to you;
   (ii)   you do any tests, including bloods, urinalysis, X-ray or ECG, even if they are normal;
   (iii)   you make a new diagnosis;
   (iv)   you start new medication, or change or stop an existing treatment regime;
   (v)   you refer the patient back to the GP for further care and review, including removing sutures or changing dressings;
   (vi)   you refer the patient to outpatients;
   (vii)   the patient is admitted, or a patient is brought in dead (or dies in the department).

(3) Give the patient the letter to deliver by hand, but assume it is likely to be opened and read, so fax, post or email letters containing sensitive information and when you have any doubt about the reliability or capacity of the patient to transfer the letter on.

CONSENT

(1) Patients over the age of 16 years may sign or with-hold their own informed consent either under common law principles or as set out in legislation.

(2) The doctor must explain the details of the proposed procedure, and warn of any possible complications, and the patient must understand the implications and nature of the treatment proposed.

(3) In cases of emergency to save life, the doctor should proceed even if consent was not obtained.

(4) Patients under the age of 16 years may be able to consent for treatment provided they have the ability to understand what is proposed, although for major treatment it is preferable to seek consent from the parent or guardian (or teacher in an emergency). If the latter refuse, it is again appropriate to proceed to life-saving treatment, such as a blood transfusion in a Jehovah's

Witness minor, having contacted the hospital administration, the paediatric team and at least commenced
application for a court order.
(5) Conversely, medical information should not then be supplied to others, including parents, without permission.

SELF-DISCHARGE AND REFUSAL OF TREATMENT

(1) Patients who refuse admission to hospital and a recommended treatment plan may be permitted to discharge
themselves providing they are competent and informed,
i.e. understand fully the consequences of their actions.
(2) Make meticulous notes of exactly what was said to the
patient and their response, demonstrating that they
understood the issues. They may sign the appropriate
form, accepting responsibility for their own action, again
providing it is documented what they understood.
(3) If the patient refuses, or disappears before the form is
signed, this should be recorded and countersigned by a
witness, such as a senior nurse or a second doctor.
(4) Patients with conditions that preclude comprehension of
the nature and implications of proposed treatment may
be given emergency treatment without consent to save
life or to prevent serious damage to health.
(5) Similarly, patients suffering from a mental illness may be
detained against their will under the relevant Mental
Health Act if they are a danger to themselves or others
(see p. 382).

POLICE

The police are involved within the emergency department in a
number of ways.

REQUEST FOR INFORMATION CONCERNING A PATIENT

(1) All medical information concerning the care of a patient in the A&E department is confidential and must not be divulged without the patient's written consent, except on behalf of a coroner (or procurator fiscal).

(2) Traffic police investigating an accident may be told the name, address and age of any patient involved, a brief description of the injury, the severity and disposal, e.g. whether the accident is likely to prove fatal or whether the patient is to be admitted or sent home.

(3) If a patient is suspected of being involved in a serious arrestable offence, such as murder, rape, child abuse or armed robbery, the doctor may disclose this information to a senior police officer, thereby acting in the public interest for the safety of the lives of others.

(4) Obtain the advice of the senior A&E physician or hospital administration if there is any doubt as to the appropriateness of releasing non-clinical information to the police.

REQUEST TO INTERVIEW A PATIENT

(1) Permission may be granted if the patient is in a fit state medically to be seen, after informing the patient.

(2) The doctor may suggest a time limit.

REQUEST FOR AN ALCOHOL BREATH TEST OR BLOOD SAMPLE

(1) The doctor must first give the police permission to perform these, providing the patient's clinical condition would not be adversely affected.

(2) In certain circumstances, permission cannot be granted: if the patient is unconscious, critically ill, or incapable of cooperating, possibly due to a facial injury.

(3) If permission is granted, inform the patient that you have allowed the police to be involved, and record on the A&E record that in your opinion the patient was fit to be seen at the time and understood what was happening.

(4) The police officer or police surgeon must take the sample, using all their own equipment, and will not involve the hospital facilities at any stage.

REQUEST FOR A POLICE MEDICAL STATEMENT

(1) The purpose of this statement is to act as a record to be read out in court without requiring the doctor to be present.

(i)   The patient must always provide written consent before you may disclose confidential medical information.

(ii) Use the preprinted forms supplied by the police.

(iii) State your full name, age, contact address and telephone number, medical qualifications, job status, employing health authority, and duration of that employment.

(iv) State the date you were on duty in the department, the hospital name, and the time you examined the patient.

(v)   Continue with the full name, age, sex, occupation and address of the patient, and record the time and date of any subsequent attendances in the A&E department.

(vi) The history (as told to you) should be recounted without making personal inferences, and the physical findings recorded using language a non-medical person can understand.

(vii) The actual size of abrasions, bruises and lacerations should be stated where possible, and a comment made as to whether the injuries found are consistent with the use of a particular weapon or implement as suggested by the patient's history.

(viii) List all the investigations performed, such as X-rays and laboratory tests, and their results, including relevant negatives.

(ix) State the treatment given, including sutures and their number, and record the time the patient spent in hospital or attending outpatients.

(x)   Finally, end the report where possible with a prognosis. The report is then signed where indicated on each separate page.

(2) Always keep a photocopy of your report, and note the name and number of the police officer requesting the statement, and his or her police station.

BREAKING THE NEWS OF SUDDEN DEATH

(1) Breaking the news of sudden death to a relative, especially when unexpected as in trauma or cardiac arrest, must be done in the privacy of a quiet relatives' room.

(2) Be accompanied by an experienced nurse, introduce yourself, identify the patient's nearest relative, and sit by them.

(3) Come to the point avoiding any preamble or euphemisms, and use the words 'dead' or 'death' early on, followed by a brief account of events.

(4) Be prepared to touch or hold the relative's hand and do not be afraid to show concern or empathy yourself. Allow a period of silence, avoiding platitudes or false sympathy, but encourage and answer any questions.

(5) Understand that the relative's reaction may vary from numbed silence, disbelief, acute distress to anger, denial and guilt.

(6) Indicate that the nurse can stay with them. When they are ready, encourage them to see and touch the body to say goodbye to their loved one alone.

(7) Ask whether the relative wishes the hospital chaplain, social worker or bereavement counsellor to be contacted. Avoid giving sedative drugs, which will only postpone acceptance of what has happened.

(8) Phone the GP and inform the coroner as appropriate.

(9) Retain the property of the deceased, whatever its condition, for collection by the next of kin in accordance with

his or her wishes. Avoid then presenting the property in a plastic bin bag.

(10) Finally, appreciate the stress and anxiety caused to yourself and the nursing team following an unsuccessful resuscitation.

    (i)   Try to meet together briefly to talk over events and express your own feelings and emotions.

    (ii)   Thank everyone for their efforts, particularly the nurse dealing with the relatives and the nurses left to lay out the body.

CORONER

(1) The coroner (procurator fiscal in Scotland) must be informed of all sudden or unexpected deaths, and deaths involving homicide, suicide, an accident or injury, drowning, poisoning, surgery, abortion, infancy, neglect, negligence or patients in police custody or held in a mental hospital.

(2) Thus, virtually all patients brought in dead are reported to the coroner.

(3) Any patient actually dying in the department should be reported. If there are any suspicious circumstances, this should be done whatever the time of day or night, by contacting the local police station (the police are very often involved anyway).

(4) The A&E department doctor is rarely in a position to sign a death certificate.

ATTENDING AN INQUEST

An inquest takes place in the coroner's court, and is purely a fact-finding inquiry, not a trial. It is held in public, and the press may be present.

(1) The coroner's office will inform you of the date, time and place of the inquest. Arrive punctually and dress

suitably. Legal representation may be arranged for you by your medical defence organisation (MDO) if, on discussion with them, they consider it appropriate.

(2) Take the medical notes and a copy of your statement with you. Read both thoroughly beforehand so you have the facts readily available.

(3) The oath is taken, then the coroner will take you through your statement and ask questions.

(4) Your replies should be concise, clear and factual, indicating whether they are factual or based on hearsay.

(5) Following this, you may be examined by any 'properly interested persons' or usually their lawyer. You are not obliged to answer any questions that may incriminate you.

(6) After the inquest, the coroner's officer will pay you the appropriate witness fee and expenses.

RETRIEVAL AND TRANSFER

(1) Retrieval is the transport of a sick or injured patient by specially trained staff from a lesser-equipped (sending) hospital to a higher-level (receiving) hospital for further care.

(2) The sending doctor should speak directly to the receiving hospital doctor or retrieval specialist using a dedicated, single-point-contact, coordinated communication system.

(3) The decision to transfer, the risks involved, the benefits incurred and the patient preparation are agreed on. The sending doctor commences usual required care, such as two i.v. cannulae, nasogastric tube, in-dwelling catheter (IDC), fracture splinting and advanced airway/respiratory/cardiovascular procedures according to their ability.

(4) A transfer letter, photocopy of notes and forms, lab results, X-rays, ECGs, etc. are prepared for the retrieval team/receiving hospital.

(5) Road transport is suitable for shorter distances and helicopter beyond these. Helicopters require expert

crew and landing areas, incur high costs, need dedicated equipment, and involve flight physiology considerations such as altitude hypoxia and trapped gas expansion, e.g. in a pneumothorax.

(6) Retrieval equipment must be compact, portable, light, robust and reliable, and have adequate battery capacity. Special ventilators, monitors, suction equipment, alarms, defibrillator, mattress and equipment frame 'bridge' are essential.

(7) Retrieval staff will spend time assessing, stabilising and packaging the patient at the sending hospital, pre-empting any potential complications during transfer. It is not a time to rush.

(8) The aim is to improve the level of care at each stage, particularly during high-risk times such as loading, unloading and inter-hospital travel.[2]

THE MAJOR INCIDENT

(1) Each hospital will have its own plan for coping with large numbers of casualties, known as a major disaster plan. This should be linked to regional and state plans for mass casualty situations in any location, however remote.

(2) Portions of the major disaster plan pertinent to individual members of staff are summarised on documents known as action cards. Those concerned with the medical and nursing staff within the A&E department should be distributed to, and read by, all new members of staff.

(3) All new A&E doctors must also make certain that:
   (i)   switchboard have a reliable contact telephone number for the purpose of an emergency call-out;
   (ii) they know the call-out procedure, the different states of alert, and the significance of being the designated hospital or the supporting hospital;

(iii)   they understand their role within the department, which senior doctor they are responsible to, and from whom they should receive advice;

(iv)   they can operate any equipment reserved for use in a major incident, including that used by the mobile medical team;

(v)   they are familiar with the special stationery and records used in a major incident, including the significance of the triage labels and where to find details of any pre-hospital care given, particularly drugs and fluids;

(vi)   they know how to obtain social and psychological support following the incident to minimise the potential for post-traumatic stress.

(4) Some incidents pose an additional danger to staff themselves.

    (i)   *Radiation contamination*

        (a)   Patients requiring urgent treatment are taken to the nearest major A&E department.

        (b)   Advice and help are usually given by a radiation physicist or by contacting the local National Arrangements for Incidents involving Radioactivity (NAIR) staff.

        (c)   A&E staff attending these patients will be assigned to a predetermined isolation and decontamination area, and expected to wear caps, theatre clothes, aprons, double gloves and boots, which they should be familiar with in advance.

    (ii)   *Toxic chemical contamination*

        (a)   The fire brigade are responsible for identifying toxic chemical spillage and for decontaminating on site, usually with large volumes of water.

        (b)   Similar designated decontamination areas and protective clothing are used by staff as in radiation contamination.

        (c)   Hypothermia from wet protective blankets must be excluded in all cases, and standard resuscitation procedures adopted without delaying for the arrival of specific antidotes.

(d) Most patients require admission for a period of observation, even if asymptomatic. Inhalation injury and absorption through skin, e.g. of phenol, may cause delayed toxic effects, which should be anticipated in advance.

REFERENCES

1   Wilson LL, Fulton M. Risk management: how doctors, hospitals and MDOs can limit the costs of malpractice litigation. *Med J Aust* 2000;172:77–80.
2   Faculty of Intensive Care, Australian and New Zealand College of Anaesthetists, Australasian College for Emergency Medicine. Minimum standards of transport of the critically ill. http://www.acem.org.au/open/documents/transport.htm (Accessed 6/2/2001.)

FURTHER READING

Advanced Life Support Group. *Advanced Paediatric Life Support: the practical approach*, 3rd edn. BMJ Books, London; 2001.

Browne GJ, Choong RKC, Gaudry PL, Wilkins BH. *Principles and Practice of Children's Emergency Care*. MacLennan and Petty, Sydney; 1997.

Bull PD. *Lecture Notes on Diseases of the Ear, Nose and Throat*, 8th edn. Blackwell Scientific Publications, Oxford; 1996.

Cameron P, Jelinek G, Kelly A-M, *et al. Textbook of Adult Emergency Medicine*. Churchill Livingstone, Edinburgh; 2000.

Colquhuon MC, Handley AJ, Evans TR. *ABC of Resuscitation*, 4th edn. BMJ Books, London; 1999.

Driscoll P, Skinner D, Earlham R. *ABC of Major Trauma*, 3rd edn. BMJ Books, London; 2000.

Dunn R, Dilley S, Brookes J, *et al. The Emergency Medicine Manual*, 2nd edn. Robert Dunn, West Beach; 2000.

Evans R, Burke D. *Key Topics in Accident and Emergency Medicine*, 2nd edn. Bios Scientific Publishers, Oxford; 2001.

Fulde GWO. *Emergency Medicine: the principles of practice*, 3rd edn. MacLennan and Petty, Sydney; 1998.

Harwood-Nuss A, Wolfson A, Linden C, Shepherd SM, Stenklyft PH. *The Clinical Practice of Emergency Medicine*, 3rd edn. Lippincott Williams & Wilkins, Philadelphia; 2001.

Huckstep RL. *A Simple Guide to Trauma*, 5th edn. Churchill Livingstone, Edinburgh; 1995.

James B. *Lecture Notes on Ophthalmology*, 8th edn. Blackwell Scientific Publications, Oxford; 1997.

Jenkins JL, Braen R, Richard G. *Manual of Emergency Medicine*, 4th edn. Lippincott Williams & Wilkins, Philadelphia; 1999.

Keats TE. *Atlas of Normal Roentgen Variants That May Simulate Disease*, 6th edn. Mosby – Year Book Medical Publishers, Chicago; 1996.

London PS. *The Anatomy of Injury and Its Surgical Implications*. Butterworth-Heinemann, Oxford; 1991.

Martin T, Burgess J. *Dreisbach's Handbook of Poisoning*, 13th edn. Parthenon Publishing, Carnforth; 2001.

Mattox KL. *Complications of Trauma*. Churchill Livingstone, New York; 1994.

McLatchie GR. *Essentials of Sports Medicine*, 2nd edn. Churchill Livingstone, Edinburgh; 1993.

McRae R. *Practical Fracture Treatment*, 3rd edn. Churchill Livingstone, Edinburgh; 1994.

Mengert T, Eisenberg MS, Copass MK. *Emergency Medical Therapy*, 4th edn. W.B. Saunders Co., Philadelphia; 1995.

Mirvis SE, Young JWR. *Imaging in Trauma and Critical Care.* Williams and Wilkins, Baltimore; 1992.

Moulton C, Yates D. *Lecture Notes on Emergency Medicine*, 2nd edn. Blackwell Science, Oxford; 1999.

Oh TE. *Intensive Care Manual*, 4th edn. Butterworth-Heinemann, Oxford; 1997.

Raby N, Berman L, de Lacy G. *Accident and Emergency Radiology.* W.B. Saunders Co., Philadelphia; 1995.

Ramrakha P, Moore K. *Oxford Handbook of Acute Medicine.* Oxford University Press, Oxford; 1997.

Roberts JR, Hedges JR. *Clinical Procedures in Emergency Medicine*, 3rd edn. W.B. Saunders Co., Philadelphia; 1997.

Rosen P, Barkin R, *et al. Emergency Medicine: concepts and clinical practice*, 4th edn. Mosby Year Book, St Louis; 1997.

Rosen P, Barkin RM, Hayden SR, *et al. The 5 Minute Emergency Medicine Consult.* Lippincott Williams & Wilkins, Philadelphia; 1999.

Royal Children's Hospital, Melbourne. *Paediatric Handbook*, 6th edn. Blackwell Science Asia, Melbourne; 2000.

Rubenstein D, Wayne D, Bradley D. *Lecture Notes on Clinical Medicine*, 5th edn. Blackwell Scientific Publications, Oxford; 1997.

Rushman GB, Davies NJ, Cashman JN. *Lee's Synopsis of Anaesthesia*, 12th edn. Butterworth-Heinemann, Oxford; 1999.

Settle JAD. *Burns – The First Five Days.* Smith and Nephew Pharmaceuticals Ltd, Romford; 1987.

Skinner D, Swain A, Peyton R, Robertson C. *Cambridge Textbook of Accident and Emergency Medicine.* Cambridge University Press, Cambridge; 1997.

Sprigings D, Chambers J. *Acute Medicine: a practical guide to the management of medical emergencies*, 2nd edn. Blackwell Scientific Publications, Oxford; 2001.

Steedman DJ. *Environmental Medical Emergencies.* Oxford University Press, Oxford; 1994.

Tintinalli J, Kelen G, Stapczynski S. *Emergency Medicine: a comprehensive study guide*, 5th edn. McGraw-Hill, New York; 2000.

Trunkey DD, Lewis FR. *Current Therapy of Trauma*, 4th edn. Mosby Year Book, St Louis; 1998.

Webb LA. *Eye Emergencies Diagnosis and Management.* Butterworth-Heinemann, Oxford; 1995.

Willatts SM, Winter RJ. *Principles and Protocols in Intensive Care.* Farrand Press, London; 1992.

Wyatt J, Illingworth R, Clancy M, *et al. Oxford Handbook of Accident and Emergency Medicine.* Oxford University Press, Oxford; 1999.

ELECTRONIC INFORMATION

www.acem.org.au
www.baem.org.uk
www.bestbets.org
www.cdc.gov/travel
www.emedicine.com
www.trauma.org
www.spib.axl.co.uk

GLOSSARY

A&E	accident and emergency
ABG	arterial blood gases
AC	alternating current
ACE	angiotensin-converting enzyme
ACTH	adrenocorticotropic hormone
ACS	acute coronary syndromes
A/H	after-hours
AIDS	acquired immune deficiency syndrome
ANF	antinuclear factor
AP	anteroposterior
APTT	activated partial thromboplastin time
ATLS	advanced trauma life support
b.d.	*bis die* (twice daily)
BNF	British National Formulary
BP	blood pressure
C1:C7	first and seventh cervical vertebrae
C7/T1	seventh cervical and first thoracic vertebrae
CAP	community-acquired pneumonia
CCU	coronary care unit
CD4+	cluster designation (of antigen) 4+
CDC	Centers for Disease Control and Prevention
CK	creatine kinase
CK-MB	creatine kinase MB isoenzymes
Cl	chloride
CNS	central nervous system
CO_2	carbon dioxide
COPD	chronic obstructive pulmonary disease
CPR	cardiopulmonary resuscitation
CPAP	continuous positive airways pressure
CSF	cerebrospinal fluid
CT	computerised (axial) tomography
CTPA	computerised tomography pulmonary angiogram
cTnI	cardiac troponin I
cTnT	cardiac troponin T
CVA	cerebrovascular accident
CVP	central venous pressure

CXR	chest X-ray
D&C	dilation and curettage
DC	direct current
DCI	decompression illness
DHF	dengue haemorrhagic fever
DIC	disseminated intravascular coagulation
DKA	diabetic ketoacidosis
DNA	deoxyribonucleic acid
DNW	did not wait
DPL	diagnostic peritoneal lavage
DVT	deep vein thrombosis
ECG	electrocardiogram
ED	emergency department
EMD	electromechanical dissociation
ENT	ear, nose and throat
ERPC	evacuation of retained products of conception
ESR	erythrocyte sedimentation rate
ET	endotracheal
FAST	focussed abdominal sonogram for trauma
FBC	full blood count
FEV_1	forced expiratory volume in 1 s
F_iO_2	inspired oxygen concentration
GA	general anaesthesia
G&S	group and save (blood)
GCS	Glasgow Coma Scale
GI	gastrointestinal
Glucostix	enzyme-impregnated reagent strips for measuring capillary blood glucose
GP	general practitioner
GTN	glyceryl trinitrate
h	hour
H_1/H_2	histamine type 1, histamine type 2
Hb	haemoglobin
HCG	human chorionic gonadotrophin
HCO_3	bicarbonate
HIV	human immunodeficiency virus
HLA	human leucocyte antigen
ICS	intercostal space
IDC	in-dwelling catheter

IgE	immunoglobulin E
i.m.	intramuscular
ITP	idiopathic thrombocytopoenic purpura
ITU	intensive therapy unit
IU	international units
IUCD	intrauterine contraceptive device
i.v.	intravenous
IVU	intravenous urogram
JVP	jugular venous pressure
K	potassium
KCl	potassium chloride
KUB	kidneys, ureters, bladder
LBBB	left bundle branch block
LFTs	liver function tests
LMWH	low-molecular-weight heparin
LP	lumbar puncture
LSD	lysergic acid diethylamide
MAP	mean arterial pressure
MAST	military antishock trousers
MDO	medical defence organisation
mEq/l	milliequivalents per litre
MHA	Mental Health Act
MI	myocardial infarction
mm Hg	millimetres of mercury
MCP	metacarpophalangeal
MSU	midstream specimen of urine
Mu	megaunit
Na	sodium
NAA	nucleic acid amplification
NAI	non-accidental injury
NAIR	National Arrangements for Incidents involving Radioactivity
NGT	nasogastric tube
normal saline	isotonic 0.9% sodium chloride solution
NSAID	nonsteroidal anti-inflammatory drug
o.d.	*omni die* (once daily)
O&G	obstetrics and gynaecology
OM	occipitomental
OPG	orthopantomogram
PA	postero-anterior

P_aCO_2	partial pressure of carbon dioxide (arterial)
PCR	polymerase chain reaction
PCV	packed cell volume
PE	pulmonary embolus
PEF	peak expiratory flow
PGL	persistent generalised lymphadenopathy
pH	negative logarithm of the hydrogen ion concentration
P_aO_2	partial pressure of oxygen (arterial)
PTA	post-traumatic amnesia
PTI	prothrombin index
p.r.	per rectum
q.d.s.	*quater in die sumendus* (four times daily)
RBBB	right bundle branch block
RNA	ribonucleic acid
ROSC	return of spontaneous circulation
r-PA	recombinant plasminogen activator
rt-PA	recombinant tissue-type plasminogen activator
s	second
S_aO_2	oxygen saturation
s.c.	subcutaneous
SCIWORA	spinal cord injury without radiological abnormality
SIADH	syndrome of inappropriate ADH secretion
SLR	straight-leg raising
SNP	sodium nitroprusside
TB	tuberculosis
t.d.s.	*ter in die sumendus* (three times daily)
TIA	transient ischaemic attack
TURP	transurethral resection of the prostate
u	unit
U&E	urea and electrolytes
UTI	urinary tract infection
VF	ventricular fibrillation
V/Q	ventilation perfusion (lung scan)
VT	ventricular tachycardia
WCC	white cell count
X-match	cross-match blood

CRITICAL CARE AREAS DRUG INFUSION GUIDELINES

These infusion guidelines were developed for use in critical care areas only. Most require close monitoring with titration to response, and are thus inappropriate for general ward areas. All calculations assume a standard adult weight of 70–80 kg. Drug doses for paediatrics are available in paediatric texts (see Further reading).

Drug	Loading dose	Paediatric infusion range (<30 kg)	Dilution			Standard adult dose (range 70–80 kg)	
			Volumetric concentration	Syringe pump		Dose per hour	Volume per hour
Adrenaline	According to condition 1–100 µg/kg	0.05–1.0 µg/kg/min	6 mg in 100 ml DS	3 mg in 50 ml DS	60 µg/ml	2–20 µg/min	2–20 ml/h
Aminophylline (standard)	5.0 mg/kg in 100 ml DS over 20 min by IP	0.5–0.9 mg/kg/h	1000 mg in 500 ml DS	–	2 mg/ml	0.5–0.9 mg/kg/h	17.5–30 ml/h
Aminophylline (transport)	5.0 mg/kg in 100 ml DS over 20 min by IP	0.5–0.9 mg/kg/h	500 mg in 100 ml DS	250 mg in 50 ml DS	5 mg/ml	0.5–0.9 mg/kg/h	7–13 ml/h
Amiodarone (standard)	2–5 mg/kg in 100 ml DW over 30 min by IP	5–15 µg/kg/min	600 mg in 500 ml DW glass bottle Discard at 12 h	–	1.2 mg/ml	20–60 mg/h Max: 15 mg/kg/24 h	17–52 ml/h
Amiodarone (transport)	2–5 mg/kg in 100 ml DW over 30 min by IP	5–15 µg/kg/min	300 mg in 100 ml DW	150 mg in 50 ml DW	3 mg/ml	20–60 mg/h Max: 15 mg/kg/24 h	7.5–22 ml/h
Clonazepam	1.0–2.0 mg	5–10 µg/kg/h	10 mg in 100 ml DS	5 mg in 50 ml DS	0.1 mg/ml	0.35–0.7 mg/h	3.5–7.0 ml/h
Dobutamine	–	2–30 µg/kg/min	250 mg in 100 ml DS	125 mg in 50 ml DS	2.5 mg/ml	2–30 µg/kg/min	2–30 ml/h
Dopamine	–	Renal: 0.5–2.5 µg/kg/min Inotrope: 5–20 µg/kg/min	200 mg in 100 ml DS	100 mg in 50 ml DS	2 mg/ml	Renal: 0.5–2.5 µg/kg/min Inotrope: 5–20 µg/kg/min	Renal: 1–5 ml/h Inotrope: 10–40 ml/h
Fentanyl	1–5 µg/kg	1–10 µg/kg/h	1000 µg in 100 ml DS	500 µg in 50 ml DS	10 µg/ml	50–200 µg/h	5–20 ml/h

Drug	Dose	Preparation	Preparation	Concentration	Dose rate	ml/h
GTN (standard)	–	200 mg in 500 ml DW Use glass bottle/low-absorption set	–	400 µg/ml	0.4–8 mg/h	1–20 ml/h
GTN (transport)	–	50 mg in 100 ml DW	25 mg in 50 ml DW	500 µg/ml	0.5–10 mg/h	1–20 ml/h
Insulin (Actrapid)	2–20 units	100 units in 100 ml NS	50 units in 50 ml NS	1 unit/ml	2–20 units/h	2–20 ml/h
Isoprenaline (low dose)	1–10 µg/kg/min	1 mg in 100 ml DS	0.5 mg in 50 ml DS	10 µg/ml	0.5–7.5 µg/min	2–30 ml/h
Isoprenaline (high dose)	–	6 mg in 100 ml DS	3 mg in 50 ml DS	60 µg/ml	2–20 µg/min	2–20 ml/h
Ketamine	IV: 1–2 mg/kg IM: 5–10 mg/kg	1000 mg in 100 ml DS	500 mg in 50 ml DS	10 mg/ml	0.3–1.2 mg/kg/h	2–10 ml/h
Lignocaine (standard)	1–2 mg/kg	Premixed: 2 g in 500 ml DW	Premixed: 2 g in 500 ml DW	4 mg/ml	8 mg/min 4 mg/min 2 mg/min	120 ml/h (20 min) 60 ml/h (60 min) 30 ml/h (24 h)
Lignocaine (transport)	1–2 mg/kg	2 g in 100 ml DW	1 g in 50 ml DW	20 mg/ml	8 mg/min 4 mg/min 2 mg/min	24 ml/h (20 min) 12 ml/h (60 min) 6 ml/h (24 h)
Magnesium sulphate Amp: 5 ml 49.3% soln = 10 mmol = 2.47 g	0.15–0.3 mmol/kg = 10–20 mmol (adult) Dilute in 50 ml DS Infuse: 2 min (VT) to 20 min (pre-eclampsia) 0.05–0.1 mmol/kg/h	40 mmol in 100 ml DS 4 × 5-ml amps	20 mmol in 50 ml DS 2 × 5-ml amps	0.4 mmol/ml 0.1 g/ml	2–8 mmol/h 0.5–2.0 g/h	5–20 ml/h
GTN (standard) [Methyl prednisolone (spinal injury)]	1–10 µg/kg/min					
GTN (transport)	1–10 µg/kg/min					
Isoprenaline (low dose)	50–100 µg increments					
Ketamine	15–50 µg/kg/min					
Methyl prednisolone (spinal injury)	30 mg/kg over 30 min by IP 5.4 mg/kg/h	4 g in 100 ml Reconstitute in water BP Dilute in DS	2 g in 50 ml Reconstitute in water BP Dilute in DS	40 mg/ml	5.4 mg/kg/h for 23 h	10 ml/h (70 kg)

Drug	Loading dose	Paediatric infusion range (<30 kg)	Dilution		Standard adult dose (range 70-80 kg)	
			Volumetric concentration	Syringe pump	Dose per hour	Volume per hour
Midazolam	0.05–0.1 mg/kg in 1–2.5 mg increments	10–100 µg/kg/h	50 mg in 100 ml DS	25 mg in 50 ml DS · 0.5 mg/ml	2.5–10 mg/h	5–20 ml/h
Morphine	2.5–15 mg in 2.5-mg increments	10–50 µg/kg/h	100 mg in 100 ml DS	50 mg in 50 ml DS · 1 mg/ml	2–10 mg/h	2–10 ml/h
Naloxone	0.4–2.0 mg Max: 10 mg	10 µg/kg/h	4 mg in 100 ml DS	2 mg in 50 ml DS · 40 µg/ml	0.5–1.0 mg/h	12.5–25 ml/h
Nimodipine	–	6–30 µg/kg/h	10 mg in 50 ml dispensed	10 mg in 50 ml dispensed · 0.2 mg/ml	0.4–2.0 mg/h Titrate to maintain MAP	Start 2 ml/h Increase 2 ml/h every h to max. 10 ml/h
Noradrenaline	–	0.05–1.0 µg/kg/min	6 mg in 100 ml DS	3 mg in 50 ml DS · 60 µg/ml	2–20 µg/min	2–20 ml/h
Octreotide	50–200 µg	3–5 µg/kg/h	1000 µg in 100 ml DS	500 µg in 50 ml DS · 10 µg/ml	25–100 µg/h	2.5–10 ml/h
Phenobarbitone	15–25 mg/kg in 100 ml DS over 20–30 min (max: 50 mg/min) in IP					
Phenytoin	15–18 mg/kg in 100 ml NS over 20–30 min (max: 50 mg/min) in IP					

Procainamide	10 mg/kg (max 1000 mg) in 100 ml DW over 30 min by IP	20–80 µg/kg/min	1000 mg in 100 ml DW	500 mg in 50 mg DW	10 mg/ml	2–6 mg/min	12–36 ml/h
Propofol	Sedation: 0.5–1.0 mg/kg Induction: 2–3 mg/kg	1–10 mg/kg/h		500 mg in 50 ml (dispensed as 20-ml and 50-ml amps, both with 10 mg/ml)	10 mg/ml	Sedation: 1–2 mg/kg/h Anaesthesia: 5–10 mg/kg/h	Sedation: 7–15 ml/h Anaesthesia: 35–70 ml/h
rt-PA (alteplase)	15-mg bolus (15 ml)	–	100 mg in 100 ml water BP	–	1 mg/ml	(a) 15-mg bolus (b) 0.75 mg/kg (max 50 mg) (c) 0.5 mg/kg (max 35 mg)	Over 30 min Over 60 min
r-PA (reteplase)	10-U bolus in 2 min After 30 min: second 10-U bolus in 2 min	–	–	2 vials/prefilled syringes/ reconstitution devices and needles			
Salbutamol (asthma)	5–10 µg/kg in 100 ml DS over 10 min	1.0–5.0 µg/kg/min	6 mg in 100 ml DS	3 mg in 50 ml DS	60 µg/ml	5–50 µg/min	5–50 ml/h
Salbutamol (obstetric)	5–10 µg/kg in 100 ml DS over 10 min	0.2–1.0 µg/kg/min	6 mg in 100 ml DS	3 mg in 50 ml DS	60 µg/ml	10–50 µg/min	10–50 ml/h
Sodium nitroprusside	–	0.05–10 µg/kg/min	100 mg in 500 ml DW in glass bottle Protect from light Discard at 24 h		200 µg/ml Max: 800 µg/min	0.05–10 µg/kg/min Max: 1.5 mg/kg/24 h	1–210 ml/h 500 ml/24 h

Drug	Loading dose	Paediatric infusion range (<30 kg)	Dilution: Volumetric concentration	Dilution: Syringe pump	Standard adult dose (range 70–80 kg): Dose per hour	Standard adult dose (range 70–80 kg): Volume per hour
Streptokinase (AMI)	1.5 million units in 100 ml NS over 45 min by IP	–	–	–	2.5 ml/min	150 ml/h
Streptokinase (PE, DVT, etc.)	250 000 units in 100 ml NS over 30 min by IP	1500–2000 units/kg/h	500 000 units in 100 ml NS	–	100 000 units/h	20 ml/h
Thiopentone	3–6 mg/kg 0.5 mg/kg in shock	1–5 mg/kg/h	2500 mg in 100 ml water BP Protect from light	1250 mg in 50 ml water BP Protect from light	75–350 mg/h	3–15 ml/h
Vecuronium	0.1 mg/kg	0.05–0.1 mg/kg/h	100 mg in 100 ml Reconstitute in water BP Dilute in DS	50 mg in 50 ml Reconstitute in water BP Dilute in DS	4–8 mg/h	4–8 ml/h

DS, dextrose saline, or any isotonic crystalloid. DW, 5% dextrose in water; IP infusion pump; MAP, mean arterial pressure; NS, normal saline; Standard, use in A&E department; Transport, use for retrievals/inter-hospital transfers.
Reproduced by kind permission of Dr CT Myers, Senior Staff Specialist, Department of Emergency Medicine, Royal Brisbane Hospital, Brisbane, Australia (current as at April 2001).

Index